Memorix

CW00537169

Memorix

The *Memorix* series consists of easy to use pocket books in a number of different medical and surgical specialities. They contain a vast amount of practical information in very concise form through the extensive use of tables and charts, lists and hundreds of clear line diagrams, often in two colours.

Memorix will give students, junior doctors and some of their senior colleagues a handy and comprehensive reference in their pockets.

Titles in the series include:

Obstetrics
Thomas Rabe

Gynecology
Thomas Rabe

Neurology
Peter Berlit

Emergency Medicine
Sönke Müller

Surgery
Jürgen Hussmann and Robert Russell

Clinical Medicine
Conrad Droste and Martin von Planta

Pediatrics
Dieter Harms and Jochem Scharf

Physiology
Robert Schmidt, W.D. Willis and L. Reuss

Memorix

Clinical Medicine

Conrad Droste and Martin von Planta

Translated and adapted by
Dennis Guttmann MA, BM BCh, BSc, FRCP

A member of the Hodder Headline Group
LONDON • NEW YORK • NEW DELHI

English language edition 1997

First published in Great Britain in 1997 by Chapman & Hall
This impression reprinted in 2002 by
Arnold, a member of the Hodder Headline Group,
338 Euston Road, London NW1 3BH

http://www.arnoldpublishers.com

Co-published in the United States of America by
Oxford University Press Inc.,
198 Madison Avenue, New York, NY 10016
Oxford is a registered trademark of Oxford University press

Original German Language edition-Memorix Konstanten der Klinischen Medizin. Third edition
© 1993, VCH Verlagsgesellschaft mbH, D-6940 Weinheim, Germany

Typeset in Times by Best-set Typesetter Ltd, Hong Kong
Printed and bound in India by Replika Press Pvt. Ltd., 100% EOU, Delhi 110 040

ISBN 0 412 56050 X

A catalogue record for this book is available from the British Library

Library of Congress Catalog Card Number: 96-83979

CONTENTS

CONTENTS

Chest medicine   105

Emergencies, acid–base balance and disturbances, electrolytes   117

Gastroenterology

CONTENTS

CONTENTS

CONTENTS

PD Dr André Aeschlimann
Chefarzt
Rheumaklinik
CH-8437 Zurzach
(**Rheumatology and the locomotor
system**)

Prof. Dr Peter Berlit
Neurologische Klinik
Alfried-Krupp-Krankenhaus
Alfried-Krupp-Straße 21
D-4300 Esssen 1
(**Neurology**)

Prof. Dr Klaus Bross
Abteilung Innere Medizin I
Medizinische Klinik I
der Universität
Franz-Josef-Strauß-Allee
D-8400 Regensburg
(**Haematology and oncology**)

Dr Michael Droste
Internist und Endokrinologe
Elisenstraße 12
D-2900 Oldenburg
(**Diabetology**)

PD Dr Walter Haefeli
Klin. Pharmakologie
Kantonsspital
Petersgraben 4
CH-4031 Basel
(**Clinical pharmacology**)

Dr Michael Henke
Medizinische Universitätsklinik
Freiburg
Hugstetter Straße 55
D-7800 Freiburg
(**Haematology and oncology**)

Dr Beat Huser
Dialysestation
Kantonsspital
CH-6000 Luzern 16
(**Nephrology**)

Dr Rolf Kroidl
Internist, Lungenarzt, Allergologe
Hökerstraße 37
D-2160 Stade
(**Chest medicine**)

PD Dr Thomas Schürmeyer
Medizinische Hochschule
Hannover
Krankenhaus Oststadt
Podbielskistraße 380
D-3000 Hannover 51
(**Endocrinology**)

PD Dr Brigitte Volk
Abteilung Innere Medizin II
Medizinische Universitätsklinik
Hugstetter Straße 55
D-7800 Freiburg
(**Gastroenterology**)

Dr Christian Wussler
Arzt für Radiologie
Basler Straße 78a
D-7850 Lörrach
(**Radiology**)

Prof. Dr Werner Zimmerli
Infektiologie
Kantonsspital
Petersgraben 4
CH-4031 Basel
(**Infections**)

Preface

This third edition of *Memorix – Clinical Medicine* offers a compact pocket reference manual of constants of clinical medicine which will be of value to the busy practitioner in hospital and doctors in general practice.

The authors decided on a complete revision of *Memorix* in view of the profusion of similar publications that have appeared recently. Thus, over half of the information included in this edition is completely new. Representatives of sub-specialities of internal medicine were enrolled as co-authors in order to improve the topicality and clinical relevance of the volume.

As a result of close collaboration between the publishers, authors and users of *Memorix*, many critical suggestions have been considered. We were stimulated by this feedback from students, graduates in pre-registration year, practising doctors and many others to refine the choice of important and often essential anatomical and radiological diagrams, international classifications, treatment strategies and tables of differential diagnoses. It thus became possible to bring *Memorix* up to date without increasing the size of the volume. It still fits into the coat pocket, so that it is readily available at the bedside, in the office and in the interpretation of results. The format of the volume, its tabular style and the keyword presentation of the data, however, have inevitably led to some deficiencies.

Conrad Droste
Martin von Planta

Preface to the first and second editions

Most doctors carry a small notebook in their coat pocket in which they have recorded important data for quick reference as necessary.

We have looked at many of these books and have found that in the main they contain the same information: established and expanded tables, schedules and plans which one knows in outline but which are so complex that one cannot commit them to memory in detail.

The purpose of *Memorix* is to compile a systematic aide memoire for the coat pocket.

This book offers the reader important and often essential anatomical and radiological schedules, international classifications, medication summaries, treatment plans and tables of differential diagnoses for everyday use in the clinic and in practice.

The book has been kept deliberately small enough to fit into the coat pocket. It is designed to permit a rapid orientation at the bedside, when composing medical reports and when evaluating findings, and to act as a prompt and as a check to ensure that nothing has been forgotten.

Our book cannot, of course, replace personal observations and notes, but, where appropriate, it should complement personal interpretation, preferred preparations and local normal values.

The authors are aware that the limitation of the scope, the tabular format and the keyword presentation of the material may not make the volume fully comprehensive.

We were delighted with the concept of a book of this kind and we hope that our readers will share our enthusiasm.

This book was developed during our joint clinical activity in the Canton Hospital in Basle. We would like to thank our Chief, Dr W. Stauffacher, Director of the Department of Internal Medicine, for the generous support of our work. The realization of *Memorix* would not have been possible without the support and generous production of the publishers, VCH. We would like to express our sincere thanks to all those involved, the publisher's management, Mrs Sylvia Osteen and Mrs Myriam Nothacker. We are particularly grateful to Mr Jorg Kuhn, Heidelberg, for his splendid illustrations, and to Mrs Doris Engel, Biengen, for the frequently tedious secretarial work on the manuscripts.

Conrad Droste
Martin von Planta

Translator's note

In order to preserve the intention of providing a convenient and comprehensive pocket reference book, I have kept to the format of the Swiss original as far as possible. Some alterations have been required to conform to British clinical practice. These include the diagnosis of brain death, the treatment of tuberculosis, immunization schedules and vaccination for travellers. Drugs not available in the UK have been omitted, and dosage recommendations have been modified where they differed from those in the *British National Formulary*, which should in any case be consulted as a revised edition appears every six months.

In a volume that attempts to cover all clinical disciplines, there will inevitably be some omissions, and the reader working in a specialty may find it helpful to consult one of the specialized companion volumes.

My thanks are due to Drs B.F. Millet, N.E. Williams, J.M. Roland and D.B. Rowlands for helpful suggestions with the radiology, rheumatology, endocrinology and cardiology sections.

Dennis Guttmann
Peterborough
October, 1996

Symbols used in this volume

−	Not available/not known
n	normal (unchanged)
=	unchanged (equivalent)
+ ++ +++	present (positive)
− −− −−−	absent (negative)
↑ ↑↑ ↑↑↑	increased
↓ ↓↓ ↓↓↓	reduced
<	less than (below)
>	greater than (above)
∅	diameter

Symbols for recording a family history

Example:

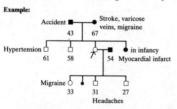

Symbols:

✒	Patient
■	male, deceased/affected
●	female, deceased/affected
□	male, living/not affected
○	female, living/not affected
♦	abortion
⊡	male carrier
⊙	female carrier
□—○	consanguinous marriage

Short contents

Nomogram for determination of body surface area of adults from height and weight[a]

(From Lentner (1977))

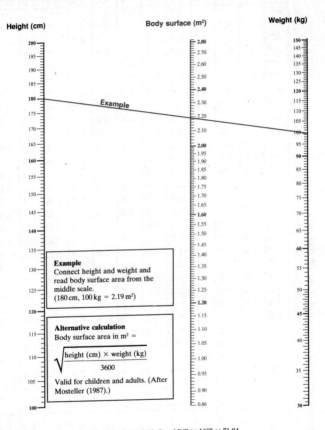

Height (cm) · **Body surface (m²)** · **Weight (kg)**

Example

Example
Connect height and weight and read body surface area from the middle scale.
(180 cm, 100 kg = 2.19 m²)

Alternative calculation
Body surface area in m² =

$$\sqrt{\frac{\text{height (cm)} \times \text{weight (kg)}}{3600}}$$

Valid for children and adults. (After Mosteller (1987).)

[a] After the formula of Du Bois and Du Bois (1916) $O = M^{0.425} \times L^{0.725} \times 71.84$
or $\log O = \log M \times 0.425 + \log L \times 0.725 + 1.8564$.
(O = body surface area (in cm²), M = weight (in kg), L = height (in cm))

Determination of expected date of delivery

Expected date of delivery is found in the lower row below the date of the first day of the last menstrual period in the upper row.

LMP / start month	1	2	3	4	5	6	7	8	9	10	11	12	13	14	15	16	17	18	19	20	21	22	23	24	25	26	27	28	29	30	31	LMP / end month
January / October	8	9	10	11	12	13	14	15	16	17	18	19	20	21	22	23	24	25	26	27	28	29	30	31	1	2	3	4	5	6	7	**January / November**
February / November	8	9	10	11	12	13	14	15	16	17	18	19	20	21	22	23	24	25	26	27	28	29	30	1	2	3	4	5				**February / December**
March / December	6	7	8	9	10	11	12	13	14	15	16	17	18	19	20	21	22	23	24	25	26	27	28	29	30	31	1	2	3	4	5	**March / January**
April / January	6	7	8	9	10	11	12	13	14	15	16	17	18	19	20	21	22	23	24	25	26	27	28	29	30	31	1	2	3	4		**April / February**
May / February	5	6	7	8	9	10	11	12	13	14	15	16	17	18	19	20	21	22	23	24	25	26	27	28	1	2	3	4	5	6	7	**May / March**
June / March	8	9	10	11	12	13	14	15	16	17	18	19	20	21	22	23	24	25	26	27	28	29	30	31	1	2	3	4	5	6		**June / April**
July / April	7	8	9	10	11	12	13	14	15	16	17	18	19	20	21	22	23	24	25	26	27	28	29	30	1	2	3	4	5	6	7	**July / May**
August / May	8	9	10	11	12	13	14	15	16	17	18	19	20	21	22	23	24	25	26	27	28	29	30	31	1	2	3	4	5	6	7	**August / June**
September / June	8	9	10	11	12	13	14	15	16	17	18	19	20	21	22	23	24	25	26	27	28	29	30	1	2	3	4	5	6	7		**September / July**
October / July	8	9	10	11	12	13	14	15	16	17	18	19	20	21	22	23	24	25	26	27	28	29	30	31	1	2	3	4	5	6	7	**October / August**
November / August	8	9	10	11	12	13	14	15	16	17	18	19	20	21	22	23	24	25	26	27	28	29	30	31	1	2	3	4	5	6		**November / September**
December / September	7	8	9	10	11	12	13	14	15	16	17	18	19	20	21	22	23	24	25	26	27	28	29	30	1	2	3	4	5	6	7	**December / October**

Skin alterations

Primary eruptions

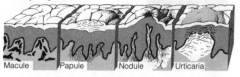

Macule | Papule | Nodule | Urticaria

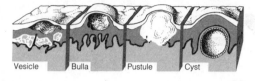

Vesicle | Bulla | Pustule | Cyst

Secondary eruptions

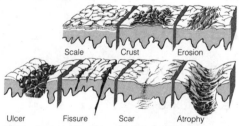

Scale | Crust | Erosion

Ulcer | Fissure | Scar | Atrophy

Clinical classification of skin lesions

Stratum	Within the skin plane	Above the skin plane	Below the skin plane
Epidermis Melanocytes	Hypomelanotic and hypermelanotic (brown) macule		
Keratinocytes	Macule	Papule, vesicle, bulla, pustule, plaque, hyperkeratosis excematous dermatitis, exudative (impetiginous) lesion	Atrophy Fissure
Dermis Connective tissue	Atrophy Sclerosis	Papule, nodule, oedema	Ulcer, sclerosis atrophy, excoriation
Vessels	Telangiectasia Purpura	Urticaria, erythema multiforme, morbilliform, scarlatiniform	
Adipose layer		Nodule, erythema nodosum	Atrophy

Eye test chart

95

874

2843

638   ЕШЄ   XOO

8745   ЄПШ   OXO

63925   ПЕЄ   XOX

428365   ШЕП   OXO

374258   ЄШЄ   x x o

937826   шпЕ   x o o

   ешп   o o x

Point	Jaeger	Equivalent distance
		0.025
		0.05
26	16	0.1
14	10	0.2
10	7	0.29
8	5	0.4
6	3	0.5
5	2	0.67
4	1	0.8
3	1+	1.0

View at a distance of 35 cm under good illumination. Test with and without spectacles, ensuring that long-sighted patients look through the close-vision segment of the lens. Short-sighted patients are tested only with spectacles. (After Rosenbaum, J.G., Graham-Field Surgical, New Hyde Park, NY11040)

Hearing tests

Conductive (usually middle ear) or **perceptive** (usually inner ear) **deafness?**

1. Weber test:

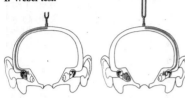

Place a tuning fork on the vertex of the skull. The patient indicates whether the tone is heard centrally or is **lateralized** to one ear.

Conductive (middle ear) deafness: lateralization into the **affected** (deafer) ear

Perceptive (inner ear) deafness: lateralization into the healthy (better) ear

Tuning fork is placed on mastoid process (bone conduction). If no sound is heard, hold the tuning fork in front of the ear

2. Rinne's test:

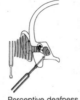

Conductive deafness right

Perceptive deafness left

Evaluation:
Rinne's test **normal** (= **positive**): Air conduction is heard about twice as long as bone conduction (30 s longer)

Rinne's test **abnormal** (= **negative**): Air conduction is briefer than bone conduction

Conductive (middle ear) deafness: Rinne **abnormal** (negative)

Perceptive (inner ear) deafness: Rinne **normal** (positive)

Lesion of	Weber	Rinne
Middle ear	Lateralization to abnormal ear	Abnormal (= negative)
Inner ear	Lateralization to healthy ear	Normal (= positive)

Adult dentition

View from in front of the patient

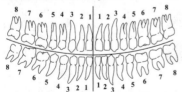

Two-digit dental scheme (after the Fédération Dentaire Internationale, London, 1970); **now universally accepted**.

Each quadrant of the permanent dentition receives a reference number (1 to 4), clockwise: right upper – left upper – left lower – right lower

	Reference Number 1								Reference Number 2							
	18	17	16	15	14	13	12	11	21	22	23	24	25	26	27	28	
Right	48	47	46	45	44	43	42	41	31	32	33	34	35	36	37	38	Left
	Reference Number 4								Reference Number 3							

Catheter and needle sizes

Gauge (gg.)	External diameter mm	inch
35	0.13	0.005
34	0.18	0.007
33	0.20	0.008
32	0.23	0.009
31	0.25	0.010
30	0.30	0.012
29	0.33	0.013
28	0.36	0.014
27	0.41	0.016
26	0.46	0.018
25	0.51	0.020
24	0.56	0.022
23	0.64	0.025
22	0.71	0.028
21	0.81	0.032
20	0.89	0.035
19	1.07	0.042
18	1.27	0.050
17	1.50	0.059
16	1.65	0.065
15	1.83	0.072
14	2.11	0.083
13	2.41	0.095
12	2.77	0.109
11	3.05	0.120
10	3.40	0.134
9	3.76	0.148
8	4.19	0.165
7	4.57	0.180
6	5.16	0.203

French	mm
34	11.3
32	10.7
30	10.0
28	9.3
26	8.7
24	8.0
22	7.3
20	6.7
19	6.3
18	6.0

French	mm
3	1.0
4	1.35
5	1.67
6	2.0
7	2.3
8	2.7
9	3.0
10	3.3
11	3.7
12	4.0
13	4.3
14	4.7
15	5.0
16	5.3
17	5.7

For an **oval-shaped** instrument: lay a strip of paper around the circumference of the instrument and read the value from the scale

0 5 10 15 20 25 30 35 40

Calculation of the drip rate of infusions

Calculation of number of drops per minute (drip rate)

Given:
Required infusion volume in litres (l)
Desired infusion duration in hours (h)

Explanation of the use of the graph:
(Example: 1.5l to be infused in 6h)

1. Find 1.5 on the **lower horizontal** scale (infusion volume).

2. Draw a vertical line from this point to the intersection with the diagonal line 'Infusion duration 6 h' (scale above and on right).

3. Draw a horizontal line from this intersection to the scale on the **left**, where the **answer**, '65 drops per minute', can be read.

Valid for 1 ml liquid = 16 drops

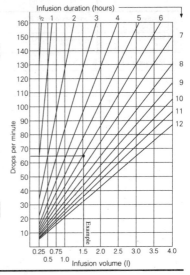

Calculation:	Number of drops per minute (drip rate)
Given:	Desired infusion volume in millilitres (ml)
	Desired infusion volume in hours (h)

| Milli- | Hours | | | | | | | | | | | | | | | | | | | |
litres	0.5	1	2	3	4	5	6	7	8	9	10	11	12	14	16	18	20	24	48
100	66	33	16	11	8	6	5	4	3	–	–	–	–	–	–	–	–	–	–
200	133	66	33	22	16	13	11	10	9	7	–	–	–	–	–	–	–	–	–
250	166	83	42	24	17	16	14	13	11	10	9	–	–	–	–	–	–	–	–
300	200	100	50	33	25	20	17	15	13	12	11	–	.	–	–	–	–	–	–
400	266	133	66	44	33	27	22	19	17	14	13	12	11	–	–	–	–	–	–
500	333	166	83	55	41	33	28	24	21	19	17	15	14	12	10	9	8	7	–
1000	666	333	166	111	83	66	56	48	42	37	33	30	28	24	21	19	16	14	7
2000	–	667	333	222	166	133	111	95	83	74	67	61	56	48	42	37	33	28	14
3000	–	–	500	333	250	200	167	142	125	111	100	91	83	71	63	56	50	42	21
4000	–	–	666	444	333	267	222	190	167	148	133	121	111	95	83	74	67	56	28
5000	–	–	833	555	417	333	278	238	208	185	167	152	139	119	104	93	83	69	35

Table valid for: 1 ml liquid = 20 drops

Formula:

$$\frac{\text{Infusion volume in millilitres}}{\text{Infusion duration in hours} \times K} = \text{Drops per minute}$$

K for 16 drops/ml: 3.75
K for 20 drops/ml: 3

Patient population

		Ill	Healthy
T E S T	Positive	Correct-positive (CP) Sensitivity	False-positive (FP)
	Negative	False-negative (FN)	Correct-negative (CN) Specificity

The character of a test is defined as follows:

Specificity	$\dfrac{CN}{FP + CN}$	Sensitivity	$\dfrac{CP}{CP + CN}$
Pos. prediction	$\dfrac{CP}{CP + FP}$	Neg. prediction	$\dfrac{CN}{FN + CN}$

Normal distribution

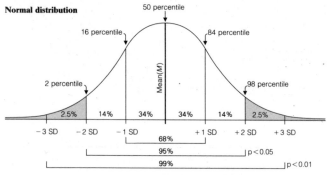

M ± 2 standard deviations (SD) = 95% of the values in a 'normal' population

$$\text{Mean } (M) = \frac{\text{sum of } x}{n} \qquad \text{SEM} = \frac{\text{SD}}{\sqrt{n}}$$

Null hypothesis (H_o)	Is correct	Is false
Is disproved	Error of the first kind Probability of error α (α-error)	No error Probability $1 - \alpha$
Is confirmed	No error Probability $1 - \beta$*	Error of the second kind Probability of error β (β-error)

Epidemiological and demographic parameters

Mortality = $\dfrac{\text{Number of deaths}}{\text{Average total population}}$	Incidence = $\dfrac{\text{Number of new cases}}{\text{Average total population}}$
Lethality = $\dfrac{\text{Number of deaths}}{\text{Number of completed cases}}$	Prevalence = $\dfrac{\text{Number of cases**}}{\text{Average total population}}$

* = 'Power'   ** Number at a particular point in time

SI units

Measurement	Unit	Symbol	Equivalents
Length	metre	m	
Area	square metre	m^2	
Volume	cubic metre	m^3	$= 1000\,dm^3 = 1000\,l$
	litre	l	
Mass	kilogram	kg	
Amount of substance	mole	mol	
Concentration (molarity)	mole per cubic metre	mol/m^3	$= 10^3 \times mol/l$
Catalytic activity	catal	cat	$= mol/s$
Force	newton	N	$= 0.102\,kgf$
Power	watt	W	$= J/s$
Energy, work, amount of heat	joule	J	$= 0.239\,cal_{th}$
	kilojoule	kJ	$= 0.239\,kcal_{th}$
Thermodynamic temperature	kelvin	K	$1\,K = 1°C$
	celsius	°C	$0°C = 273.15\,K$
Pressure	pascal	Pa	$= 0.0075\,mmHg$
	kilopascal	kPa	$= 7.5\,mmHg$
	bar	bar	$= 100\,kPa$
	standard physical atmosphere	atm	$= 101.3\,kPa$
Velocity	metres per second	m/s	
Acceleration	metres per second²	m/s^2	
Frequency	hertz	Hz	
Electric current	ampère	A	
Electric charge	coulomb	C	
Electric potential difference	volt	V	
Electric capacity	farad	F	
Electric resistance	ohm	Ω	
Electric conductivity	siemen	S	
Luminous intensity	candela	cd	
Illuminance	lux	lx	
Wavelength	ångström	Å	$= 0.1\,nm = 10^{-10}\,m$
Radioactivity	becquerel	Bq	$= 0.27 \times 10^{-10}\,Ci$
	curie	Ci	$= 3.7 \times 10^{10}\,Bq$
Absorbed dose	gray	Gy	$= 100\,rd$
	rad	rd	$= 0.01\,Gy$
Exposure	röentgen	R	$= 2.58 \times 10^{-4}\,C/kg$
Dose equivalent	sievert	Sv	$= 100\,rem$
	rem	rem	$= 0.01\,Sv$

Prefixes for SI units

Factor	Prefix	Symbol	Factor	Prefix	Symbol	Factor	Prefix	Symbol
10^{18}	exa	E	10^6	mega	M	10^{-9}	nano	n
10^{15}	peta	P	10^3	kilo	k	10^{-12}	pico	p
10^{12}	tera	T	10^{-3}	milli	m	10^{-15}	femto	f
10^9	giga	G	10^{-6}	micro	μ	10^{-18}	atto	a

Normal chemical values

Determination	Normal Values		
	Conventional	SI units	In-house
Albumin (p. 201)	3.5–5.0 g/dl	35–50 g/l	
Ammonia	80–110 ug/dl	47–65 µmol/l	
Anion gap (p. 126)	8–12 meq/l	8–12 mmol/l	
Bilirubin: total (p. 149)	0.3–1.0 mg/dl	5–17 µmol/l	
indirect	0.2–0.7 mg/dl	3.4–12 µmol/l	
direct	0.1–0.3 mg/dl	1.7–5.0 µmol/l	
Blood coagulation (p. 218)			
Blood count (p. 208)			
Blood gases (p. 128)			
Calcium: total	8.5–10.6 mg/dl	2.12–2.65 mmol/l	
ionized	4.0–5.0 mg/dl	1.0–1.25 mmol/l	
Cerebrospinal fluid (p. 178)			
Chloride	95–105 meq/l	95–105 mmol/l	
Cholesterol (p. 100)	140–250 mg/dl	3.6–6.4 mmol/l	
Cholesterol HDL (p. 100)	30–75 mg/dl	0.78–1.94 mmol/l	
Complement CH50	150–250 U/ml	1.5–2.5 g/l	
C3	55–120 mg/dl	0.55–1.2 g/l	
C4	20–50 mg/dl	0.2–0.5 g/l	
C-reactive protein	< 10 mg/l		
Creatinine (p. 162)	0.6–1.5 mg/dl	60–130 µmol/l	
Drug assay (pp. 298–326)			
Ferritin	15–200 ng/ml	15–200 µg/l	
Folic acid	6–15 ng/ml	14–34 nmol/l	
Glucose	70–110 mg/dl	4.0–6.0 mmol/l	
Glucose load (p. 245)			
Hormones (p. 235)			
Iron	70–140 µg/dl	13–25 µmol/l	
Ketones/acetoacetate	0.3–2.0 mg/dl	< 0.3 mmol/l	
Lactate	0.6–1.8 meq/l	0.6–1.8 mmol/l	
Lipid electrophoresis (p. 100)			
Magnesium	1.5–2.1 meq/l	0.75–1.05 mmol/l	
Osmolarity	285–295 mosm/l	285–298 mosm/l	
Phosphate (inorganic)	3.0–4.5 meq/l	1.0–1.5 mmol/l	
Potassium	3.5–5.0 meq/l	3.5–5.0 mmol/l	
Protein (total) (p. 201)	6–8.5 g/dl	60–80 g/l	
Sodium	135–145 meq/l	135–145 mmol/l	
Triglycerides	50–250 mg/dl	0.6–3.0 mmol/l	
Tumour markers (p. 227)			
Urea	15–40 mg/dl	2.5–6.7 mmol/l	
Uric acid	3.0–7.0 mg/dl	180–420 µmol/l	
Urine (p. 163)			
Vitamin B$_{12}$	40–150 mg/dl	0.45–1.5 mmol/l	

Note: Commonly used laboratory results are listed with average normal values. The interpretation of normal values must include consideration of the following parameters: method of sample collection, analytical technique, transport time, and age and sex of the patient.

Normal enzyme values

Due to the large number of analytical methods, it is not possible to give normal values.

Abbreviation	Determination	Conversion
	Aldolase	
	α-Amylase	
	Cholinesterase	
CK	Creatine phosphokinase	
CK-MB	Cardiac isoenzyme of CK	
γ-GT	γ-Glutamyl transferase	
HBDH	Hydroxybutyrate dehydrogenase	
LAP	Leucine aminopeptidase	
LDH	Lactate dehydrogenase	
	Lipase	
	5'-Nucleotidase	
AP	Phosphatase: alkaline	
	acid	
	prostate specific	
SGOT/ASAT	Aspartate aminotransferase	
SGPT/ALAT	Alanine aminotransferase	

Conversion scale: μkat / U / nkat / U

$\leftarrow \times 0.016\,67$ $\times 60.0 \rightarrow$

$\leftarrow \times 16.67$ $\times 0.060 \rightarrow$

Plasma alcohol (blood alcohol) determination

Conversion of g/l to mmol/l:

Factor = 21.71

$(0.8\,g/l \times 21.71 = 17.37\,mmol/l)$

Conversion of mmol/l to g/l:

Factor = 0.04607

$(17.37\,mmol/l \times 0.04607 = 0.8\,g/l)$

Alcohol intoxication

Degree of intoxication	mg/dl	mmol/l	g/l
Mild	80–200	17–43	0.8–2.0
Moderate	200–400	43–87	2.0–4.0
Severe	>400	>87	>4.0

Antabuse reaction

Disulfiram-like reactions have been described with the following drugs:
cefamandol, cefmenoxim, cefoperazon, chloral hydrate, chloramphenicol, chlorpropamide, disulfiram, moxalactam, metronidazole, nitrofurantoin, tinidazole, tolbutamide.

Estimation of the alcohol concentration:

Men:
$$\text{alcohol (in \%)} = \frac{0.8 \times ml\ alcohol}{0.68 \times weight\ (kg)}$$

Women:
$$\text{alcohol (in \%)} = \frac{0.8 \times ml\ alcohol}{0.55 \times weight\ (kg)}$$

Conversion factor: 1 mg/l = 0.1% by weight
Breakdown per hour: 0.015–0.02 %/h

Conversion scales 1 (From Deom (1992))

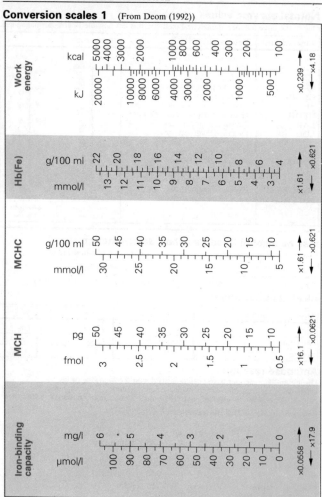

Conversion scales 2 (From Deom (1992))

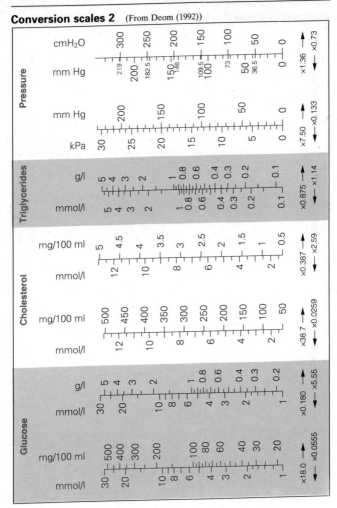

Conversion scales 3 (From Deom (1992))

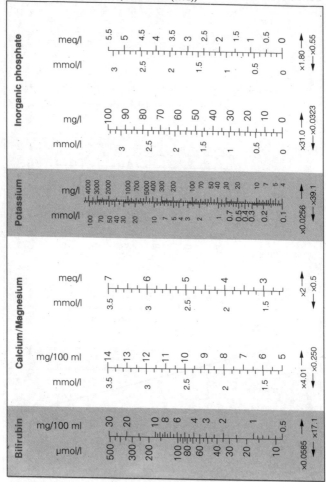

Conversion scales 4 (From Deom (1992))

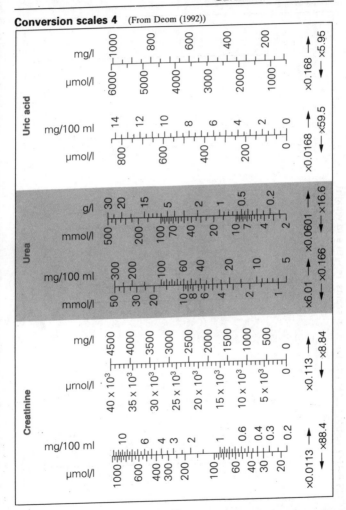

US & UK/metric system conversion scales: length and weight

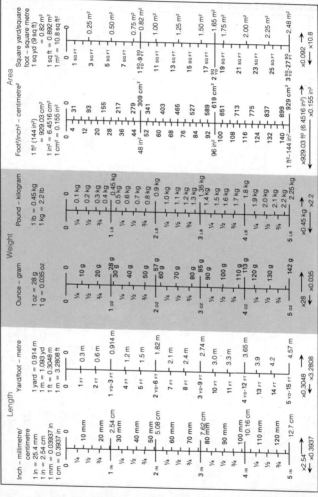

US/metric system conversion scales: volume and temperature

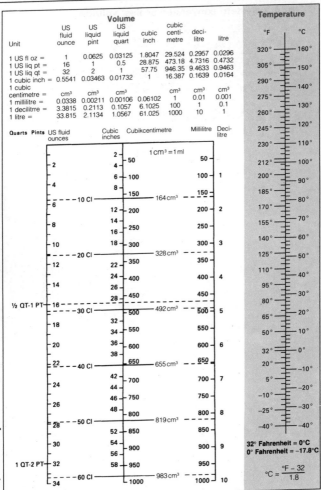

Unit	US fluid ounce	US liquid pint	US liquid quart	cubic inch	cubic centimetre	deci-litre	litre
1 US fl oz =	1	0.0625	0.03125	1.8047	29.524	0.2957	0.0296
1 US liq pt =	16	1	0.5	28.875	473.18	4.7316	0.4732
1 US liq qt =	32	2	1	57.75	946.35	9.4633	0.9463
1 cubic inch =	0.5541	0.03463	0.01732	1	16.387	0.1639	0.0164
1 cubic centimetre =	cm³ 0.0338	cm³ 0.00211	cm³ 0.00106	0.06102	1	cm³ 0.01	cm³ 0.001
1 millilitre =	3.3815	0.2113	0.1057	6.1025	100	1	0.1
1 decilitre =	33.815	2.1134	1.0567	61.025	1000	10	1
1 litre =							

Temperature

32° Fahrenheit = 0°C
0° Fahrenheit = −17.8°C

$$°C = \frac{°F - 32}{1.8}$$

UK/metric system conversion scales: volume

Unit	UK fluid ounce	UK liquid pint	Volume UK liquid quart	Cubic inch	Cubic centi-metre	Deci-litre	Litre
1 UK fl oz =	1	0.0625	0.01732	1.7339	28.413	0.2841	0.0284
1 UK liq pt =	20	1	0.5	34.677	568.26	5.683	0.5682
1 UK liq qt =	40	2	1	69.355	1136.5	113.65	1.1365
1 cubic inch =	0.5767	0.02883	0.01442	1	16.39	0.1639	0.0164
1 cubic centimetre =	cm³ 0.0352	cm³ 0.00176	cm³ 0.00088	cm³ 0.06102	1	cm³ 0.01	cm³ 0.001
1 millilitre =	0.0352	0.00176	0.00088	0.06102	1	0.01	0.001
1 decilitre =	3.5195	0.17596	0.08799	6.1024	100	1	0.1
1 litre =	35.195	1.7596	0.87987	61.024	1000	10	1

Radiological unit conversion scales

Röntgen – Curie – Becquerel

Rad – Gray

Röntgen – Curie – Becquerel

R/s $\begin{cases} mA/kg \\ \mu A/g \end{cases}$ $\updownarrow$ R $\begin{cases} mC/kg \\ \mu C/g \end{cases}$

2.6 2.4 2.2 2.0 1.8 1.6 1.4 1.2 1.0 0.8 0.6 0.4

10 9 8 7 6 5 4 3 2 1 — 0.258

3.876 4 — 1.0

1 R = 0.258 mC/kg
1 mC/kg = 3.876 R

R/min — $\begin{cases} \mu A/kg \\ nA/g \end{cases}$

40 35 30 25 20 15 10 5

10 9 8 7 6 5 4 3 2 1 — 5

2.326 — 10

mR/h $\begin{cases} pA/kg \\ pA/g \end{cases}$ $\updownarrow$ R/h $\begin{cases} nA/kg \\ pA/g \end{cases}$

700 600 500 400 300 200 100 — 71.67

10 9 8 7 6 5 4 3 2 1.395

1 R/h = 71.7 nA/kg
1 nA/kg = 13.95 R/h
= 0.2326 R/min
= 3.876 mR/s

kCi $\begin{cases} TBq \\ GBq \\ MBq \end{cases}$ Ci $\begin{cases} mCi \\ \mu Ci \\ nCi \end{cases}$ $\begin{cases} kBq \\ Bq \end{cases}$

350 300 250 200 150 37 100 50

10 9 8 7 6 5 4 3 2.703 1

1 Ci = 37 GBq
1 Bq = 27 pCi

rd $\begin{cases} mGy \\ mJ/min \end{cases}$ mrd/h $\begin{cases} mGy/min \\ \mu Gy/h \end{cases}$

100 90 80 70 60 50 40 30 20 10

10 9 8 7 6 5 4 3 2 1

1 rd = 10 mGy
1 Gy = 100 rd

rd/min $\begin{cases} mW/kg \\ \mu W/g \end{cases}$

1.6 1.4 1.2 1.0 0.8 0.6 0.4 0.2 — 0.1667

10 9 8 7 6 5 4 3 2 1.2 1

mrd/h $\begin{cases} pW/kg \\ nW/g \\ nW/g \\ \mu W/kg \end{cases}$ — 2.78

25 20 15 10 5

10 9 8 7 6 5 4 3 2 1 — 0.36

Patient positions for X-rays

supine recumbent, face up
prone recumbent, face down
erect sitting or standing

Projection determined by the direction which the X-rays take through the patient
(from X-ray tube to cassette)

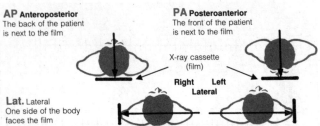

AP Anteroposterior
The back of the patient
is next to the film

PA Posteroanterior
The front of the patient
is next to the film

X-ray cassette
(film)

Right **Left**
Lateral

Lat. Lateral
One side of the body
faces the film

Oblique Any position between AP or PA and lateral (for special purposes, e.g. coronary
arteriography, the angle is commonly specified)

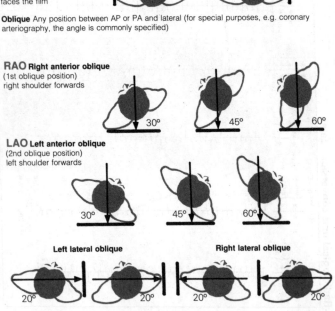

RAO Right anterior oblique
(1st oblique position)
right shoulder forwards

30°   45°   60°

LAO Left anterior oblique
(2nd oblique position)
left shoulder forwards

30°   45°   60°

Left lateral oblique   **Right lateral oblique**

20°   20°   20°   20°

Checklist for assessing a chest X-ray

Method
Routine diagnostic chest X-rays should be taken with at least 120 kV. The thorax should preferably be examined in two planes (i.e. also a lateral view). Advantages afforded by lateral views: atelectases often only visible in one plane; retrocardiac and retrosternal lesions and hilar changes often only seen on lateral films.

Technical evaluation
- Centring (symmetrical sternoclavicular joints, central spinous processes)
- Exposure (4th intervetrebral space just visible behind cardiac shadow)
- The lungs should be demonstrated to the periphery (subpleural)
- Degree of inspiration (with adequate inspiration the diaphragms should lie between the 10th and 11th ribs dorsally)
- The whole lung is demonstrated (pleural apices and costophrenic angles)
- Sharp outlines (no respiratory movement)
- Patient: age, sex, position, PA/AP, lateral

Chest X-rays: diagnostic procedure

- **Systematic analysis of the X-ray according to morphological structures**
  Attempt to follow the course of all important lines and structures and to interpret them
- A viewing distance of 2 metres is advantageous
- **Free analysis**, diagnosis by general impression
- Negative findings should be checked after an interval

Chest X-ray sectors in which diagnosis may be easy or difficult

1 few diagnostic errors
4 common diagnostic errors

Common sources of diagnostic errors

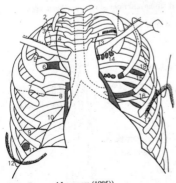

1 Cervical rib
2 Sternomastoid outline
3 1st and 2nd rib shadow
4 Azygos lobe
5 Bony articulation between 1st and 2nd ribs anteriorly
6 Bone bridge between 5th and 6th ribs posteriorly
7 Bifid 3rd rib
8 Horizontal fissure between upper and middle lobes
9 Low-lying accessory fissure of apical segment of lower lobe
10 Cardiac lobe
11 Nipple
12 Breast shadow
13 Subclavian artery
14 Calcified costal cartilage
15 Costal groove
16 Fissure of accessory left middle lobe
17 Pectoralis shadow
18 Edge of scapula

(From Freye and Lammers (1985))

Systematic analysis of morphological structures in chest X-rays

Bony thorax: harmonious, coniform, symmetrically sloping ribs; emphysematous subjects: barrel shaped; ribs widely spread, running horizontally, vertebral, sternal, rib deformity; cervical rib; fractures

Soft tissues neck/thorax: subcutaneous emphysema, foreign bodies, calcification

Pleura: pneumothorax, effusion, thickening, tumours, interlobar fissures, sinus

Diaphragm: dome (right higher than left in 90% of subjects); smooth surfaces, flattening, adhesions

Mediastinum: widening, displacement, emphysema

Trachea: position, lumen, stenosis (natural narrowing in laryngeal region, slight deviation to right in region of aortic arch), angle of bifurcation (normal 56°, range 41–71°)

Thoracic aorta: size, dilated, elongated? Normally reaches to 1 finger's breadth below clavicle in adequate inspiration; calcification; ectasia; stenoses

Heart: size, outline (p. 27), valves (see below), coronary calcification, pacing electrode, prosthetic valve

Differential diagnosis: calcification of aortic or mitral valve: line between heart apex and hilum on lateral view → aortic above, mitral below

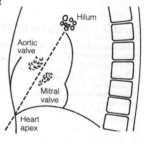

Hila: (p. 24): size, shape
- Pulmonary arteries, main and branches (normal r. pulmonary artery < 15 mm)
- Pulmonary veins (open below arteries in 1st atrium; arteries and veins parallel in upper lobes; veins lateral to arteries)
- Left hilum higher than right in 97% (range 0.75–2.25 cm)
- Lymph node enlargement
- Calcified lymph nodes

Pulmonary vessels (p. 30)
Distribution alteration – especially well seen in lateral view; alteration of calibre

Identifiable mediastinal lines

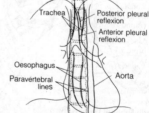

(From Burgener and Kormano (1985))

Lungs: parenchyma and interstitial tissues
Air bronchogram, outlines, calcification, interstitial/alveolar infiltrates (see below), Kerley lines (pp. 30, 31), double track phenomenon in bronchitis

Differentiation between interstitial and alveolar shadowing

Shadow pattern of interstitial disorders:
1. Ground glass appearance, uniform opalescence
2. Increased reticular lung markings
   (see ILO classification: symbols 's', 't', 'u'; p. 116)
3. Macular opacities, micronodular, nodular
   (see ILO classification: symbols 'p', 'q', 'r'; p. 116)
4. Hila usually not enlarged, often blurred
5. Elevation of diaphragm
6. Cysts (honeycombing)
7. Cardiac shadow may be deformed (right ventricular strain)

Alveolar shadowing:
1. Blurred contours
2. Tendency to confluence
3. Segmental/lobar distribution
4. Symmetrical left and right parahilar butterfly pattern
5. Air bronchogram
6. Peribronchial acinar rounded consolidations
7. Rapid evolution

General remarks:
Round opacities are recognizable early and are often overdiagnosed.
Linear opacities are recognized late and therefore often underdiagnosed.
In the normal chest X-ray one does not find rounded opacities, but numerous linear opacities may be seen.

Lung alterations

Topography
Position, shape, boundaries, one or more lobes, single segments (pp. 25, 26)

Character

Opacification (relative reduction of air content)
- **Zonal** (esp. parenchyma: infiltrates, neoplasms, atelectases)
  homogeneous – mottled sharp – blurred borders
  (round-/wedge-shaped opacity)

- **Linear**/streaky reticular: (esp. changes of the lung framework, blood/lymph vessels, bronchi)

- **Patchy:** (parenchyma or interstitium)

Translucencies (relative increase of air content)
Hyperplasia, malformation, reduced perfusion, expanded bronchial tree, bronchiectasis, Cysts, reduced lung parenchyma (emphysema)
Condensation of lung tissues

Diagnosis of lymph node enlargement

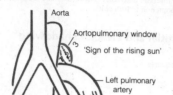

Aorta

Aortopulmonary window

'Sign of the rising sun'

Left pulmonary artery

Lymph nodes in aortopulmonary window
Fold between descending aorta and right pulmonary artery
- is concave (1): normal
- is straight (2): suspicion of lymph node enlargement
- is convex (3): definite lymph node enlargement ('sign of the rising sun')

Topography of the hila
(lateral chest X-ray)

The first branches of the pulmonary vessels can be identified on a technically satisfactory film.

If this is not possible, a pathological condition can be assumed, e.g. neoplasm, lymphadenopathy, vascular enlargement

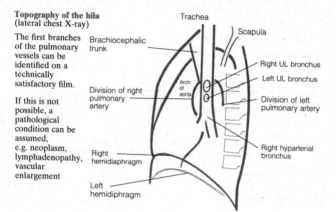

Trachea

Scapula

Brachiocephalic trunk

Division of right pulmonary artery

Arch of aorta

Right UL bronchus

Left UL bronchus

Division of left pulmonary artery

Right hyparterial bronchus

Right hemidiaphragm

Left hemidiphragm

Differential diagnosis: prominent azygos vein or lymph gland?

Problem: On PA film a spherical opacity in the position of the azygos vein.
→ Lymphadenopathy or prominent (engorged) vein?

Solution:
Attempt to identify the opacity on the lateral film: lymph node lies **in front** of the trachea.
A lymph node can be identified in both planes, but a vessel cannot be.

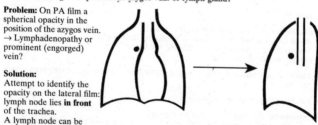

Bronchopulmonary segments – CT

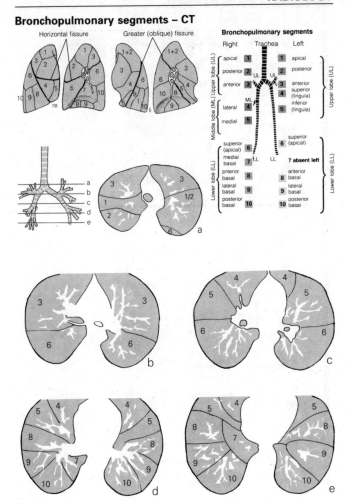

Horizontal fissure

Greater (oblique) fissure

Bronchopulmonary segments

Right	Trachea	Left
apical **1**		**1** apical
posterior **2**		**2** posterior
anterior **3**		**3** anterior
		4 superior (lingula)
lateral **4**		**5** inferior (lingula)
medial **5**		
superior (apical) **6**		**6** superior (apical)
medial basal **7**		**7** absent left
anterior basal **8**		**8** anterior basal
lateral basal **9**		**9** lateral basal
posterior basal **10**		**10** posterior basal

25

Radiological appearance of opacification of individual bronchopulmonary segments

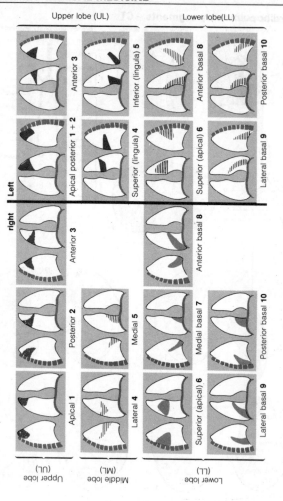

Cardiac outlines in the four standard radiological positions

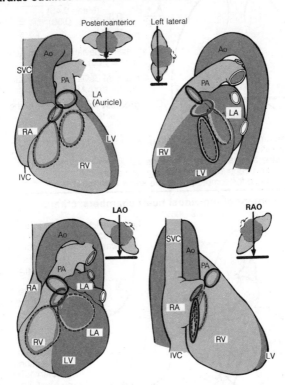

◯ Aortic valve position

◌ Mitral valve position

◯ Pulmonary valve position

◌ Tricuspid valve position

Ao   Aorta
PA   Pulmonary artery
LA   Left atrium
LV   Left ventricle
RA   Right atrium
RV   Right ventricle
SVC   Superior vena cava
IVC   Inferior vena cava

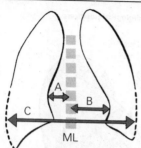

Cardiothoracic ratio

$$\frac{A + B}{C} < 0.5 \quad \begin{array}{l}\text{(Mean 0.45)}\\ \text{(0.39–0.50)}\end{array}$$

ML   midline

A   maximal deviation of right heart border from ML

B   maximal deviation of left heart border from ML

C   **greatest** inner diameter of thorax, internal to ribs

Measurements are valid only with good positioning and maximal inspiration.

Cardiothoracic ratio has no absolute validity as it is dependent on body build and concurrent illnesses (emphysema).

Very suitable for comparison **in the same individual**.

Enlargement of individual heart chambers: criteria
(From Burgener and Kormano (1985))

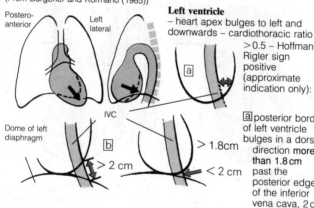

Left ventricle
– heart apex bulges to left and downwards – cardiothoracic ratio

> 0.5 – Hoffmann–Rigler sign positive (approximate indication only):

[a] posterior border of left ventricle bulges in a dorsal direction **more than 1.8 cm** past the posterior edge of the inferior vena cava, 2 cm above their intersection

and/or

[b] posterior border of left ventricle crosses posterior border of inferior vena cava **less than 2 cm** above the dome of the left diaphragm

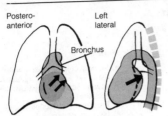

Postero-anterior | Left lateral

Bronchus

Left atrium

Displacement of oesophagus posteriorly (barium swallow) – prominent left auricle – heavy shadow (superimposed projection of right and left atria) – double contour on right (r./l. atria) – elevated left main bronchus – carina angle widened, normal 56° (41–71°) → collapse of left lower lobe with extreme enlargement, due to obstruction of left lower lobe bronchus

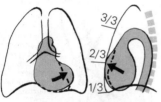

3/3
2/3
1/3

Right ventricle

Cardiac enlargement to left with elevated, often rounded, cardiac apex (due to displacement of left ventricle) – filling of retrosternal space (> 1/3) – right atrium can be displaced to right – left ventricle can be displaced posteriorly – seldom an isolated finding. Exception: pulmonary stenosis, Fallot's tetralogy, etc.

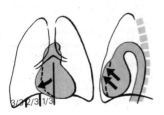

3/3 2/3 1/3

Right atrium

Cardiac shadow occupies more than a third of right hemithorax – rounded right cardiac contour – retrosternal space can be filled – seldom an isolated finding

Pulmonary venous congestion

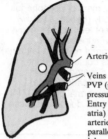

Arteries

Veins
PVP (pulmonary venous pressure) < 10 mmHg
Entry of pulmonary veins (into atria) lower than pulmonary arteries. Arteries and veins run parallel to each other in upper lobes, veins **lateral** to arteries

Normal

- Vessels at lung bases wider than at apices (greater volume due to hydrostatic pressure)
- Progressive reduction of calibre to periphery
- Vessels no longer recognizable as individual structures in peripheral third of lung field

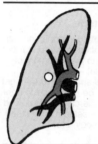

Early division

Dilatation of upper lobe veins → vessels in upper and lower lung equally filled

PVP 10–15 mmHg

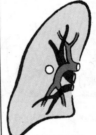

Diversion

Basal pulmonary veins narrowed with distinctly dilated upper lobe veins (vein diameter >3 mm in first intercostal space)

PVP 15–20 mmHg

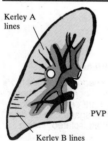

Kerley A lines

PVP 20–25 mmHg

Kerley B lines

Diversion and interstitial oedema

- Perivascular oedema, near hilum and/or peripherally
- Blurred vascular shadows
- Cuff formation around bronchi and vessels (peribronchial oedema)
- Ground glass-like shadowing
- Possibly pleural effusion (costophrenic, interlobular)
- Development of **Kerley A and B lines**

(Modified from Burgener and Kormano (1985))

Kerley lines:

oedematous interlobar septa, denser than vascular structures, no branching

Kerley B lines:

peripheral, near pleura (mostly basal, posterior), horizontal distinct lines, perpendicular to pleura, up to 1 cm in length

Kerley A lines:

radiating from hila, possibly curved, up to 4 cm in length

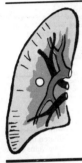

PVP
25–35 mmHg

Intra-alveolar oedema:

- Homogeneous, confluent macular shadows

- Positive bronchogram in region of shadowing (air becomes visible due to fluid filling of adjacent alveoli)

Additional, non-pathognomonic indications: pleural effusion, haemosiderosis (nodular), fibrosis, aneurysmal pulmonary veins, right heart hypertrophy

Radiological signs of pulmonary hypertension

(Pulmonary arterial hypertension, e.g. primary, after pulmonary embolus, response to persistent pulmonary venous hypertension)

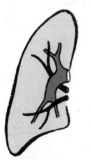

PAP
(pulmonary arterial pressure)
>50 mmHg

(PVP <
10 mmHg)

Pulmonary arterial hpertension

- Dilatation of pulmonary artery main stem and main branches (normal right pulmonary artery <15 mm)

- Transition in calibre centrally to peripheral pulmonary vessels (ratio usually more than 7:1): pruning of vessels, increased translucency of peripheral lung fields

PVP pulmonary venous pressure
PAP pulmonary arterial pressure

Summary of skeletal radiology

(Modified from Voegeli (1981))

Osteopenia **Quantitative reduction** of bone tissue, increased X-ray transradiency (however, beware the use of poor technique or overexposure)

Osteoporosis

- **Increased transradiency** of bone ('brilliance')
- Reduced number of trabeculae of spongiosa (coarse-stranded spongiosa) outside the lines of stress (**spongiolysis**)
- Splintering of the cortex from within
- **Enhanced prominence of cortex** ('frame' appearance of vertebrae)
- Reduced load-bearing capacity of bone → **incomplete fractures** (spine: wedging, collapse of vertebrae)

Osteomalacia

- Radiological signs mainly similar to those of osteoporosis

Differences:

- **Looser zones** (pseudofractures, incomplete fatigue fractures, often symmetrical in pelvis, e.g. pubis, ischium, neck of femur, ribs, running perpendicular to cortex. If numerous and symmetrical: Milkman's syndrome)
- **Bone deformity** (bell-shaped rib cage, 'ace of hearts' pelvis, kyphoscoliosis, biconcave vertebrae ('cod-fish spine'))
- Hazy, indistinct outlines of trabeculae

Hyperparathyroidism

- Subperiosteal bone resorption (early: radial side of middle phalanx of 2nd and 3rd digits)
- Distal osteolysis (tuft erosions)
- Osteoporosis (see above, esp. in primary hyperparathyroidism)
- Brown tumours (esp. in secondary hyperparathyroidism)
- Calcification in arteries, soft tissues and articular cartilage (chondrocalcinosis)
- Band sclerosis of vertebrae
- 'Pepper pot' mottling of skull

Osteolysis **Destruction of bone** (neoplastic: primary, metastatic; inflammatory)

- Spongy bone destroyed more quickly than compact bone
- Bone destruction visible on X-ray after about 10 days

Types of osteolysis
- Geographical (sharp boundary to surrounding bone)
- Moth-eaten (indistinct boundary)
- Infiltrating (boundary between affected and healthy bone difficult to determine)

Osteosclerosis New bone formation, increased bone density, reduced transradiency

1 **Reactive new bone formation** by pre-existing bone-forming elements (osteoblasts) as reaction to diverse irritants (inflammation, tumour, trauma) is a non-specific sign
   - Condensation of pre-existing bone elements (spongiosa, compacta) follows original organization of the bone

1a **Endosteal reactive new bone formation**
   (e.g. geographic lysis with sclerotic borders)

1b **Periosteal reactive new bone formation**
   Solid
   Interrupted
   - Lamellar
   - Radial (ray-like, sunburst)
   - Amorphous

2 **New bone formation by tumour cells**
   (chondrogenic, osteogenic tumours)
   Calcification of tumour matrix
   - Disorganized nests of new bone formation independent of the original organization of the bone

Osteonecrosis Bone death
(Ischaemic, e.g. trauma, embolism, compression of blood vessels)
- Alteration of bone density → increased transradiency
- In surrounding osteoporosis or repair (sequestrum)
- Patchy picture of osteolysis and osteosclerosis

Osteoarthritis/inflammatory arthritis

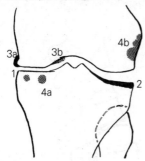 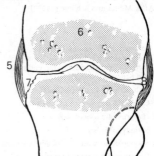

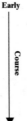

Osteoarthritis of knee	**Early**	**Inflammatory arthritis of knee**

Osteoarthritis of knee

1   Joint space reduction
2   Subchondral sclerosis
3a Osteophytes
3b Inner margin pad
4a Subchondral/periarticular cystic erosions
4b Marginal erosions

Course

Inflammatory arthritis of knee

5   Soft-tissue swelling (distension of the joint capsule by effusion or synovial swelling)
6   Periarticular osteoporosis
7   Erosions, destruction
8   Joint space reduction

Late

NB: Radiological signs of arthritis may only be visible after days or weeks.
Scintigraphy (bone scan) is more sensitive and enables earlier diagnosis.

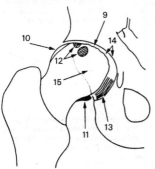

Osteoarthritis of hip
(After Freye and Lammers (1982))

9   Wavy outline of joint line
10 Reduplication of joint line
11 Calcification of joint capsule
12 Cystic defects
13 Reactive new bone or cartilage formation
14 Incongruence of joint surfaces
15 Deformation of femoral head Joint space reduction

Radiological signs of non-inflammatory changes of the spine
(After Müller and Schillung (1982))

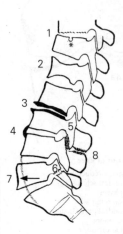

1 Juvenile developmental defect (Scheuermann's disease) with wedged vertebra, irregularities of the end plates and Schmorl's nodes*

2 Fish vertebra in osteoporosis

3 Osteochondrosis with spondylosis

4 Hyperostotic spondylosis

5 Spondylarthrosis

6 Spondylolysis with 7 Spondylolisthesis

8 Baastrup's syndrome ('kissing osteophytes')

Radiology of the vertebra
(After Schinz *et al.* (1979))

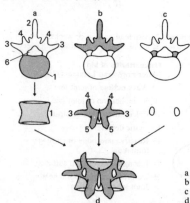

1 Body
2 Spinous process
3 Transverse process
4 Superior articular process
5 Inferior articular process
6 Vertebral foramen

a Projection of the vertebral body
b Projection of the region of the arch
c Pedicles which connect a with b
d Superimposed view of a–c

Bone metastases

- **Sclerotic (osteoblastic)** metastases (common in carcinoma of prostate, breast, stomach, pancreas, etc.)
- **Osteolytic (osteoclastic)** metastases (common in carcinoma of bronchus, thyroid, breast, ovary, colon, gall bladder; renal cell carcinoma, primary carcinoma of liver)
- Mixed osteolytic–osteoblastic metastases

Primary tumour in:	Bone metastases (% of cases)
Breast	61
Prostate	50
Lung (carcinoma of bronchus)	33
Kidney	25
Thyroid	20
Liver	17
Pancreas	14
Bladder	12
Stomach	12
Body and cervix of uterus	11

Preferred sites
- Spine   70% (lumbar > thoracic > cervical)
- Femur   50%
- Humerus   17%
- Ribs   10%
- Cranial vault   9%
- Pelvis   9%
- Shoulder girdle   6%
- Tibia   1%

Solitary bone metastases ~25%

Typical distribution of bone metastases

Individual regions of the skeleton are affected by bone metastases with different frequencies.
In patients with carcinoma of the breast, bone metastases involve pelvis, spine, femur, ribs and skull in decreasing order of frequency. Patients with carcinoma of the prostate show skeletal metastases (in decreasing order of frequency) in the lumbar spine, sacrum, pelvis, upper half of femur and humerus, ribs, scapula and skull.

Typical distribution of bone metastases

Very frequent	▓▓▓ : pelvis, spine, femur
Frequent	▒▒▒ : ribs, skull
Infrequent	███ : extremities

Lateral skull

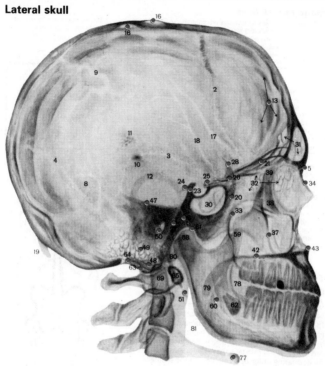

1 Sagittal suture
2 Coronal suture (partly calcified)
3 Squamous suture
4 Lambdoid suture
5 Nasofrontal suture
6 Spheno-occipital
   cartilaginous joint*
7 Frontozygomatic suture
8 Sutural bone*
9 Diploetic canals
10 Calcified pineal*
11 Calcification in choroid
   plexus*
12 External ear

13 Impressions of cerebral gyri
14 Calcification of falx*
15 Frontal emissary*
16 Arachnoid granulations*
17 Sphenoparietal sulcus
18 Groove for middle
   meningeal artery
19 Occipital protuberance*
20 Anterior wall of middle
   cranial fossa
21 Roof of orbit
22 Floor of posterior
   cranial fossa
23 Dorsum sellae

24 Calcification at insertion
   of tentorium*
25 Anterior clinoid process
26 Sphenoidal plane
27 Clivus
28 Greater and lesser wings
   of sphenoid
29 Crista galli
30 Sphenoidal sinus
31 Frontal sinus
32 Ethmoidal air cells
33 Wall of maxillary sinus
* Inconstant or variable

(After Gerlach J., Viehweger G. and Pupp J.S. With permission of Boehringer, Ingelheim)

Skull AP

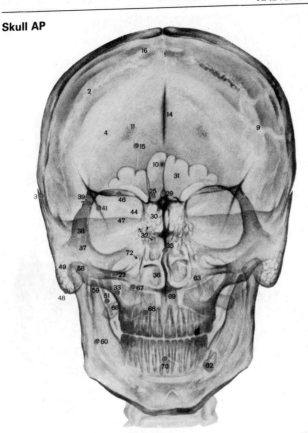

34 Nasal bone
35 Nasal septum
36 Inferior turbinate
37 Zygomatic bone
38 Frontosphenoidal
  process of zygoma
39 Zygomatic process of
  frontal bone

40 Margin of orbit
41 Innominate line
42 Hard palate
43 Anterior nasal spine
44 Superior orbital fissure
45 Optic foramen
46 Lesser wing of sphenoid

47 Petrous part of temporal bone
48 Mastoid process
49 Mastoid air cells
50 External auditory meatus
51 Styloid process
52 Arcuate eminence
* Inconstant or variable

(After Gerlach J., Viehweger G. and Pupp J.S. With permission of Boehringer, Ingelheim)

37

Sinuses

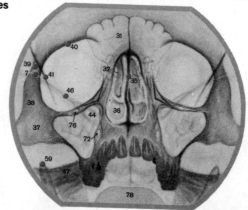

Nasal sinuses

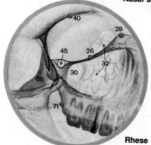

Rhese   **Stenvers**

53 Internal auditory meatus
   and foramen
54 Cochlea
55 Vestibulum
56 Upper and lateral
   semicircular canals
57 Trigeminal notch
58 Head of mandible
59 Muscular process of
   mandible
60 Mandibular canal
61 Temporomandibular joint

64 Foramen magnum
65 Anterior arch of atlas
66 Transverse process of atlas
67 Atlanto-occipital joint
68 Atlantoaxial joint
69 Odontoid process of axis
70 Split vertebral spine
71 Pterygoid process
72 Foramen rotundum
73 Foramen ovale
74 Foramen spinosum

75 Foramen lacerum
76 Infraorbital foramen
77 Hyoid bone with
   greater cornua
78 Tongue
79 Uvula
80 Ear lobe
81 Pharyngeal cavity
82 Trachea
* Inconstant or variable

(After Gerlach J., Viehweger G. and Pupp J.S. With permission of Boehringer, Ingelheim)

CT cross-sectional topography

(From Wegener, O.H. Ganzkörper-Computertomographie. With permission of the author and Schering AG, Berlin)

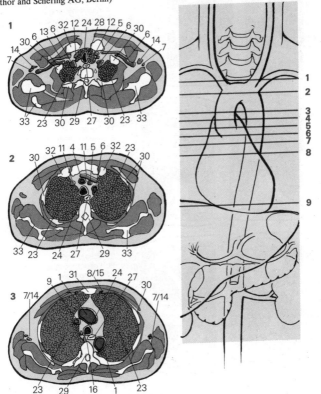

Hounsfield units (HU).

Water	0 HU	Blood, clotted	50–100 HU
Cerebrospinal fluid	10 HU	Bone	>500 HU
Brain	30–40 HU	Fat	–50 to –100 HU
Blood, liquid	40–50 HU		

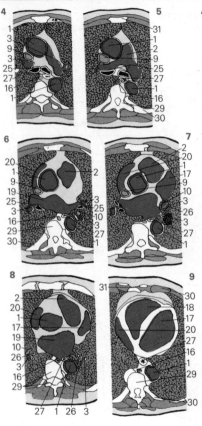

Arteries

1 Aorta
2 Pulmonary trunk
3 Pulmonary artery
4 Innominate artery
5 Common carotid artery
6 Subclavian artery
7 Axillary artery
8 Internal mammary artery

Veins

9 Superior vena cava
10 Pulmonary vein
11 Innominate vein
12 Internal jugular vein
13 Subclavian vein
14 Axillary vein
15 Internal mammary vein
16 Azygos vein

Organs

17 Heart, left ventricle
18 Heart, right ventricle
19 Heart, left atrium
20 Heart, right atrium
21 Interventricular septum
22 Pericardium
23 Lung
24 Trachea
25 Main bronchus
26 Lobar bronchus
27 Oesophagus
28 Thyroid gland

Skeleton

29 Spinal column
30 Rib(s)
31 Sternum
32 Clavicle
33 Scapula

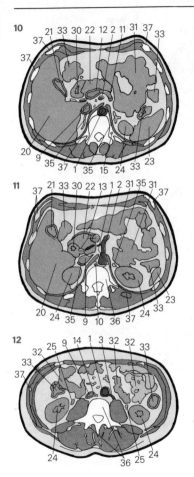

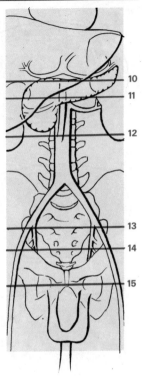

Arteries
1. Abdominal aorta
2. Superior mesenteric artery
3. Lumbar artery
4. Internal iliac artery
5. External iliac artery
6. Femoral artery
7. Pudendal artery
8. Dorsalis penis artery

41

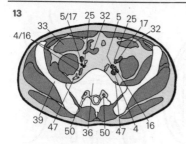

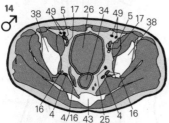

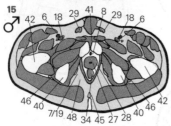

Veins

9 Inferior vena cava
10 Azygos vein
11 Splenic vein
12 Portal vein
13 Superior mesenteric vein
14 Lumbar vein
15 Vertebral vein
16 Internal iliac vein
17 External iliac vein
18 Femoral vein
19 Pudendal vein

Organs

20 Liver
21 Gall bladder
22 Pancreas
23 Spleen
24 Kidney
25 Ureter
26 Urinary bladder
27 Urethra
28 Prostate
29 Spermatic cord
30 Duodenum
31 Jejunum
32 Ileum
33 Colon
34 Rectum
35 Adrenal gland

Skeleton, etc.

36 Spinal column
37 Rib(s)
38 Hip bone
39 Ilium
40 Ischial tuberosity
41 Symphysis pubis
42 Femur
43 Sacrum
44 Sacroiliac joint
45 Coccyx
46 Sciatic nerve
47 Lumbosacral plexus
48 Ischiorectal fossa
49 Lymph nodes
50 Spinal nerve root

CT retroperitoneal spaces and pelvis

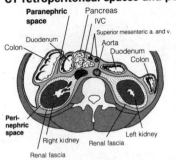

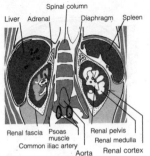

Retroperitoneal fascial spaces

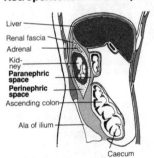

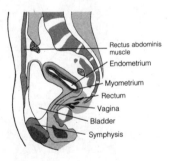

CT anatomy of (left) acetabulum – axial section

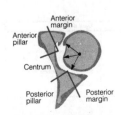

CT skull

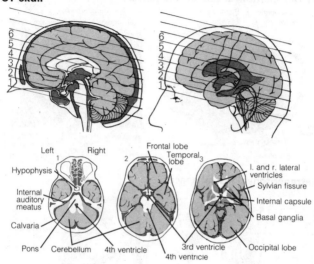

Left   Right   Frontal lobe
Temporal lobe

1   2   3

Hypophysis
l. and r. lateral ventricles
Internal auditory meatus
Sylvian fissure
Internal capsule
Calvaria
Basal ganglia
Pons   Cerebellum   4th ventricle
3rd ventricle
Occipital lobe
4th ventricle

Body of lateral ventricle   Calcar avis
Corpus callosum

4   5   6

Insula
Falx cerebri
Falx cerebri   Thalamus   Pre-central gyrus

Lesions

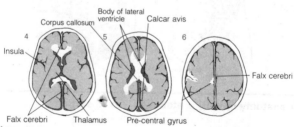

More dense	Less dense	Equal density
Fresh haemorrhages Calcification Bones Metastases Meningiomata	Infarcts (from 3rd day) Tumours Inflammatory foci Foci of demyelinization Fat Air Old haemorrhages Cerebral oedema Consequences of trauma	Cerebral infarct (first 3 days, 2nd week with contrast, dependent on the collateral supply over weeks) Subacute haematoma Astrocytoma

Magnetic resonance imaging – indications

Brain

Demyelinating lesions	Primary imaging procedure in cases of uncertain clinical diagnosis
	Second examination with unremarkable first examination and persisting symptoms
	In first episode (patient aged < 40 years)
Tumours	After unremarkable or non-diagnostic CT examination (with contrast)
	Primary indication in brain stem region with therapeutic possibility
Temporal lobe epilepsy	After unremarkable or non-diagnostic CT examination (with contrast)
	Primary indication if treatment resistance
Vascular lesions	After unremarkable or non-diagnostic CT examination (with contrast)
	Primary indication in region of brain stem

Mediastinal tumours

Primary and secondary tumours ⎫	After unremarkable or non-diagnostic CT examination
⎬	Before CT if vascular infiltration demonstrated
Inflammatory lesions ⎭	Possibly primary for determination of operability

Abdomen

Upper abdomen	
Liver	Haemangioma, adenoma, focal nodular hyperplasia
Retroperitoneal organs	Tumours for preoperative clarification after CT (selection of free planes)
	Vascular diagnosis in case of intolerance of contrast media
Pelvis	Tumour staging (after CT)

Spinal column

Intramedullary conditions	Primary imaging procedure
Extramedullary conditions	With intraspinal masses primary imaging procedure (before CT and myelography)
	With smaller lesions possibly Gd-DTPA
Disc lesions	In clinically unequivocal segmental association primary CT
	In discrepancy between clinical symptomatology and CT → MR
	With unclear segmental association MR possible as diagnostic procedure

Vessels

Aneurysms	Alternative to CT with contrast	⎫
Dissections	Primary indication	⎬ Large- and medium-calibre vessels
Thrombi	Alternative to CT with contrast	⎪
Coarctation of the aorta	Primary indication	⎭

Musculoskeletal system

Joints	Cartilage	MR best non-invasive imaging procedure	Temporomandibular arthropathy
			MR if therapeutically relevant
			Articular cartilage and menisci of other joints
			MR only after conventional investigation and if therapeutically relevant
	Ligaments	Non-invasive demonstration of the ligaments	Knee
			MR if therapeutically relevant and in cases not clarifiable with other non-invasive procedures
Bones	Necroses	MR most sensitive imaging procedure	MR for early recognition if therapeutically relevant, in cases inexplicable by other procedures and clinical examination
	Tumours	MR highly sensitive, but not specific (no DD between malignant and benign)	MR if therapeutic relevance, if not explicable by other procedures (after conventional radiography including tomography, but before CT)
	Metastases	Demonstration of bone marrow	MR with negative conventional radiography and nuclear scintigraphy with positive clinical findings and therapeutic relevance
Muscle		Demonstration of neuromuscular disorders, MR for planning of biopsy	

(Modified from Lissner and Seiderer (1990))

Magnetic resonance imaging – head

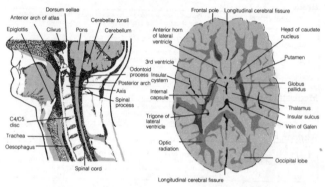

Cervical spine (T₁ image)

Axial skull (proton density image)

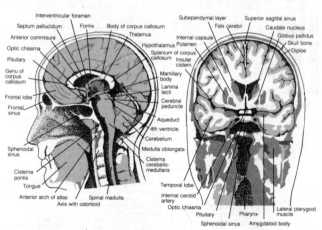

Saggital skull (spin-echo image)

Coronal skull (T₁ image)

MRI appearances of brain structures

	T_1 image	Proton density	T_2 image
Fluid space	Dark	Grey	Light
Vessel	Dark	Dark	Dark
Grey matter	Grey	Light grey	Light grey
White matter	Light grey	Grey	Grey
Fat	White	Light	Light
Bone/air	Dark	Dark	Dark

Image planes

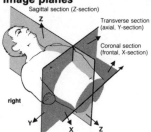

Sagittal section (Z-section)

Transverse section (axial, Y-section)

Coronal section (frontal, X-section)

right

Female pelvis – normal anatomy

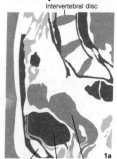

Intervertebral disc

Symphysis   Bladder   Uterus

1a: T_1, **1b**: proton density **1c**: T_2

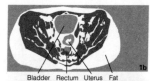

Bladder   Rectum   Uterus   Fat

1b

1c

Rectum

Retroperitoneal space, gradient echo

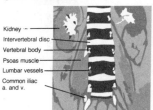

Kidney
Intervertebral disc
Vertebral body
Psoas muscle
Lumbar vessels
Common iliac a. and v.

Knee joint – sagittal (T_1)

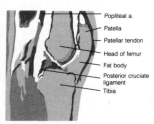

Popliteal a.
Patella
Patellar tendon
Head of femur
Fat body
Posterior cruciate ligament
Tibia

NYHA criteria

NYHA grade	Criteria
Grade I	**Exercise tolerance is uncompromised** (exceptionally strenuous physical effort can produce symptoms)
Grade II	**Exercise tolerance is slightly compromised** Symptoms with increased but not unusual effort (e.g. **walking uphill**). Mild effort without symptoms
Grade III	**Exercise tolerance is moderately compromised** Symptoms with mild effort (e.g. walking **on the level**), no symptoms at rest
Grade IV	**Exercise tolerance is severely compromised** Symptoms **at rest**: none of the effort above possible

Assessment of cardiovascular risk before non-cardiac operation

(After Goldman *et al.* (1977))

		Points
History	a) Age > 70 years b) Myocardial infarct < 6 months previously	5 10
Clinical examination	a) Grade 3 hypertension, distended neck veins b) Significant aortic stenosis	11 3
ECG	a) Not in sinus rhythm, or supraventricular ES in last preoperative ECG b) More than 5 VES/min at any time preoperatively	7 7
Poor general condition	$pO_2 < 8\,kPa$ or $pCO_2 > 6.7\,kPa$ K < 3.0 or $HCO_3 < 20\,mmol/l$ Urea > 8.3 mmol/l or creatinine > 300 µmol/l SGOT ↑, signs of chronic liver disease or patient bedridden for non-cardiac reasons	3
Nature of intended operation	a) Intraperitoneal, intrathoracic or on aorta b) Emergency surgery	3 4
Greatest possible point count		53

Severe complications to be expected*

Grade	Point count	Risk	e.g. perioperative infarct, pulmonary oedema, non-fatal ventricular tachycardia	Cardiac death
I	0–5	Small	0.5–0.7%	0.2%
II	6–12	Small to moderate	2–5%	1–2%
III	13–25	Moderate to high	11–12%	2–4%
IV	>25	Very high	to 22%	26–56%

* Approximate data from various references.

Central venous pressure

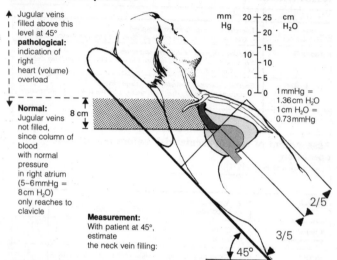

▲ Jugular veins
| filled above this
| level at 45°
| **pathological:**
| indication of
| right
| heart (volume)
| overload
|
▼ **Normal:**
Jugular veins
not filled,
since column of
blood
with normal
pressure
in right atrium
(5–6 mmHg =
8 cm H_2O)
only reaches to
clavicle

8 cm

mm Hg 20 — 25 cm H_2O
20
15
10 — 15
10
— 5
0 — 0 1 mmHg =
1.36 cm H_2O
1 cm H_2O =
0.73 mmHg

2/5

3/5

45°

Measurement:
With patient at 45°,
estimate
the neck vein filling:

Raised central venous pressure (jugular veins filled at 45°). Causes: raised right atrial pressure = **manifest** right heart failure; Differential diagnosis: constrictive pericarditis, superior vena cava obstruction, etc. The pressure can be estimated by increasing or decreasing the angle and determining the distance from the baseline to the height of the jugular vein filling.

Determination of baseline (level of right atrium):
4th intercostal space, perpendicular through the thorax, level at border between 2nd and 3rd fifths of diameter of thorax.

Hepatojugular reflux

Examination: Patient positioned with upper body at 45°, apply pressure with palm of hand (about 30–60 s) to right upper quadrant of abdomen or epigastrium; patient should be informed and should continue to breathe quietly.

Interpretation:

Volume loading by pressure on splanchnic region

Normal: **Correction** within a few heart beats, neck veins no longer visible **or** collapsed on inspiration (negative intrathoracic pressure → improved venous return)

Positive: **(pathological):** Neck veins continuously visible, remain engorged even in inspiration

Causes: **Latent** right heart failure

Differential diagnosis: constrictive pericarditis, superior caval obstruction

Auscultation areas
(After Shah, Slodki and Luisada (1964))

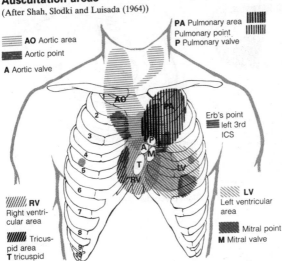

PA Pulmonary area
Pulmonary point
P Pulmonary valve

AO Aortic area
Aortic point
A Aortic valve

Erb's point
left 3rd
ICS

RV Right ventricular area

**Tricuspid area
T** tricuspid valve

LV Left ventricular area

Mitral point
M Mitral valve

Heart sounds and extra sounds

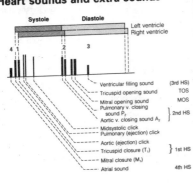

Systole	Diastole
	Left ventricle
	Right ventricle

Ventricular filling sound (3rd HS)
Tricuspid opening sound TOS
Mitral opening sound MOS
Pulmonary v. closing sound P_2
Aortic v. closing sound A_2 } 2nd HS
Midsystolic click
Pulmonary (ejection) click
Aortic (ejection) click
Tricuspid closure (T_1)
Mitral closure (M_1) } 1st HS
Atrial sound 4th HS

Sound intensity
Degree
1/6: only just heard with concentration
2/6: heard immediately at beginning of auscultation, not through hand laid on chest
3/6: heard distinctly (also through hand)
4/6: loud, accompanied by faint thrill, conducted to wrist
5/6: very loud with strong thrill, only heard with stethoscope applied to chest wall
6/6: very loud, still heard when stethoscope is a few centimetres from chest wall

ECG – electrode positions

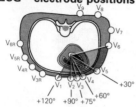

1st rib not palpable (under clavicle)

2nd rib: first palpable rib

Chest leads
(unipolar)

V_1 – 4th r. ICS parasternal
V_2 – 4th l. ICS parasternal
V_3 – between V_2 and V_4
V_4 – 5th ICS in l. midclavicular line (normally heart apex)
V_5 – l. anterior axillary line at height of V_4
V_6 – l. midaxillary line at height of V_4

Special chest leads

V_7 – posterior axillary line at height of V_4
V_8 – l. middle scapular line at height of V_4
V_9 – l. paravertebral line at height of V_4

Right precordial leads:

V_{3R}, V_{5R} } at positions corresponding to
V_{4R}, V_{6R} } those of the left-sided leads

Extremity leads:

right arm: red (or 1 ring)
left arm: yellow (or 2 rings)
left leg: green (or 3 rings)
(right leg: black [earth])

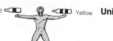

Red ▬ Yellow
Black (earth) Green

Bipolar extremity leads
after Einthoven

lead I   left arm → right arm
lead II   left leg → right arm
lead III left leg → left arm

Unipolar leads after Golberger
(a: augmented)

aVR – right arm potential
aVL – left arm potential
aVF – left foot potential

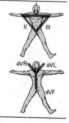

Frequently used leads in
Long-term ECG

(positive [+] and negative [−] bipolar electrode positions [usually designated C])

M	Manubrium sterni (or close to right or left)
S	Left, infraclavicular
B	Infrascapular on back
C	r. 5th ICS, anterior axillary line
V_1, V_3, V_5	Standard leads (see above)
aVF_1	Left costal margin, anterior axillary line
aVF_2	In xiphoid region

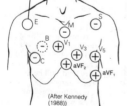

Earth

(After Kennedy (1988))

Recording of ischemia	Anterior	Inferior
	$CM – V_5$	$CS – aVF_1$
	$CM – V_3$	$CM – aVF_2$
	$CC – V_5$	$CS – V_1$
	$CB – V_5$	$CM – V_1$

ECG – normal values

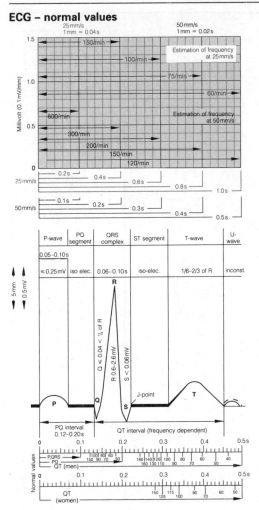

P-wave	PQ segment	QRS complex	ST segment	T-wave	U-wave
0.05–0.10 s		0.06–0.10 s			
≤ 0.25 mV	iso-elec.		iso-elec.	1/6–2/3 of R	inconst.

Q ≤ 0.04 < ¼ of R
R 0.6–2.6 mV
S < 0.06 mV

PQ interval 0.12–0.20 s

QT interval (frequency dependent)

ECG – ruler

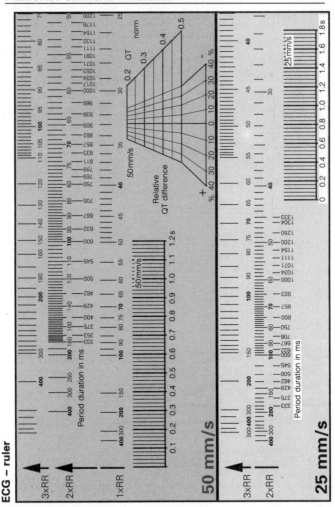

ECG axes/QT duration

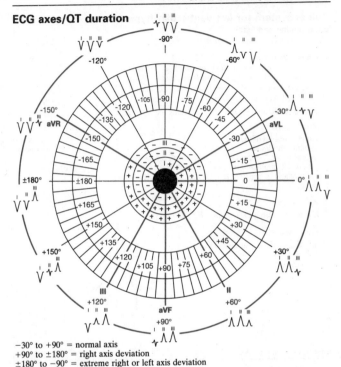

−30° to +90° = normal axis
+90° to ±180° = right axis deviation
±180° to −90° = extreme right or left axis deviation
−30° to −90° = left axis deviation

Deviation of QT duration from normal value

Method:

1. Read off normal value of QT duration
   (QT_{norm}) for relevant pulse rate (p. 53).

2. Align the isoelectric line with the horizontal
   line relating to the determined QT_{norm} value,
   so that the end of the T-wave lies under the
   numbered oblique line. The origin of Q
   then indicates the desired percentage value.
   (Example in illustration: $QT_{norm} = 0.4$s,
   relative QT difference = +10%).

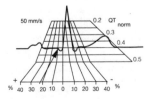

Points system for left ventricular hypertrophy
after Romhilt and Estes
(After Csapo and Kalusche (1989))

1. Amplitude criteria   3 points

a) greatest R or S wave in the extremity leads $\geq 2\,mV$
    (20 mm; typically an increase of R in I and/or aVL)
b) greatest S wave in V_1, V_2 or $V_3 \geq 2.5\,mV$ (25 mm)
c) greatest R wave in V_4, V_5 or $V_6 \geq 2.5\,mV$ (25 mm)

The presence of **one** or more criteria fulfills the three points.

2. ST-T criteria

In patients **not on digitalis**   3 points
In patients **on digitalis**   1 point
ST segment and T-wave shift in opposite direction to QRS complex
(typically: ST depressed in I, aVL or aVF; V_{5-6} [ST elevation in V_{2-3}, also
T flat, biphasic or negative in I, aVL, V_{5-6}] possibly aVF; QT interval
prolonged)

3. Axis criteria

Left axis deviation greater than $-15°$ 2 points

4. QRS criteria

a) left bundle delay: intrinsicoid
deflection (ID) begins at
$> 0.04\,s$ in V_6 1 point

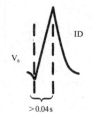

b) QRS duration $> 0.9\,s$ **1** point

Maximum points:	**10** points
Left ventricular hypertrophy	≥ 5 points
Suspicion of left ventricular hypertrophy	4 points

In patients in sinus rhythm, a leftward shift of P-wave axis (P mitrale) provides 3
additional points (provided that mitral stenosis has been excluded).

Conventional indices for left ventricular hypertrophy (all amplitudes are counted as
positive)

Sokolow–Lyon index:
S in V_1 or V_2 (whichever is greater) + R in V_5 or $V_6 > 3.5\,mV$
Lewis index:
R in I + S in III $> 2.5\,mV$

Points system for right ventricular hypertrophy

1. Amplitude criteria   3 points
a) V_1: R high (>0.7 mV), S small (<0.2 mV);
   with incomplete right bundle-branch block V_1: R > 1.0 mV;
   with complete right bundle-branch block V_1: R > 1.5 mV
b) V_{5-6}: R small, S deep (>0.7 mV)

2. ST-T criteria   3 points
ST-T in opposite direction to QRS in V_{1-3}: ST segment depressed,
T-wave negative or biphasic

3. Axis criteria   2 points
Right axis: QRS > 120° (if >150°, II predominantly negative)

4. QRS criteria
a) Right bundle delay: ID begins at >0.03 s in V_1 1 point
b) QRS duration between 0.09 and 0.11 s   1 point

Maximum points	10 points
Right ventricular hypertrophy	≥5 points
Suspicion of right ventricular hypertrophy	4 points

Sokolow–Lyon index: for right ventricular hypertrophy: R in V_2 or V_3 + S in V_5 or V_6
(whichever is greater) >1.05 mV

Atrial strain	Alteration of the P-wave configuration	Representative lead (where esp. obvious)	Lead V_1
Left (P mitrale = sinistroatrial P)	Widened, notched (>0.11 s)	I, II, aVL, V_{4-6} Macruz quotient (measured in II) = $\dfrac{\text{Duration of P (ms)}}{\text{Duration of PR (ms)}}$ >1.6 (normal 1.0–1.6)	Negative 2nd part
Right (P pulmonale = dextroatrial P)	Pointed, high (>3 mm)	II, III, aVF	Positive
Both atria (P cardiale = biatrial P)	Widened and/or pointed, high	I, II, III, aVL, aVF, V_{4-6}	Biphasic (pointed and widened)

Stress testing

Nomogram for determination of target performance (75% of maximal performance) for women and men in relation to age and weight (**WHO nomogram**) (especially for progressive stress test in recumbent patient)

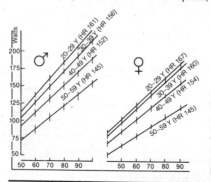

Alternatively: Calculation (maximal target performance in watts)(100%):

(Men): 3 W/kg body weight for age 20–30, subtract 10% per decade of life.

(Women): 2.5 W/kg body weight, subtract 10% per decade of life.

Alternatively: Nomogram for determination of target value of work capacity. The identified values indicate the **maximal** target performance (**100%**)

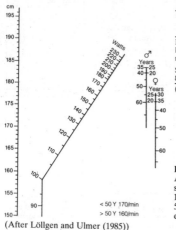

(After Löllgen and Ulmer (1985))

	Age (years)				
	20–29	30–39	40–49	50–59	60–69
Maximal heart rate	190	182	179	171	164
Submax. 85%	162	155	152	145	139

(Ellestad *et al.* (1979))

Rule of thumb for blood pressure:
At **100** W the arterial blood pressure should not exceed **200/100** lying and **210/105** sitting in patients aged 30–50. Above 50 years of age the pressure should not exceed **215/105** (sitting)

Coronary arteries – nomenclature

(International Nomenclature Commission, Leningrad, 1970; after Kaltenbach and Roskamm (1980))

Abbreviations

RCA	Right coronary artery
Bca	Branch to conus arteriosus
San	Sinoatrial node branch
Ra	Right atrial branch
Rv	Right ventricular branch
Rm	Right marginal branches
Pd	Posterior descending branch
Ps	Posterior septal branch
Avn	Atrioventricular node branch
Rpl	Right posterolateral branch
Rav	Right atrioventricular branch

LCA	Left coronary artery

CXA	Circumflex artery
La	Left atrial branch
Lav	Left atrioventricular branch
Lpl	Left posterolateral branch
Piv	Posterior interventricular branch
Lm	Left marginal branch
Ps	Posterior septal branch
Ll	Left lateral branch
Avn	Atrioventricular node branch

LAD	Left anterior descending artery
Db	Diagonal branch
As	Anterior septal

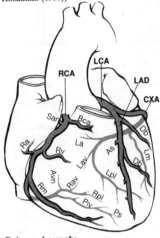

Balanced supply

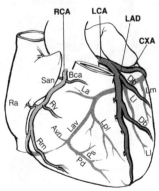

Left-sided supply

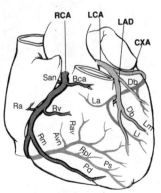

Right-sided supply

Myocardial scintigram

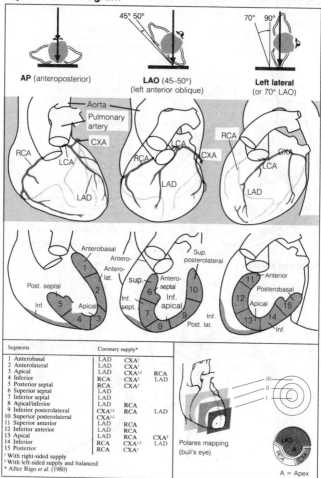

AP (anteroposterior)

LAO (45–50°)
(left anterior oblique)

Left lateral
(or 70° LAO)

Segments	Coronary supply*		
1 Anterobasal	LAD	CXA[1]	
2 Anterolateral	LAD	CXA	
3 Apical	LAD	CXA[1,2]	RCA
4 Inferior	RCA	CXA[2]	LAD
5 Posterior septal	RCA	CXA[2]	
6 Superior septal	LAD		
7 Inferior septal	LAD		
8 Apical/inferior	LAD	RCA	
9 Inferior posterolateral	CXA[1,2]	RCA	LAD
10 Superior posterolateral	CXA[1,2]		
11 Superior anterior	LAD	RCA	
12 Inferior anterior	LAD	RCA	
13 Apical	LAD	RCA	CXA[2]
14 Inferior	RCA	CXA[1,2]	LAD
15 Posterior	RCA	CXA[1]	

[1] With right-sided supply
[2] With left-sided supply and balanced
* After Rigo et al. (1980)

Polares mapping
(bull's eye)

A = Apex

X-ray ventriculogram

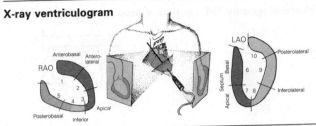

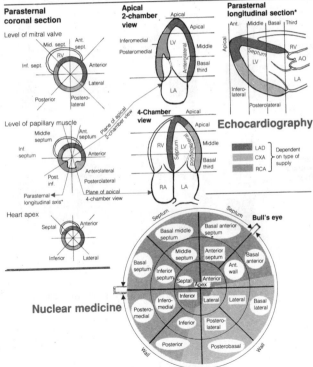

Parasternal coronal section

Level of mitral valve

Level of papillary muscle

Heart apex

Apical 2-chamber view

Parasternal longitudinal section*

4-Chamber view

Echocardiography

LAD
CXA } Dependent
RCA } on type of supply

Nuclear medicine

Bull's eye

Echocardiography TM – normal values

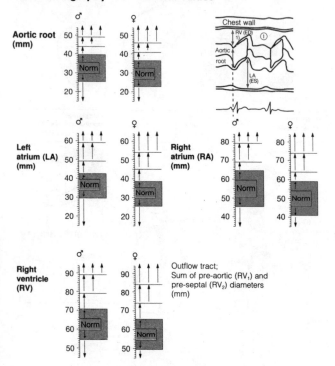

Aortic root (mm)

Left atrium (LA) (mm)

Right atrium (RA) (mm)

Right ventricle (RV)

Outflow tract;
Sum of pre-aortic (RV_1) and pre-septal (RV_2) diameters (mm)

'Leading edge method': measurement from leading edge to leading edge of the respective echo structures.

Echocardiography TM – ventricle

Left ventricular (LV) diameter
ED end-diastolic (measured at beginning of QRS)
ES end-systolic

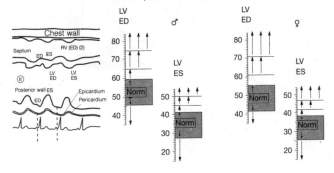

$$\text{(Segmental) shortening fraction} = \frac{LV_{ED} - LV_{ES}}{LV_{ED}}$$

Myocardial thickness (ED): septum and posterior wall (mm)

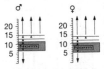

Systolic increase in thickness (%)

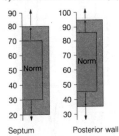

Septum   Posterior wall

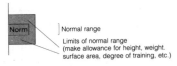

] Normal range

Limits of normal range
(make allowance for height, weight,
surface area, degree of training, etc.)

Modified after Bubenheimer (1982)

ECG changes in infarct

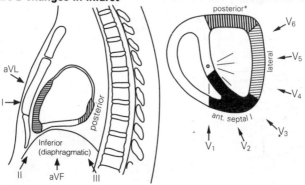

Infarct localization	Coronary findings to be expected (p. 59)	ECG changes in:													
		I	II	III	aVR	aVL	aVF	V_1	V_2	V_3	V_4	V_5	V_6	V_7	V_8
Large anterior wall infarct	Proximal occlusion of LAD														
Anteroseptal infarct	Occlusion of peripheral parts of LAD and As														
Apical anterior wall infarct	Occlusion of peripheral parts of LAD														
Anterolateral infarct	Occlusion of peripheral parts of LAD and inclusion of Db														
Inferolateral infarct	Occlusion of Lm														
Inferior (diaphragmatic) posterior wall infarct	Occlusion of peripheral parts of RCA or CXA														
Posterior (basal) posterior wall infarct	Occlusion of peripheral parts and branches of CXA, especially of Lav							(*)	*	(*)					

▨ always involved, unequivocal criteria (Q)

▨ often additionally involved, criteria not unequivocal (T wave inversion)

* posterior infarct → indirect signs: especially high R waves in (V_1) V_2 (V_3) (relation of R to S > 1) together with tall pointed positive T-waves

Time course of typical changes after acute myocardial infarct

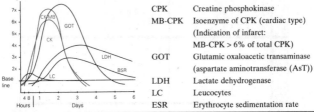

CPK	Creatine phosphokinase
MB-CPK	Isoenzyme of CPK (cardiac type)
	(Indication of infarct:
	MB-CPK > 6% of total CPK)
GOT	Glutamic oxaloacetic transaminase
	(aspartate aminotransferase (AsT))
LDH	Lactate dehydrogenase
LC	Leucocytes
ESR	Erythrocyte sedimentation rate

	Beginning of significant change in activity (h)	Greatest value of change in activity	Average greatest multiple of normal value	Average time to normalization
CPK	4–8	16–36	7 (2–25)	3rd to 6th day
MB-CPK	4–8	16–32	7 (–30)	2nd to 3rd day
GOT	4–8	16–48	7 (2–25)	3rd to 6th day
LDH	6–12	24–60	3.3 (2–8)	7th to 15th day
HBDH	6–12	30–72	3.5 (2–8)	10th to 20th day

Indication of infarct on ECG	1st to 3rd hour ~40%	4th to 6th hour ~50%	7th to 9th hour ~90%	10th to 12th hour up to 100%

Killip classification of cardiac insufficiency in acute infarct (after Killip and Kimball (1967))

I: No signs of cardiac insufficiency (no moist Rs (rales), no 3rd HS (heart sound))
II: Mild to moderate cardiac insufficiency: Rs over up to 50% of both lung fields or 3rd HS
III: Severe cardiac insufficiency, often pulmonary oedema: Rs over 50% of both lung fields, 3rd HS
IV: Cardiogenic shock

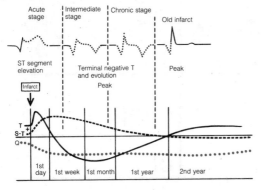

Heart valve abnormalities

Abnormality	Clinical examination	Auscultation	Maximal intensity	ECG	X-ray
Aortic stenosis	Plateau pulse, thrill (jugular fossa, 2nd r. ICS, 4th l. ICS)	**Systolic crescendo/decrescendo murmur, distinct from 1st HS, often early systolic click** The more marked, the later the max. sound, A₂ becomes softer, paradoxical splitting of 2nd HS **Mild grade** **Higher grade** 	2nd r. ICS, parasternal, heart apex, jugular fossa, supraclavicular	Often normal, l. hypertrophy, l. strain, P mitrale, seldom l. bundle-branch block	Often normal, l. heart enlargement (l. ventricle), calcified valve, pulmonary congestion
Aortic incompetence	High pulse pressure, diastolic pressure lower, waterhammer pulse, capillary pulsation, palpable finger pulsation, visible carotid pulse	**High-frequency diastolic decrescendo murmur.** **Mild:** 1st HS NAD, possibly early systolic click, soft early systolic bruit, 2nd HS normal or accentuated, early diastolic decrescendo murmur. **Severe: 1st and 2nd HS softer,** early–midsystolic crescendo/decrescendo murmur, 3rd, 4th HS, possibly presystolic murmur at apex (Austin Flint) **Low grade** **Higher grade** 	At base, esp. sitting, leaning forward (apex)	Only in high grade – left axis, P mitrale, l. hypertrophy, T-wave changes, l. strain	With progression l. ventricle↑, aortic dilatation, later l. atrium↑ (mitralization), pulmonary congestion, valve calcification

Mitral stenosis	Occasionally late systolic/early diastolic thrill at heart apex		**Accentuated 1st HS** systole clear. **2nd HS normal, OS** followed by rumbling low-frequency decrescendo murmur; in SR presystolic crescendo murmur; the earlier the OS, the more marked the valve lesion. **Signs of pulmonary hypertension:** P₂ accentuated, **murmur of pulmonary insufficiency**	Apex (L. lateral position)	P mitrale, atrial flutter/fibrillation, vertical heart, L. axis, incomplete r. bundle-branch block, seldom R cardiac hypertrophy, repolarization changes	**L. atrium ↑, signs of pulmonary congestion (pp. **) Signs of pulmonary hypertension:** pulmonary arch ↑, r. ventricle ↑ **Valve calcification**
Mitral incompetence	Apex beat diffuse, lateralized, lifting, systolic thrill at apex		**Pansystolic murmur starting at 1st HS** (band shaped), possibly 3rd HS **Mild:** Early–midsystolic murmur, high-frequency, blowing, diastole clear, 1st and 2nd HS normal **Higher grade:** **1st HS diminished** medium/low-frequency pansystolic murmur (rougher), wide splitting of 2nd HS; **early diastolic low-frequency crescendo/decrescendo murmur** (relative mitral stenosis) 3rd, 4th HS	Left 5th ICS parasternal, apex, conduction → L. lateral in midaxillary line	If mild, usually normal. L. axis, P mitrale, atrial fibrillation, L. hypertrophy, sometimes r. hypertrophy	If mild, usually normal; L. ventricle ↑, L. atrium ↑, pulmonary congestion

1st HS	1st heart sound
2nd HS	2nd heart sound
C	Click
EC	Ejection click
Palm EC	Pulmonary ejection click
OS	Opening snap
TOS	Tricuspid opening sound

67

Abnormality	Clinical examination	Auscultation	Maximal intensity	ECG	X-ray
Mitral valve prolapse		1st HS — C — 2nd HS — 1st HS. **Very variable**, one or more midsystolic clicks, often contiguous systolic murmur. Changes with posture: standing → displacement into early systole; squatting → late systole	2nd to 5th ICS, heart apex	Mostly normal, ventricular, supraventricular extrasystoles, sometimes T negative in II, III, aVF	Changes only with significant mitral incompetence
Pulmonary stenosis	Possibly systolic thrill, l. 1st–3rd ICS parasternal	**Mild grade** 1st HS — Pulm. EC — 2nd HS A P. **Higher grade** 1st HS — Pulm. EC — 2nd HS A — P. 1st HS normal, **diamond-shaped systolic murmur separated from 1st HS** pulmonary ejection click. Higher grade — systolic murmur reaches beyond A_2, greater interval A_2–P_2	Left 1st–3rd ICS parasternal, conduction to left and laterally	Often normal, incomplete right bundle-branch block, r. hypertrophy; higher grade: r. axis, dextroposition, P pulmonale	**Pulmonary arch accentuated** even with mild forms; **higher grade**: r. ventricle ↑↑, r. and r. pulmonary artery dilated, pulmonary arch +++, reduced peripheral lung vessels
Pulmonary incompetence		1st HS — A — P — 2nd HS — 1st HS. 1st HS normal, soft early-midsystolic murmur, split 2nd HS, P_2 accentuated, separate from early-middiastolic murmur. The higher the stenosis, the closer the systolic murmur to P_2	3rd–4th left ICS	Incomplete right bundle-branch block	Right ventricle ↑, pulmonary arch ↑, pulmonary hypertension, mitral stenosis
Tricuspid stenosis (usually accompanying other abnormalities)	**Upper and lower inflow obstruction** (mostly simultaneous mitral stenosis), dyspnoea on exertion, presystolic **jugular vein pulsation**	1st HS — 2nd HS TOS — 1st HS. Presystolic crescendo, 1st HS accentuated. TOS with joining decrescendo diastolic murmur, louder in inspiration	4th–5th left ICS	Often atrial fibrillation, P pulmonale	Right atrium ↑

68

	Clinical signs	Phonocardiogram	Auscultation	Location	ECG	X-ray/Imaging
Tricuspid incompetence (usually accompanying other abnormalities)	Upper and lower inflow obstruction, systolic liver/venous pulsation, ascites, right heart insufficiency	1st HS — 2nd HS Ap — 1st HS	High-frequency pansystolic murmur, absent in severe forms or r. heart insufficiency, louder in inspiration	Left 4th–5th ICS, if dilatation of r. ventricle up to apex	Depending on accompanying heart valve abnormality, atrial fibrillation	Right ventricle ↑, r. atrium ↑, superior vena cava ↑, azygos vein ↑
Atrial septal defect		**Small defect:** 1st HS — 2nd HS Ap — 1st HS **Larger defect:** 1st HS — 2nd HS Ap — 1st HS	1st HS unremarkable, early/midsystolic diamond-shaped murmur, **fixed splitting of 2nd HS** — Larger defect: early/middiastolic diamond-shaped murmur	Left 2nd–4th ICS	Mostly **incomplete r. bundle-branch block** (complete r. bundle-branch block), possibly P pulmonale, P biatriale, r. hypertrophy. **Ostium Primum defect:** (abnormal) l. axis **Ostium secundum defect:** mostly vertical or r. axis	Right ventricle ↑, widened peripheral lung vessels, 'dancing hila' on fluoroscopy
Ventricular septal defect	Higher grade: cyanosis, clubbing, drumstick fingers	1st HS — 2nd HS P — 1st HS	1st HS unremarkable, high-frequency protosystolic crescendo–decrescendo murmur. No fixed splitting of 2nd HS (possibly relative mitral stenosis)	Left 3rd–5th ICS parasternal, l. lateral	Left hypertrophy, P mitrale	With medium-sized defect: cardiac enlargement, r. ventricle ↑, l. atrium ↑, 'dancing hila' on fluoroscopy
Patent ductus arteriosus	Diastolic blood pressure low, drumstick fingers, clubbing	1st HS — 2nd HS P — 1st HS	Medium/high-frequency systolic/diastolic (**machinery**) murmur. Higher grade: accentuated P_2	Left 1st–2nd ICS parasternal, l. lateral	Left hypertrophy, P mitrale, atrial fibrillation; **pulmonary hypertension:** r. strain, r. hypertrophy	Only with large shunt: l. atrium ↑, l. ventricle ↑, peripheral lung vessels widened

Heart valve prostheses

Valve type	Ball valve prosthesis	Lifting disc valve prosthesis	Tilting disc valve prosthesis	Double wing prosthesis	Bioprosthesis
Illustrated model					
Illustrated model	Starr-Edwards	Kay-Shiley	Björk-Shiley	St Jude Medical	Carpentier-Edwards
Similar models	Harken, Cooley-Cutter, Smeloff-Cutter. McGovern, Braunwald-Cutter, De Bakey	Cross-Jones, Hufnagel, Kay-Suzuki, Kay-Shiley, Starr-Edwards (Model 6500) Beall, Harken, Cooley-Bloodwell, Cooley-Cutter	Wada-Cutter, Lillehei-Kaster, Hall-Kaster Omniscience, Omnicarbon, Medtronic-Hall	Duromedics	Hancock, Ionescu-Shiley, Mitroflow, Liotta, Xenomedica, Angel-Shiley
Illustration of blood flow					
Mitral position Auscultation	2nd HS-MOS interval 0.07–0.11 (to 0.15) s MOS louder than MCS 2–3/6 ejection murmur No diastolic murmur	Ball valve ('ball in cage') Lifting disc valve ('disc in cage') identical on auscultation	2nd HS-MOS interval 0.05–0.09s MOS very audible 2/6 systolic ejection murmur usual 1–2/6 diastolic flow murmur 'Rumble' not uncommon	MOS seldom audible (0.09 ± 0.02s after 2nd HS) 2/6 systolic ejection murmur common Soft diastolic flow murmur possible	2nd HS-MOS interval 0.01s MOS audible in 50% of patients 1–2/6 apical ejection murmur in 50% Diastolic rumble in 50–70%
Echo Δp mean (mmHg) tp2 (ms) MOP (cm²)	3–10 80–170 2.8–1.3		2–5 60–120 3.7–1.8	2–4 50–110 4.4–2.0	3–8 70–150 3.1–1.5

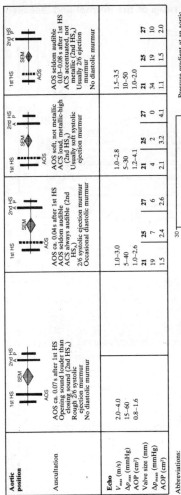

Aortic position				
Auscultation	AOS ca. 0.07s after 1st HS Opening sound louder than closing sound (2nd HS$_A$) Rough 3/6 systolic ejection murmur No diastolic murmur	AOS ca. 0.04s after 1st HS AOS seldom audible ACS always audible (2nd HS$_A$) 2/6 systolic ejection murmur Occasional diastolic murmur	AOS soft, not metallic ACS loud, metallic-high (2nd HS$_A$) Usually soft systolic ejection murmur	AOS seldom audible 0.03–0.08s after 1st HS ACS accentuated, not metallic (2nd HS$_A$) Usually 2/6 ejection murmur No diastolic murmur
Echo				
V_{max} (m/s)	2.0–4.0	1.0–3.0	1.0–2.8	1.5–3.5
Δp_{max} (mmHg)	15–60	5–40	5–30	10–50
AOP (cm²)	0.8–1.6	1.0–2.6	1.2–4.1	1.0–2.0
Valve size (mm)		21 **25** 27	21 **25** 27	21 **25** 27
Δp_{mean} (mmHg)		19 7 6	4 2 0	34 19 10
AOP (cm²)		1.5 2.4 2.6	2.1 3.2 4.1	1.1 1.5 2.0

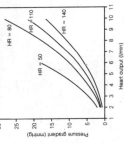

Echo measurements for illustrated valve (modified after Bubenheimer (1990) and Harrison *et al.* (1988))

Pressure gradient at an aortic valve prosthesis of 1.5cm² in relation to heart rate (HR) and cardiac output (CO)

Abbreviations:
1st HS 1st heart sound
2nd HS 2nd heart sound ⟨ 2nd HS$_A$ Aortic closing sound
                          2nd HS$_P$ Pulmonary component of 2nd HS

AOS Aortic opening sound   MCS Mitral closing sound
ACS Aortic closing sound   SEM Systolic ejection murmur
MOS Mitral opening sound   DM   Diastolic murmur

Δ   Pressure gradient at valve
$t_{1/2}$ Pressure half time
MOP Mitral opening plane
AOP Aortic opening plane

Systolic and diastolic flow rates of the normal and diseased heart

(Modified after Bubenheimer and Kneissl (1990))

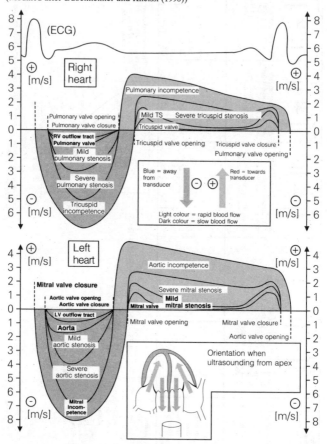

Endocarditis prophylaxis

Prevention of endocarditis in patients with heart valve lesions, septal defect, patent ductus or prosthetic valve:

Dental procedures that require antibiotic prophylaxis are:

> *Extractions*
> *Scaling*
> *Surgery involving gingival tissues*

Antibiotic prophylaxis for dental procedures may be supplemented with *chlorhexidine gluconate gel 1%* or *chlorhexidine gluconate mouthwash 0.2%*, used 5 minutes before procedure.

> *Note.* Oral clindamycin now replaces oral erythromycin (which caused nausea and vomiting); if clindamycin is used, periodontal or other multistage procedures should not be repeated at intervals of less than 2 weeks.

Dental procedures *under local or no anaesthesia.*
1. Patients who have not received a penicillin more than once in the previous month, including those with a prosthetic valve (but not those who have had endocarditis): **oral amoxycillin 3 g** 1 hour before procedure; CHILD under 5 years, quarter adult dose; 5–10 years, half adult dose.
2. Patients who are penicillin-allergic or have received a penicillin more than once in the preceding month: **oral clindamycin 600 mg** 1 hour before procedure; CHILD under 5 years, quarter adult dose; 5–10 years, half adult dose.
3. Patients who have had endocarditis, **amoxycillin + gentamicin**, as under general anaesthesia.

Dental procedures *under general anaesthesia.*
1. *No special risk* (including patients who have not received a penicillin more than once in the previous month):
either i.m. or i.v. amoxycillin 1 g at induction, then **oral amoxycillin 500 mg** 6 hours later; CHILD under 5 years, quarter adult dose; 5–10 years, half adult dose
or oral amoxycillin 3 g 4 hours before induction then **oral amoxycillin 3 g** as soon as possible after procedure; CHILD under 5 years quarter adult dose; 5–10 years, half adult dose
or oral amoxycillin 3 g + **oral probenecid 1 g** 4 hours before procedure.
2. *Special risk* (patients with a prosthetic valve of who have had endocarditis): **i.m. or i.v. amoxycillin 1 g + i.m. or i.v. gentamicin 120 mg** at induction, then **oral amoxycillin 500 mg** 6 hours later; CHILD under 5 years, **amoxycillin** quarter adult dose, **gentamicin 2 mg/kg**; 5–10 years, **amoxycillin** half adult dose, **gentamicin 2 mg/kg**.
3. Patients who are penicillin-allergic or who have received a penicillin more than once in the preceding month:
either i.v. vancomycin 1 g over at least 100 minutes then **i/v gentamicin 120 mg** at induction or 15 minutes before procedure; CHILD under 10 years, **vancomycin 20 mg/kg, gentamicin 2 mg/kg**
or i.v. teicoplanin 400 mg + **gentamicin 120 mg** at induction or 15 minutes before procedure; CHILD under 14 years, **teicoplanin 6 mg/kg, gentamicin 2 mg/kg**
or i.v. clindamycin 300 mg over at least 10 minutes at induction or 15 minutes before procedure then **oral or i.v. clindamycin 150 mg** 6 h later; CHILD under 5 years, quarter adult dose; 5–10 years, half adult dose.

Upper respiratory-tract procedures
as for dental procedures; postoperative dose may be given parenterally if swallowing is painful.

Genito-urinary procedures
as for *special risk* patients undergoing dental procedures under general anaesthesia except that clindamycin is not given, see above; if urine infected, prophylaxis should also cover infective organism.

Obstetric, gynaecological and gastrointestinal procedures
(prophylaxis required for patients with prosthetic valves or those who have had endocarditis only), as for genito-urinary procedures.

(After *BNF*)

Cardiac cycle

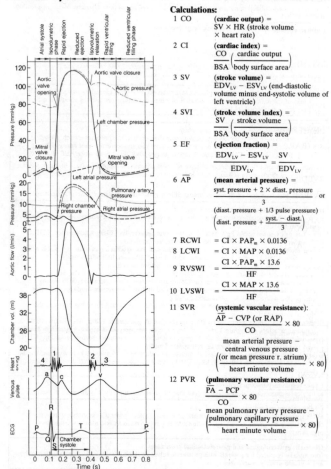

Calculations:

1 CO   **(cardiac output)** =
$SV \times HR$ (stroke volume × heart rate)

2 CI   **(cardiac index)** =
$$\frac{CO}{BSA} \left(\frac{\text{cardiac output}}{\text{body surface area}} \right)$$

3 SV   **(stroke volume)** =
$EDV_{LV} - ESV_{LV}$ (end-diastolic volume minus end-systolic volume of left ventricle)

4 SVI   **(stroke volume index)** =
$$\frac{SV}{BSA} \left(\frac{\text{stroke volume}}{\text{body surface area}} \right)$$

5 EF   **(ejection fraction)** =
$$\frac{EDV_{LV} - ESV_{LV}}{EDV_{LV}} = \frac{SV}{EDV_{LV}}$$

6 $\overline{AP}$ **(mean arterial pressure)** =
$$\frac{\text{syst. pressure} + 2 \times \text{diast. pressure}}{3} \text{ or}$$
(diast. pressure + 1/3 pulse pressure)
$$\left(\text{diast. pressure} + \frac{\text{syst.} - \text{diast.}}{3} \right)$$

7 RCWI $= CI \times PAP_m \times 0.0136$

8 LCWI $= CI \times MAP \times 0.0136$

9 RVSWI $= \dfrac{CI \times PAP_m \times 13.6}{HF}$

10 LVSWI $= \dfrac{CI \times MAP \times 13.6}{HF}$

11 SVR   **(systemic vascular resistance):**
$$\frac{\overline{AP} - CVP \text{ (or RAP)}}{CO} \times 80$$
$$\left(\frac{\substack{\text{mean arterial pressure} - \\ \text{central venous pressure} \\ \text{(or mean pressure r. atrium)}}}{\text{heart minute volume}} \times 80 \right)$$

12 PVR   **(pulmonary vascular resistance)**
$$\frac{\overline{PA} - PCP}{CO} \times 80$$
$$\left(\frac{\substack{\text{mean pulmonary artery pressure} - \\ \text{pulmonary capillary pressure}}}{\text{heart minute volume}} \times 80 \right)$$

(After Berne and Levy (1977))

Cardiovascular normal values

Abbreviation	Parameter	Units	Normal values
Cardiac volumes			
CO	Cardiac output (1)	l/min	5–6
CI	Cardiac index (2)	l/min/m²	2.6–4.2
SV	Stroke volume (3)	ml/beat	60–70
SVI (SI)	Stroke volume index (4) (stroke index)	ml/beat/m²	30–65
EDV	End-diastolic volume	ml	–
EDVI	End-diastolic volume index	ml/m²	50–90
ESV	End-systolic volume	ml	–
ESVI	End-systolic volume index	ml/m²	9–32
EF	Ejection fraction (5)	%	60–75
Cardiac pressures			
CVP	Central venous pressure	cmH₂O	5–12
$\overline{RA}$ (RAP$_m$)	Right atrial pressure, mean	mmHg	2–8
	a-wave	mmHg	2–10
	v-wave	mmHg	2–10
RVPs	Right ventricular pressure, systolic	mmHg	15–30
RVEDP	Right ventricular end-diastolic pressure	mmHg	2–8
$\overline{PA}$ (PAP$_m$)	Pulmonary artery pressure		
	mean	mmHg	9–18
PAPs	systolic	mmHg	15–30
PAP$_{ED}$	end-diastolic	mmHg	4–12
PCP (PCWP)	Pulmonary capillary (wedge) pressure	mmHg	5–12
$\overline{LA}$ (LAP$_m$)	Left atrial pressure, mean	mmHg	2–12
	a-wave	mmHg	3–15
	v-wave	mmHg	3–15
LVPs	Left ventricular pressure, systolic	mmHg	100–140
LVEDP	Left ventricular end-diastolic pressure	mmHg	3–12
$\overline{AP}$ ($\overline{SA}$) (SAP) (MAP)	Mean (systemic) arterial pressure (6)	mmHg	70–105
SAP$_s$	Systemic arterial pressure, systolic	mmHg	100–140
SAP$_d$	Systemic arterial pressure, diastolic	mmHg	60–90
Cardiac work indices			
RCWI	Right cardiac work index (7)	kg m/min/m² BSA	0.6
LCWI	Left cardiac work index (8)	kg m/min/m² BSA	3.8
RVSWI	Right ventricular stroke work index (9)	g m/m² BSA	8–12
LVSWI	Left ventricular stroke work index (10)	g m/m² BSA	51–61
Resistances			
SVR	Systemic vascular resistance (11)	dynes sec cm⁻⁵	700–1600
PVR	Pulmonary vascular resistance (12)	dynes sec cm⁻⁵	100–230*
		*also reported in **Wood units** (1 Wood unit ≅ 80 dynes sec cm⁻⁵)	

(After Grossman (1980))

Swan-Ganz balloon catheter

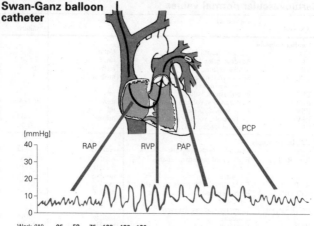

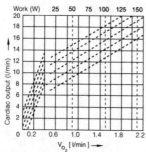

Cardiac output (CO) or oxygen consumption (V_{o_2}) in relation to work (in watts); cycle ergometer recumbent
(Values modified after Ekelund and Holmgren (1976), quoted in Görnandt (1989))

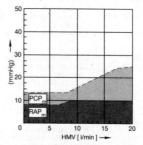

Mean pulmonary capillary pressure (PCP_m) and mean pressure right atrium (RAP_m) in relation to heart minute volume (HMV); at rest and on exercise (cycle ergometer recumbent)

   Upper limit of normal range of PVP_m

   Upper limit of normal range of RAP_m

Cardiomyopathies

Categories[a]	Congestive (dilated) (COCM)	Hypertrophic obstructive (HOCM)	Restrictive
Hypertrophy	Eccentric	Concentric, mostly asymmetric	Concentric, mostly symmetric
Systolic pump insufficiency	+++	−	+
Ejection fraction (EF)	↓↓↓	n − ↑	n − ↓
Diastolic congestive insufficiency	+	++	++
Filling pressure (PCP)	↑	↑↑	↑↑
Echo criteria			
LV$_{ED}$ (p. 63)	↑↑↑	n − (↓)	(n) − ↓
VF	↓↓(↓)	n − ↑	↓(↓)
Wall thickness			
septum	n − ↓	↑↑↑	↑(↑)
posterior wall	n − ↓	n − ↑	↑(↑)
Echo abbreviations and normal values, see pp. 62, 63		**Asymmetric** (eccentric) ≈ 90% mostly basal septum ↑↑; posterior septal wall quotient > 1.5[b] with/without obstruction[c] **Symmetric** − ≈ 5%	
LA	n (rel. MI, mitral incompetence) ↑	↑↑	↑↑
RV	↑ (advanced stage)	n	n
Mitral valve	Septum–E-point distance ↑↑ Often rel. MI due to stretching of mitral valve ring	**SAM** (systolic anterior movement) − sign of obstruction EF slope flattened	EF slope steep
Aortic valve	Reduced, delayed opening	Mid-systolic notch Muscular stenosis with obstruction	

[a] Classification after WHO/ISFC (1980, 1981)
[b] Also idiopathic hypertrophic subaortic stenosis (IHSS).
[c] Hypertrophic obstructive cardiomyopathy (HOCM).

Cardiac transplantation

Indication End-stage heart disorders (mostly, at present, cardiomyopathies ~40%, coronary heart disease ~40%, valve abnormalities, myocarditis, etc.).

End stage indicated by: despite maximal therapy, frequent and progressive clinical events such as cardiac arrest (resuscitation), recurrent heart failure, considerable effort intolerance, chronic hypotension, incipient reduction of renal or hepatic function, increasing cachexia, low heart output, supraventricular or ventricular arrhythmias, heart size ↑↑, signs of congestion, etc.

Contraindications

(After Copeland J.G. *et al.* (1987))

- **Age**
  >55–65 years, indication increasingly widened
  (also young patients), dependent on 'physiological' age

- **Severe pulmonary hypertension**
  ($PA_s > 65$–70 mmHg, PCP > 40 mmHg),
  pulmonary vascular resistance (PVR) >6 (trend to >8) Wood units
  (~500 dynes sec cm^{-5}); important whether PVR reversible

- **Irreversible renal or hepatic damage**

- **Active systemic infection**

- **Systemic disease**
  (trend: less strong)

- **History of behavioural disturbances, psychiatric illnesses**
  (trend: less strong, compliance!)

- **Pulmonary infarcts, lung disorders of undetermind origin**
  (mostly only temporary contraindication)

- **Insulin-dependent diabetes**
  (no longer a contraindication)

- **Peripheral arterial occlusive vascular disease, cerebrovascular disease**
  Relative contraindication (e.g. surgically correctable?)

- **Gastric or duodenal ulcer**
  (only temporary contraindication)

- **Inadequate psychosocial support**
  (trend: less strong, compliance!)

Conducting system of the heart

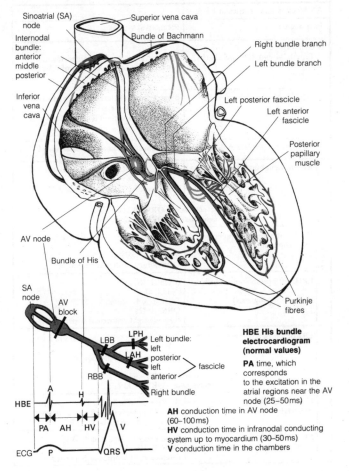

Sinoatrial (SA) node
Superior vena cava
Bundle of Bachmann
Right bundle branch
Left bundle branch
Internodal bundle: anterior middle posterior
Inferior vena cava
Left posterior fascicle
Left anterior fascicle
Posterior papillary muscle
AV node
Bundle of His
Purkinje fibres
SA node
AV block
LBB
LPH
LAH
RBB
Left bundle: left posterior left anterior } fascicle
Right bundle
HBE
A
H
V
PA
AH
HV
ECG
P
QRS

HBE His bundle electrocardiogram (normal values)

PA time, which corresponds to the excitation in the atrial regions near the AV node (25–50 ms)

AH conduction time in AV node (60–100 ms)
HV conduction time in infranodal conducting system up to myocardium (30–50 ms)
V conduction time in the chambers

79

Heart block

Type of block in ECG	Diagnostic criteria
AV block = atrioventricular block	
First degree	PR interval >0.02 s
Second degree Type 1 (Mobitz I, Wenckebach)	PR interval increases progressively to maximal value, then failure of AV conduction
Type II (Mobitz II)	Single/multiple failure of AV conduction (e.g. 2:1, 3:1, etc.) With conduction the PR interval remains constant
Third degree (complete AV block)	AV conduction completely interrupted

	Type	Diagnostic criteria
Bifascicular	**RBBB:** right bundle-branch block	Delay of largest negative deflection (>0.03 s) in V_1 (V_2) Broad positive QRS complexes in III, aVF, aVR, V_1, V_2 (R < R' in V_1) **complete – QRS ≥ 0.12 s** **incomplete – QRS < 0.12 s**
	LAH: left anterior hemiblock (very common)	Left axis deviation ($-30°$ to $-90°$) qR in I, aVL rS in II, III, aVF, V_6 QRS normal or slightly prolonged
	LPH: left posterior hemiblock (rare, poor prognosis)	qR in II, III, aVF rS in I, aVL Right axis deviation, $> +110°$ QRS < 0.12 s (exclude right ventricular hypertrophy)
Unifascicular	**LBBB:** left bundle-branch block	Broad, positive QRS complexes in I, aVL, V_5, V_6 Largest negative deflection in V_5, $V_6 > 0.055$ s **complete – QRS ≥ 0.12 s** **incomplete – QRS < 0.12 s**
	LAH + RBBB (relatively common)	RBBB picture in V_1, V_2: broad, positive QRS complexes + left axis deviation qR in I, aVL, rS in II, III, aVF
	LPH + RBBB (very rare, poor prognosis)	Right axis, $> +90°$, rS in I, aVR qR in II, III, aVF (exclude right ventricular hypertrophy)

Lown classification of VES

Lown class	Definition
0	No ventricular extrasystoles (VES)
1a 1b	Occasional VES (<1/min, <30/h) Occasional VES (>1/min, <30/h)
2	Frequent VES (>30/h)
3	Multifocal VES (some authors classify bigeminus as 3b)

4
4a
4b
	Repetitive VES
	Coupled VES
	Salvoes of VES (3 or more consecutive VES)
	    (also ventricular tachycardia or fibrillation, in original Lown
	    classification, not retained)

5	Early VES (R-on-T phenomenon, normal ventricular complexes)

WHO classification of calcium antagonists

(After Vanhoutte (1987))

Class		Type		Substances
A	Selective blockade of slow calcium channels	I	Verapamil	**Verapamil**
		II	Dihydropyridine	**Nifedipine**, amlodipine, felodipine, isradipine, lacidipine, nicardipine, nimodipine
		III	Diltiazem	**Diltiazem**
B	No selective blockade of slow calcium channels	IV	Diphenylpiperazine	Cinnarizine
		V	Prenylamine derivatives	(not in use in UK)
		VI	Others	Perhexiline

Classification of anti-arrhythmic agents (Vaughan-Williams, 1975)

Class		Principal site of action				ECG alterations			Extracardiac side effects
		SA node	Atrium	AV node	His-Purkinje/ ventricles	PR interval	QRS duration	QT interval	
			→ Retardation ↑ Sometimes also increased frequency						
I 'Membrane stabilizers' (also local anaesthetic/antifibrillation agents): direct membrane effect with specific inhibition of fast sodium inflow (fast response), thereby reduction of maximal initial (phase 0) rate of rise of AP (action potential); also, in different manner, effect on potassium flow in repolarization; subdivision following last point into:									
IA: Prolongation of the action potential	Quinidine	↓/↑	→	=/↑	↓↑	=	↑	↑↑	Gastrointestinal symptoms; cinchonism: tinnitus, vertigo, deafness, visual disturbances; haematological alterations; syncope
	Procainamide	→	=↓	→	↓/↑↓	=	↑	↑	Diarrhoea, vomiting, psychosis, leucopenia, haemolytic anaemia
	Disopyramide	↓/↑	→	=/↑↓	(=)/↓(↓)	=	↑	↑↑	Dry mouth, gastrointestinal symptoms, sedation, cholestasis, urinary retention
	Ajmaline	↓/=	→	↓/=	↓/↓↓	=/↑	↑	↑	Nausea, headache, anorexia, cholestasis, hepatic damage
IB: Shortening of the action potential	Lignocaine	=	=	=/↓	=/↓	=	=	=/↓	Drowsiness, vertigo, confusion, CNS symptoms, convulsions
	Mexiletine	=	=	=	=/↓	=	=	=	CNS symptoms, hypotension, gastrointestinal symptoms, tremor, diplopia
	Tocainide	=	=	=	(↓)	=	=	=/↓	CNS disturbances: tremor, drowsiness, hallucinations, nausea, agranulocytosis, lupus erythematosus

IC: No significant effect on action potential duration **Flecainide**	=/↑			→	←	↑↑	←	Diplopia, dizziness, headache, reduced alcohol tolerance
Propafenone	→	→	=/↓↓	↓↓↓	←	←	←	Dry mouth, salty taste, headache, gastrointestinal symptoms, postural hypotension
Aprindine (not available in UK)	=/↓	→	↓(↓)	↓↓↓	←	↑↑	←	Tremor, diplopia, psychoses, liver damage, agranulocytosis
II: Beta-blockers – blockade of catecholamine effect on impulse formation and stimulus conduction; also, in part, non-specific membrane effects, e.g. propranolol (other beta-blockers, p. 84)	→			=			→	Dizziness, nausea, diarrhoea
III(I): Prolongers of action potential and refractory phase, resting potential and phase 0 of the AP not affected Amiodarone	→	=/↓	↓↓	→	=/↑	=	↓	Hyper- or hypothyroidism, corneal deposits, photosensitivity, pulmonary fibrosis
Sotalol (beta-blocker)	→	(↓)	↓↓	(↓)	←	←	↑↑	Nausea, diarrhoea, dizziness, circulatory disturbances, nightmares, hypotension
III(II): Presynaptic beta-blocker (prevention of noradrenaline release) Bretylium	→	=	=	→	=	←	←	Hypotension, nausea, stuffy nose
IV: Calcium antagonists – specific inhibitory effect on slow (sodium) calcium inflow into myocardial cell Verapamil	↓/↑	↓/=	↓↓	=	=/↑	=	=	Hypotension, gastrointestinal symptoms
Diltiazem	=/↓	=	↓↓	=	←	=	=	Nausea, fatigue, dizziness

Beta-adrenergic blocking agents

Substance Product name	ISA	Cardioselecivity β_1	MSA	H: hydrophilic L: lipophilic	Half life (h)*
Acebutolol	+	+	+	(L)	3–4 7–13
Atenolol	–	+	–	H	6–9
Betaxolol	–	+	(+)	L	16–22
Bisoprolol	–	+	–	L/H	10–12
Celiprolol	+	+	–		4–5
Esmolol[b]	–	+	–	H	9
Labetalol[a]	–	–	+	(L)	3–4
Metoprolol	–	+	–	(L)	3–4
Nadolol	–	–	–	H	14–25
Oxprenolol	+ +	–	(+)	(L)	2–3
Penbutolol	+	–	(+)	L	4–5 1–3 20
Pindolol	+ +(+)	–	(–)	(L)	3–4
Practolol	+ +	+	–	H	6–8
Propranolol	–	–	+(+)	L	3–6
Sotalol[c]	–	–	–	H	10–15 5–12
Timolol	–/(+)	–	–	(L)	3–4

ISA intrinsic sympathomimetic activity.
MSA membrane-stabilizing activity.
* Differing data in the literature.
[a] Simultaneous α_1 blockade.
[b] Only i.v.
[c] Additional anti-arrhythmic effect.

Pacemakers

	Always specified			Possible additional data	
1	2	3	4	5	
Chamber(s) paced	Chamber(s) sensed	Mode of pacemaker response	Programmable functions	Special tachyarrhythmia functions	
V Ventricle	V Ventricle	T Triggered	P Programmable (rate and/or output only)	B Bursts Salvoes	
A Atrium	A Atrium	I Inhibited	M Multi-programmable (More than 3 functions)	N Normal rate competition	
D Dual (r. atrium + ventricle)	D Dual (r. atrium + ventricle)	D Atrium triggered, ventricle inhibited	C Communicating – possibility of non-invasive interruption	S Scanning	
O None These functions not present	O None These functions not present	O None These functions not present	E External control		
S Single chamber	S Single chamber	R Reverse Pacing reacts to tachy- rather than brady-arrhythmia	**Identification code**		

(Intersociety Commission for Heart Disease, after Parsonnet *et al.* (1981))

Pacemaker (PM) testing

ECG

Spontaneous rhythm, PM rhythm, PM impulse partially/completely effective (stimulation loss), PM rhythm (if not, → sensing defect), rate reduction, rate variation (**battery exhaustion**), parasystole, extrasystole (→ spontaneous frequency too high with fixed-frequency pacemaker, ?need for adjustment of medication) (note hysteresis: fixed prolongation of basic interval after spontaneous heart beat).

- **Possibly X-ray** if suspicion of dysfunction: battery position, electrode course, continuity, fracture, kink, displacement, disconnection of adaptor, myocardial or septal perforation
- If spontaneous frequency greater than PM frequency:
  - trial of carotid sinus massage, beta-blocker (beware side effects)
  - **Magnet ECG**: switching from demand to fixed-frequency operation (beware: occasional ventricular fibrillation → defibrillator)
  - **Function analyses** (specialized monitoring equipment)
    a) Impulse interval (= stimulation interval, = period duration) = time interval between 2 PM impulses in ms (increase = frequency reduction → **battery exhaustion**)
    b) Constancy of impulse interval (inconstancy → **battery exhaustion**)
    c) Impulse duration (= impulse width, usually 0.3–1.5 ms, prolongation → **battery exhaustion**)
- **Specialized investigations**: stimulation threshold, sensing threshold, impulse amplitude, impulse shape (oscillogram), antegrade, retrograde conduction, atrioventricular, ventriculoatrial 'crosstalk', interference signal response
- Possibly stress test
- Possibly long-term ECG

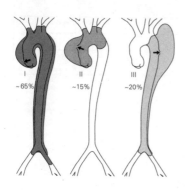

De Bakey's classification of aortic dissections

Type I: The dissection involves the ascending aorta, the aortic arch and extends distally to varying degrees.
Type II: The dissection is confined to the ascending aorta.
Type III: The dissection originates in the region of the left subclavian artery or distal to it, and extends distally to a variable degree.

The arrows point to the site of the intimal tear, with frequency in percent.

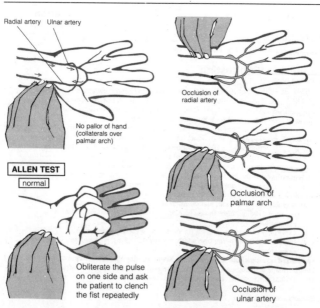

Radial artery   Ulnar artery

No pallor of hand (collaterals over palmar arch)

ALLEN TEST
normal

Obliterate the pulse on one side and ask the patient to clench the fist repeatedly

Occlusion of radial artery

Occlusion of palmar arch

Occlusion of ulnar artery

Fontaine's classification of peripheral vascular disease

Stage	Classification criteria	Subgroups by walking distance	Subgroups according to Ratschow's positioning test (see below)
I	**Objectively evident perfusion defect without subjective symptoms**		**Ia** Ratschow negative **Ib** Ratschow positive (Division into a and b in stage I not universally employed)
II	**Intermittent claudication**	**IIa** Pain-free walking distance greater than 200 m[a] **IIb** Pain-free walking distance less than 200 m[a]	**IIa** Ratschow negative **IIb** Ratschow positive
III	**Rest pain**		
IV	**Ischaemic lesion (gangrene)**		

[a] 100 m and 300 m also used for subdivision.

Ratschow's positioning test

Interpretation		Perfusion defect			
		Not present	Mild	Medium	Severe
Patient lying supine for 2 min: Alternate flexion and extension of ankle	**Pallor** of sole and toes How rapidly? (s) Uniform? Bilaterally symmetrical?	No pallor	>60	<60	Immediate on elevation of legs
Sit patient up	**Reddening** of dorsum of foot and toes How rapidly? (s) Uniform? Bilaterally symmetrical?	5–10	10–30	30–60	>60
	Filling of veins of forefoot How rapidly? (s) Bilaterally symmetrical?	up to 15	20–30	30–60	>60
	Persistent reddening	0	+	++	+++

Abdominal arteries

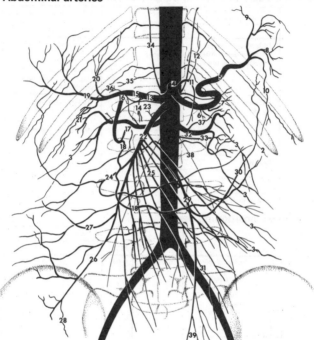

1. Intercostal a.	14. Right gastric a.	27. Right colic a.
2. Subcostal a.	15. **Hepatic a.**	28. Branch to appendix
3. Lumbar aa.	16. **Gastroduodenal a.**	29. **Inferior mesenteric a.**
4. **Coeliac a.**	17. Superior pancreaticoduodenal	30. Left colic a.
5. **Splenic a.**	a.	31. Sigmoid a.
6. Dorsal pancreatic a.	18. Right gastroepiploic a.	32. **Renal a.**
7. Arteria pancreatica magna	19. Right branch of hepatic a.	33. Accessory renal a.
8. Terminal branches of splenic a.	20. Left branch of hepatic a.	34. Inferior phrenic a.
9. Short gastric aa.	21. Cystic a.	35. Superior suprarenal a.
10. Left gastroepiploic a.	22. **Superior mesenteric a.**	36. Middle suprarenal a.
11. **Left gastric a.**	23. Inferior pancreaticoduodenal a.	37. Inferior suprarenal a.
12. Branches to oesophagus from	24. Middle colic a.	38. Testicular a. (internal spermatic
11	25. Jejunal aa.	a.) or ovarian a.
13. **Common hepatic a.**	26. Ileocaecal a.	39. Superior rectal a.

(From Muller, R.F., Figley, M.M., Rogoff, S.M. and deWeese, J.A. Arteries of the abdomen, pelvis and lower extremity. Kodak Publication No. M4-2. © Eastman Kodak Company. Reprinted courtesy of Eastman Kodak Company)

Pelvic arteries

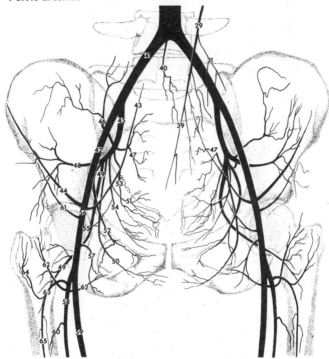

40. Middle sacral a.
41. **Common iliac a.**
42. **External iliac a.**
43. Inferior epigastric a.
44. Deep circumflex ilial a.
45. **Internal iliac** (hypogastric) **a.**
46. Iliolumbar a.
47. Lateral sacral a.
48. Superior gluteal a.
49. Inferior gluteal a.
50. Internal pudendal a.
51. Middle rectal a.
52. Obturator a.
53. Uterine a.
54. Inferior vesical a.
55. Superficial epigastric a.
56. **Femoral a.**
57. External pudendal a.
58. **Profunda femoris a.**
59. **Femoral a.**
60. Perforating aa.
61. Superficial ilial circumflex a.
62. Medial circumflex femoral a.
63. Lateral circumflex femoral a.
64. Ascending branch of lateral circumflex femoral a.
65. Descending branch of lateral circumflex femoral a.

(From Muller, R.F., Figley, M.M., Rogoff, S.M. and deWeese, J.A. Arteries of the abdomen, pelvis and lower extremity. Kodak Publication No. M4-2. © Eastman Kodak Company. Reprinted courtesy of Eastman Kodak Company)

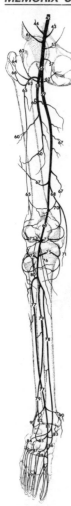

Arteries of the leg

42. **External iliac a.**
43. Inferior epigastric a.
44. Deep circumflex ilial a.
45. Internal iliac (hypogastric) a.
46. Iliolumbar a.
47. Lateral sacral a.
48. Superior gluteal a.
49. Inferior gluteal a.
50. Internal pudendal a.
51. Middle rectal a.
52. Obturator a.
53. Uterine a.
54. Inferior vesical a.
55. Superficial epigastric a.
56. **Common femoral a.**
57. External pudendal a.
58. **Profunda femoris a.**
59. **Femoral a.**
60. Perforating aa.
61. Superficial ilial circumflex a.
62. Medial circumflex femoral a.
63. Lateral circumflex femoral a.
64. Ascending branch of lateral circumflex femoral a.
65. Descending branch of lateral circumflex femoral a.
66. Transverse branch of lateral circumflex femoral a.
67. Muscular branches of femoral and profunda femoris aa.
68. Descending genicular a.
69. **Popliteal a.**
70. Articular branch of descending genicular a.
71. Saphenous branch of descending genicular a.
72. Lateral superior genicular a.
73. Medial superior genicular a.
74. Lateral inferior genicular a.
75. Medial inferior genicular a.
76. Sural a.
77. **Anterior tibial a.**
78. **Posterior tibial a.**
79. **Peroneal a.**
80. Anterior tibial recurrent a.
81. **Dorsalis pedis a.**
82. Perforating branch of peroneal a.
83. Medial tarsal a.
84. Lateral plantar a.
85. Lateral tarsal a.
86. Medial plantar a.
87. Arcuate a.
88. Deepest branch of dorsalis pedis a.
89. Dorsal and plantar metatarsal aa., dorsal and plantar digital aa.
90. Anterior medial malleolar a.
91. Anterior lateral malleolar a.

Radiological anatomy of the great veins of the leg

(deWeese, J.A., Rogoff, S.M. and Tobin, C.E. Radiographic anatomy of major veins of the lower limb. Kodak Publication M4–5. © Eastman Kodak Company. Reprinted courtesy of Eastman Kodak Company)

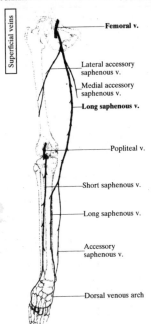

Superficial veins

- **Femoral v.**
- Lateral accessory saphenous v.
- Medial accessory saphenous v.
- **Long saphenous v.**
- Popliteal v.
- Short saphenous v.
- Long saphenous v.
- Accessory saphenous v.
- Dorsal venous arch

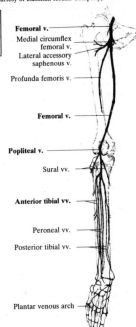

Deep veins

- **Femoral v.**
- Medial circumflex femoral v.
- Lateral accessory saphenous v.
- Profunda femoris v.
- **Femoral v.**
- **Popliteal v.**
- Sural vv.
- **Anterior tibial vv.**
- Peroneal vv.
- Posterior tibial vv.
- Plantar venous arch

Common anatomical variants

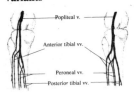

- Popliteal v.
- Anterior tibial vv.
- Peroneal vv.
- Posterior tibial vv.

Normal course of the veins

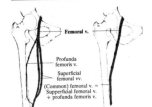

- **Femoral v.**
- Profunda femoris v.
- Superficial femoral vv.
- (Common) femoral v. = Superficial femoral v. + profunda femoris v.

Varicose veins

Trendelenburg's test
Examination of the competence of the venous valves

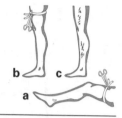

Patient stands
Find and mark the opening of the long
saphenous vein into the femoral vein

Patient recumbent
a) Lift the leg until the varicosities empty, empty
fully by stroking
Compress the opening of the long saphenous with
venous tourniquet

Patient stands up
b) Observe varicosities for 10–15s with compression
of opening
c) Then release compression

During compression (b)
Absent or only slow filling from distally:
valves of short saphenous and
communicating veins **competent**
Rapid filling from proximal to distal:
valve of short saphenous or
communicating veins **incompetent**

After release of compression (c)
No additional filling from the groin
Valve at mouth of long saphenous **competent:**
Trendelenburg negative

Rapid or additional filling from the groin:
valve at mouth of long saphenous **incompetent**
Trendelenburg positive

Perthes' test
Examination of the patency of the deep veins
Apply venous tourniquet and make patient walk about

a) **Pathological:**
Failure of emptying of varicosities with incompetent
deep veins
b) **Normal:**
Disappearance of the varicosities during walking
through drainage via intact communicating veins and
deep veins

Classification of chronic venous insufficiency of the leg

Chronic venous insufficiency Degree of severity	Symptoms (unilateral or bilateral)
I	Oedema of ankle or calf; feeling of heaviness and tension of the legs; dragging pain (possibly increased during menstruation or pregnancy) Paraplantar varicose corona
II	Symptoms of grade I also Dystrophic skin changes: Siderosclerosis, purpura jaune d'ocre, atrophie blanche, pachydermia, acroangiodermatitis, hypodermitis
III	Symptoms of Grade I and II also Florid or healed varicose ulcer

Orthostatic hypotension
Schellong test

Lying quietly	3 min elevation of legs	5–7 min standing quietly

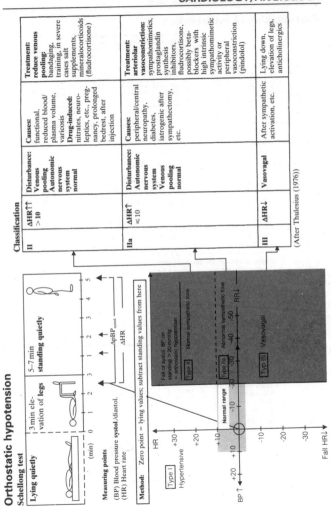

Measuring points

(BP) Blood pressure **systol.**/diastol.
(HR) Heart rate

Method: Zero point = lying values; subtract standing values from here

Classification

		Disturbance:	Causes:	Treatment:
II	ΔHR↑↑ >10	Venous pooling Autonomic nervous system normal	functional, reduced blood/ plasma volume, varicosis **Drug-induced:** nitrates, neuroleptics, etc., pregnancy, prolonged bedrest, after injection	**reduce venous pooling;** bandaging, training, in severe cases salt supplements, mineralocorticoids (fludrocortisone)
IIa	ΔHR↑ ≦10	Disturbance: Autonomic nervous system Venous pooling normal	Causes: peripheral/central neuropathy, diabetes, iatrogenic after sympathectomy, etc.	Treatment: **arteriolar vasoconstriction:** sympathomimetics, prostaglandin synthesis inhibitors, fludrocortisone, possibly beta-blockers with high intrinsic sympathomimetic activity or peripheral vasoconstriction (pindolol)
III	ΔHR↓	Vasovagal	After sympathetic activation, etc.	Lying down, elevation of legs, anticholinergics

(After Thulesius (1976))

93

Classification of hypertension

WHO classification*
(by systolic and diastolic blood pressure)

	Systolic (mmHg)	Diastolic (mmHg)***
Hypertension	≥ 160	≥ 95
Borderline	141–159	91–94
Normal	≤ 140	≤ 90

Joint National Committee Classification*
(by diastolic blood pressure only)

Diastolic (mmHg)		Frequency	Start therapy
> 115	'Severe' hypertension	20–30%	Normally at once
105–114	'Moderate' hypertension		Control and individual, start within a few days
90–104	'Mild' hypertension	70–80%	See scheme, p. 98
< 90	Normal		

Isolated systolic hypertension: systol. > 140 (>65 years >160), diastol. < 90 mmHg

Classification by degree of damage to target organs (WHO*)

Grade I   No organ changes
Grade II   At least one of the following findings:
  • Left heart hypertrophy on chest X-ray, ECG or echocardiogram
  • Hypertensive retinopathy with generalized or regional narrowing of retinal arteries (grade I–II)
  • Proteinuria
Grade III   **Hypertension-mediated target organ damage:**
  • Hypertensive heart disease, left heart failure, cerebral haemorrhage, hypertensive encephalopathy, malignant hypertensive retinopathy with haemorrhages, exudates or papilloedema (grade III–IV)
  • **Organ complications due to hypertension and other factors:**
  Coronary artery disease (angina pectoris, cardiac infarct), cerebral thrombosis, transient ischaemic attacks, dissecting aortic aneurysm, peripheral vascular disease, renal failure

Retinopathy***

Stage	Arteries	Relation artery/vein	Retina	Optic disc
Normal	Fine yellow reflex Blood column visible	3/4		
I	Mild tortuosity Broad yellow reflex Blood column visible	1/2		
II	**Arteriovenous nipping Copper wiring of arteries** (yellow reflex) Blood column visible Early wall irregularities	1/3	Isolated haemorrhages	
III	**Silver wiring of arteries** (white reflex) Blood column visible Marked wall irregularities	1/4	Multiple **haemorrhages** Cotton wool exudates	Indistinct margin (prominence)
IV	**Fibrosed cords** Blood column invisible		**Multiple haemorrhages** Cotton wool exudates	**Papilloedema** Engorged disc

* WHO (1978)
** Joint National Committee (1988)
*** After Keith, Wagener and Barker (1939)

Step scheme for treatment of arterial hypertension[a]

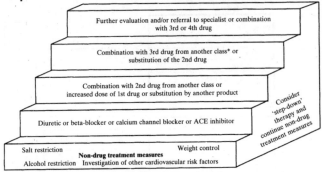

Further evaluation and/or referral to specialist or combination with 3rd or 4th drug

Combination with 3rd drug from another class* or substitution of the 2nd drug

Combination with 2nd drug from another class or increased dose of 1st drug or substitution by another product

Diuretic or beta-blocker or calcium channel blocker or ACE inhibitor

Salt restriction   **Non-drug treatment measures**   Weight control
Alcohol restriction   Investigation of other cardiovascular risk factors

Consider 'step-down' therapy and continue non-drug treatment measures

* Antihypertensives such as diuretics, beta-blockers, calcium channel blockers, ACE inhibitors, alpha-blockers, centrally acting α-agonist, and vasodilators

Recommendations for combination therapy[b]

Dual drug combination (recommended when blood pressure not below 140/90 mmHg with monotherapy)

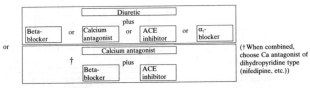

	Diuretic		
	plus		
Beta-blocker	or Calcium antagonist	or ACE inhibitor	or α₁-blocker

or

	Calcium antagonist	
	plus	
†	Beta-blocker	ACE inhibitor

(† When combined, choose Ca antagonist of dihydropyridine type (nifedipine, etc.))

Triple drug combination

or   Diuretic plus beta-blocker plus vasodilator
or   Diuretic plus ACE inhibitor plus Ca antagonist
      Diuretic plus α-agonist plus vasodilator

Alternative:
α-agonist plus diuretic

(Vasodilators: calcium antagonists, ACE inhibitors, postsynaptic α₁-blockers, hydralazine)

[a] Joint National Committee (1988)
[b] Deutsche Liga (1990)

Investigation of hypertension

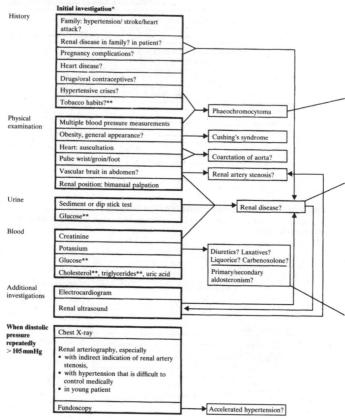

Initial investigation*

History
- Family: hypertension/ stroke/heart attack?
- Renal disease in family? in patient?
- Pregnancy complications?
- Heart disease?
- Drugs/oral contraceptives?
- Hypertensive crises?
- Tobacco habits?**

→ Phaeochromocytoma

Physical examination
- Multiple blood pressure measurements
- Obesity, general appearance? → Cushing's syndrome
- Heart: auscultation
- Pulse wrist/groin/foot → Coarctation of aorta?
- Vascular bruit in abdomen? → Renal artery stenosis?
- Renal position: bimanual palpation

Urine
- Sediment or dip stick test
- Glucose** → Renal disease?

Blood
- Creatinine
- Potassium → Diuretics? Laxatives? Liquorice? Carbenoxolone?
- Glucose** → Primary/secondary aldosteronism?
- Cholesterol**, triglycerides**, uric acid

Additional investigations
- Electrocardiogram
- Renal ultrasound

When diastolic pressure repeatedly > 105 mmHg
- Chest X-ray
- Renal arteriography, especially
  - with indirect indication of renal artery stenosis,
  - with hypertension that is difficult to control medically
  - in young patient
- Fundoscopy → Accelerated hypertension?

Suggestion of secondary hypertension/Investigation

Suggestion of phaeochromocytoma:
- Hypertensive crises (50% persistent hypertension)
- Paroxysmal somatic symptoms (headache, palpitation, pallor, sweating attacks, tremor, nausea, tachycardia)
- Grade III or IV hypertensive retinopathy
- Loss of weight, glucose intolerance
- Extreme blood pressure rise during anaesthesia or operation

→**Investigation**
- Vanillylmandelic acid/catecholamines in 24-hour urine
- Possibly estimate in plasma, stimulation or suppression tests
- CT abdomen

Suggestion of renoparenchymatous or renovascular hypertension:
- Urine protein ↑, serum creatinine ↑
- Renal history (oedema, nephritis, urinary infection, renal calculi, renal trauma, polycystic kidney, etc.)
- Age < 30, > 55 years
- Diastolic > 120 mmHg
- Lack of response to sufficiently high and combined therapy
- Grade III or IV retinopathy
- Systolic/diastolic bruit over kidneys

→**Investigation:**
- Excretion urography/early urography (difference between sides)
- Isotope renography/divided renal clearance
- Digital subtraction angiography
- Intravenous angiotomography
- Renal arteriography

Suggestion of hypertension due to mineralocorticoid excess (aldosteronism):
- Hypokalaemia (< 3.5 mmol/l)
- Exclusion of diuretic or laxative effect

→**Investigation:**
- Repeated potassium estimations after withdrawal of diuretics/laxatives (several weeks), high sodium diet
- Estimation of renin (low) and aldosterone (high) in plasma

*   Deutsche Liga (1990) (Reprinted with permission).
** Not absolutely essential for investigation of hypertension, but recommended for assessment of additional cardiovascular risk factors.

Assessment and treatment of 'mild hypertension'*

Definition: diastolic blood pressure 90–104 mmHg (cf. p. 94)
Aim: diagnostic: accurate classification of the patient
therapeutic: reduction of diastolic blood pressure below 90 mmHg (and systolic, if elevated)

```
              ┌────────────────────────┐
              │ Blood pressure recording at │
              │ least 3 times on 2 separate │
              │ occasions (days): if diast. BP │
              │      90–104 mmHg        │
              └────────────────────────┘
                         │
                         ▼
              ┌────────────────────────┐
              │ Repetition of recording on │
              │ at least 2 further days within │
              │        4 weeks          │
              └────────────────────────┘
```

After 4 weeks	**Diast. BP < 90 mmHg** → Further recordings every 3 months for 1 year

Diast. BP 90–104 mmHg
Non-drug treatment methods and supervision

After total of 3 months	Diast. BP 90–94 mmHg ndt† → Supervision	Diast. BP 95–99 mmHg Other risk factors ndt + medical treatment	Diast. BP > 100 mmHg ndt + medical treatment
After further 3 months	Diast. BP 90–94 mmHg and no other risk factors Continuation of ndt and supervision	Diast. BP 90–94 mmHg and other risk factors → Medical treatment	Diast. BP > 100 mmHg with or without other risk factors → Medical treatment

* WHO/ISH (1989)
† ndt = non-drug treatment

Differential therapy in hypertension

Differential therapy	Recomendation
Older patient (> 65 y)	Preferably Ca antagonists and diuretics
Coronary heart disease	Preferably beta-blocker and Ca antagonists
Cardiac insufficiency	Preferably diuretics and ACE inhibitors
Diabetes mellitus	Non-selective beta-blockers and diuretics not recommended
Gout	Avoid diuretics
Renal failure	Serum creatinine over 180 µmol/l: use loop diuretics Potassium-sparing diuretics can lead to hyperkalaemia Delayed excretion of several antihypertensives (e.g. atenolol, nadolol, sotalol, captopril, enalapril, lisinopril, perindopril) should be noted
Pregnancy	Methyldopa has been shown to be safe in pregnancy. Beta-blockers are safe in the third trimester but may cause intrauterine growth retardation if used earlier
Hyperlipidaemia	No long-term studies available which can justify specific therapeutic recommendations

Unwanted effects of hypertension therapy

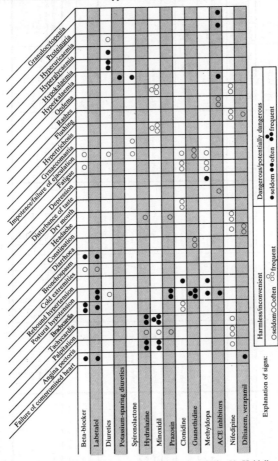

Deutsche Liga zur Bekämpfung des hohen Blutdrucks (1990) e.V., Heidelberg.
Reprinted with permission.

99

Hyperlipidaemias

Classification (after Fredrickson/WHO)	IIa	IIb	IV	I	III	V
Lipoprotein pattern (ultracentrifuge)	LDL	LDL + VLDL	VLDL	Chylomicrons	LDL + VLDL Remnants	Chylomicrons VLDL
Lipid electrophoresis	↑ Betalipoproteins	↑ Beta- + ↑ prebeta-lipoproteins	↑ Prebeta-lipoproteins	↑ Chylomicrons	↑ Beta + ↑ prebeta-lipoproteins, remnants	↑ Chylomicrons ↑ Prebeta-lipoproteins
Cholesterol	↑↑↑	↑↑↑	n – ↑	n – ↑	↑↑	n – ↑
Triglycerides	n	↑↑	↑↑↑	↑↑↑	↑↑↑	↑↑↑
Occurrence	Familial hypercholesterolaemia	Mixed hyperlipidaemia	Familial hypertriglyceridaemia	Familial lipoprotein lipase deficiency	Familial dysbetalipoproteinaemia	Mixed hyperlipidaemia
Frequency	Frequent	Frequent	Frequent	Rare	Rare	Rare
Secondary hyperlipidaemia (in each case exclude following conditions)	Cushing's syndrome Hypothyroidism Anorexia nervosa Steroid therapy Nephrotic syndrome Hepatoma	Cushing's syndrome Steroid therapy Nephrotic syndrome	Diabetes mellitus Alcoholism Acromegaly Ovulation inhibitor Uraemia Acute hepatitis Adiposity Plasmacytoma	Systemic lupus erythematosus	Plasmacytoma Hypothyroidism Diabetes mellitus	
Symptoms	Tendon xanthomata		Eruptive xanthomata	Eruptive xanthomata Pancreatitis	Tuberous palmar xanthomata	
Premature atherosclerosis	+	+	+		+	
Therapy	Diet low in cholesterol, high in polyunsaturated and low in saturated fatty acids Nicotinic acid	Weight reduction Calorie and alcohol reduction	Reduced calories, carbohydrates, alcohol Discontinue ovulation inhibitors Clofibrate	Fat-free diet, MCT, little alcohol	Weight and alcohol reduction, low-calorie diet Clofibrate	Weight reduction Low-calorie and low-alcohol diet

LDL, low-density lipoproteins; VLDL, very low-density lipoproteins; MCT, middle-chain triglycerides.

Lipid-lowering drugs

Group	Products (Selection)	Effect on lipids Cholesterol	Triglycerides	HDL-Chol.	Unwanted effects/Remarks
Ion exchange resins	Cholestyramine Colestipol	↓ 10–30%	↑ 0–20%	↑ 0–10%	Frequent gastrointestinal disturbances: nausea, flatulence, constipation. Possibly elevation of transaminases and alkaline phosphatase; reduction of fat-soluble vitamins with high dosage over prolonged periods. Drug interaction may result in reduced absorption of other drugs
Fibrates	Clofibrate Bezafibrate Ciprofibrate Fenofibrate Gemfibrozil	↓ 10–20%	↓ 25–60%	↑ 0–30%	Infrequent mild gastrointestinal disturbances: nausea, diarrhoea; myalgia, impotence and increased risk of gallstones. Possible elevation of transaminases or CPK, reduction of alkaline phosphatase possible. Drug interactions: enhanced activity of anticoagulants of coumarin type. Reduce dose in renal failure
Nicotinic acid derivatives	Nicotinic acid Nicofuranose Acipimox	↓ 15–25%	↓ 20–35%	↑ 15–20%	Flushing at onset of treatment, pruritus, epigastric pain, vomiting, diarrhoea. Possible elevation of transaminases and uric acid. Reduction of glucose tolerance
Probucol	Probucol	↓ 10–15%	0	↓ 0–30%	Infrequent mild gastrointestinal disturbances: nausea, flatulence, diarrhoea, myositis. Moderate eosinophilia possible. Prolongation of QT interval in ECG. Very long biological half life
HMG-CoA reductase inhibitors	Simvastatin Pravastatin	↓ 25–35%	↓ 10–30%	↑ 0–15%	Very infrequent gastrointestinal disturbances: nausea, abdominal discomfort. Possible elevation of transaminases and CPK. Little is known about drug interactions at present. Avoid combination with fibrates or nicotinic acid (risk of rhabdomyolisis)
Fish oils	Omega-3-marine triglycerides	(↑)	↓		Occasional nausea and flatulence

Empfehlungen der Arbeitsgruppe Lipide (1989)

Hyperlipidaemia therapy
Recommendations for treatment of hyperlipidaemia

Total cholesterol raised, triglycerides normal

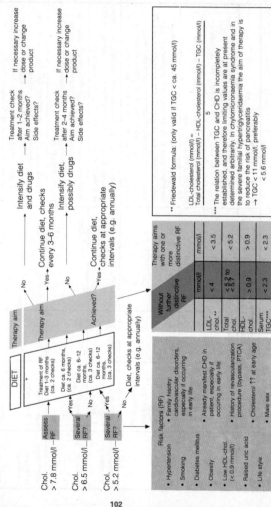

DIET

Chol. > 7.8 mmol/l — Assess RF

Treatment of RF
Diet 1–3 months (ca. 2 checks)

Chol. > 6.5 mmol/l — Several RF?
- Yes → Diet ca. 6–12 months. (ca. 2 checks)
- No → Diet ca. 6 months, (ca. 3 checks)

Chol. > 5.2 mmol/l — Several RF?
- Yes → Diet ca. 6–12 months. (ca. 3 checks)
- No → Diet, checks at appropriate intervals (e.g. annually)

Therapy aim
- No → Continue diet, checks every 3–6 months
- Yes → Intensify diet and drugs → Treatment check after 1–2 months. Aim achieved? Side effects? → If necessary increase dose or change product

Therapy aim
- No → Continue diet, checks every 3–6 months
- Yes → Intensify diet, possibly drugs → Treatment check after 2–4 months. Aim achieved? Side effects? → If necessary increase dose or change product

Achieved?
- No → Intensify diet and drugs
- Yes → Continue diet, checks at appropriate intervals (e.g. annually)

Lipid-lowering drugs (p. 101)

Risk factors (RF)
- Hypertension
- Smoking
- Diabetes mellitus
- Obesity
- Low HDL-chol. (< 0.9 mmol/l)
- Raised uric acid
- Life style
- Family history: cardiovascular disorders, especially if occurring in early life
- Already manifest CHD in patient, especially if occurring in early life
- History of revascularization procedure (bypass, PTCA)
- Cholesterol ↑↑ at early age
- Male sex

	Without further distinctive RF		Therapy aims with one or more distinctive RF	
	mmol/l		mmol/l	
LDL-chol. **	< 4		< 3.5	
Total chol.	< 5.2 to < 5.7		< 5.2	
HDL-chol.	> 0.9		> 0.9	
Serum TGC***	< 2.3		< 2.3	

** Friedewald formula: (only valid if TGC < ca. 45 mmol/l)

$$LDL\text{-cholesterol (mmol/l)} = \frac{\text{Total cholesterol (mmol/l)} - HDL\text{-cholesterol (mmol/l)} - TGC \text{ (mmol/l)}}{5}$$

*** The relation between TGC and CHD is incompletely established, and therefore limiting values are at present determined arbitrarily. In chylomicronaemia syndrome and in the severe familial hypertriglyceridaemia the aim of therapy is to reduce the risk of pancreatitis → TGC < 11 mmol/l, preferably < 5.6 mmol/l.

102

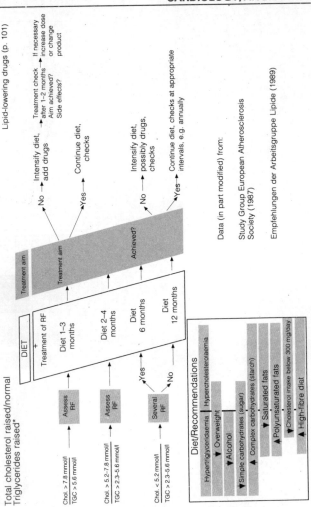

Total cholesterol raised/normal
Triglycerides raised*

Chol > 7.8 mmol/l
TGC > 5.6 mmol/l

Chol > 5.2–7.8 mmol/l
TGC > 2.3–5.6 mmol/l

Chol < 5.2 mmol/l
TGC > 2.3–5.6 mmol/l

Assess RF

Assess RF

Several RF

Yes

No

DIET
+
Treatment of RF

Diet 1–3 months

Diet 2–4 months

Diet 6 months

Diet 12 months

Treatment aim

Treatment aim

Achieved?

No — Intensify diet, add drugs

Yes — Continue diet, checks

No — Intensify diet, possibly drugs, checks

Yes — Continue diet, checks at appropriate intervals, e.g. annually

Lipid-lowering drugs (p. 101)

Treatment check after 1–2 months
Aim achieved?
Side effects?

If necessary increase dose or change product

Data (in part modified) from:

Study Group European Atherosclerosis Society (1987)

Empfehlungen der Arbeitsgruppe Lipide (1989)

Diet/Recommendations

Hypertriglyceridaemia   Hypercholesterolaemia

▶ Overweight

▶ Alcohol

▶ Simple carbohydrates (sugar)

◀ Complex carbohydrates (starch)

◀ Saturated fats

◀ Polyunsaturated fats

▶ Cholesterol intake below 300 mg/day

◀ High-fibre diet

103

Estimation of daily cigarette consumption

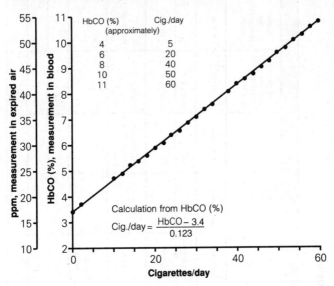

HbCO (%) (approximately) / Cig./day

HbCO (%) (approximately)	Cig./day
4	5
6	20
8	40
10	50
11	60

Calculation from HbCO (%)

$$\text{Cig./day} = \frac{\text{HbCO} - 3.4}{0.123}$$

Cigarette equivalent

1 cigarillo = 2 cigarettes
1 pipe   = 2.5 cigarettes
1 cigar   = 4 cigarettes

Estimation of cigarette consumption over the last 24–36 hours.
(Nodified after Vanuxem *et al.* (1980); see also Jarvis *et al.* (1986))

Differential diagnosis of pleural effusion

Type	Transudate	Exudate					
		Pneumonic Empyema	TB	Pulmonary embolus Pulmonary infarct	Tumour	Collagenoses, Rheumatoid arthritis SLE*	Chylothorax Tumour Thoracic duct injury
Aetiology	Heart failure Cirrhosis Nephrotic syndrome Meig's syndrome						
Appearance	Serous-clear, often right sided	Serous-turbid, purulent	Yellow	Sanguinous	Sanguinous	Yellowish	Chylous
Protein	Below 30 g/l	Over 30 g/l	> 30 g/l	> 30 g/l	> 30 g/l	> 30 g/l	
Specific gravity	Below 1016	Over 1016	>1016	>1016	>1016	>1016	>1016
Cells	0	Polymorpho-nuclear leuco-cytes	Lympho-cytes	Erythrocytes	Erythrocytes, malignant cells	Lymphocytes	0 Fat droplets
Bacteriology	0	+/– Gram stain	+ Ziehl Neelsen	0	0	0	0
Glucose	As serum	(↓)	↓↓	As serum	→	↓↓↓	
LDH	Low	High	High			High	
pH	As serum	<7.2	<7.2			<7.2	

* SLE, systemic lupus erythematosus

Lung function tests

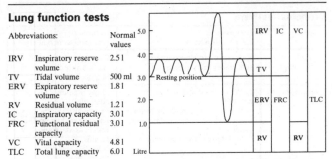

Abbreviations:		Normal values
IRV	Inspiratory reserve volume	2.5 l
TV	Tidal volume	500 ml
ERV	Expiratory reserve volume	1.8 l
RV	Residual volume	1.2 l
IC	Inspiratory capacity	3.0 l
FRC	Functional residual capacity	3.0 l
VC	Vital capacity	4.8 l
TLC	Total lung capacity	6.0 l

Normal values after EGK (Europäische Gemeinschaft für Kohle und Stahl) (Quanjer, 1983)

Tiffeneau test

Forced expiratory volume in the first second (FEV_1)
Distinction: obstructive and restrictive ventilatory disturbances

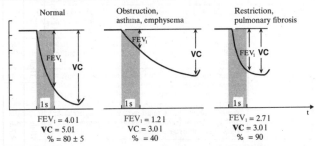

Normal	Obstruction, asthma, emphysema	Restriction, pulmonary fibrosis
$FEV_1 = 4.0$ l	$FEV_1 = 1.2$ l	$FEV_1 = 2.7$ l
VC = 5.0 l	VC = 3.0 l	**VC** = 3.0 l
% = 80 ± 5	% = 40	% = 90

Present customary representation of spirometry as flow-volume curve ($\dot{V}/V$)

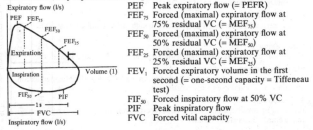

PEF	Peak expiratory flow (= PEFR)
FEF_{75}	Forced (maximal) expiratory flow at 75% residual VC (= MEF_{75})
FEF_{50}	Forced (maximal) expiratory flow at 50% residual VC (= MEF_{50})
FEF_{25}	Forced (maximal) expiratory flow at 25% residual VC (= MEF_{25})
FEV_1	Forced expiratory volume in the first second (= one-second capacity = Tiffeneau test)
FIF_{50}	Forced inspiratory flow at 50% VC
PIF	Peak inspiratory flow
FVC	Forced vital capacity

Bronchial asthma

Type	Extrinsic Exogenous allergic	Intrinsic Endogenous non-allergic
Patho-physiology	Release of bronchoconstrictor substances from mast cells	Induction of vagal reflexes via 'sensitized' receptors in mucosa
History	Onset in childhood and young adult life. Allergy common in family history; often cradle cap, neurodermatitis, rhinitis. Salicylate sensitivity common	Onset in infancy and adult life. Family history of allergy unusual; seldom cradle cap, neurodermatitis, rhinitis. Salicylate sensitivity uncommon
Clinical course	Paroxysmal (seasonal) asthma; infrequent status asthmaticus. Infrequent sinus infections or nasal polyps. Favourable course	Chronic asthma; frequent status asthmaticus. Sinus infections and nasal polyps common. Unfavourable course
Pathology	IgE elevated, skin tests positive, inhalation tests positive	IgE normal, skin tests negative, inhalation tests negative
Principal therapeutic possibilities	Desensitization effective, mast cell inhibitors (cromoglycate, ketotifen) useful	Desensitization ineffective, mast cell inhibitors little effect
	Determine aetiology, stop smoking, avoid exposure, theophylline preparations (serum assay), corticosteroids, β_2-adrenergic agents, oxygen (blood gas measurements!), adequate hydration, mucolytics, anticholinergics, sedatives (cautiously!), antibiotics (if signs of infection), inhalation therapy, physiotherapy; intubation and ventilation (seldom necessary, after consultation with chest physician and/or anaesthetist)	

Classification by clinical severity
(After Schulze-Werninghaus and Debelic (1988))

I   **Incipient asthma:**
Characterized by occasional dyspnoea or cough, also described as allergic bronchitis or allergic tracheobronchitis.

II **Mild asthma:**
Occasional paroxysmal dyspnoea with irregular need for bronchodilators.

III **Moderate asthma:**
Variable paroxysmal dyspnoea with regular need for anti-asthmatic medication, including occasional use of corticosteroids.

IV **Severe asthma:**
Frequent or continuous dyspnoea to severest asthmatic attack and continuous requirement for corticosteroids.

Management of chronic asthma in adults*

Steps	Notes
Step 1 Inhaled short-acting β_2-stimulant as required (up to once daily).	*Note*: Move to step 2 if needed more than once daily (or for night-time symptoms).
Step 2 Inhaled short-acting β_2-stimulant as required *plus* Regular standard dose inhaled corticosteroid *or try* Regular cromoglycate or nedocromil (but change to inhaled corticosteroid if control not achieved).	*Note*: Higher dose of inhaled corticosteroid may be required to gain initial control; some adults benefit from doubling for short period to cover respiratory infection.
Step 3 Inhaled short-acting β_2-stimulant as required *plus* Regular high-dose inhaled corticosteroid (large-volume spacer).	*Note*: If problems with high-dose inhaled corticosteroids, continue with standard dose *and* add regular inhaled long-acting β_2-stimulant *or* regular modified-release oral theophylline *or may try* regular cromoglycate or nedocromil. With proportionately prominent night-time symptoms (despite otherwise good control with standard or high-dose corticosteroid inhalations) a modified-release oral theophylline *or* a long-acting inhaled β_2-stimulant may be considered for administration at night.
Step 4 Inhaled short-acting β_2-stimulant as required with Regular high-dose inhaled corticosteroid (large-volume spacer) *plus sequential therapeutic trial of one or more of* Inhaled long-acting β_2-stimulant Modified-release oral theophylline Inhaled ipratropium or oxitropium Modified release oral β_2-stimulant High-dose inhaled bronchodilators Cromoglycate or nedocromil	*Note*: High doses of inhaled bronchodilators should only be considered if the patient does not respond to standard doses; β_2-stimulants and ipratropium (or oxitropium) can be given using a nebulizer (or by multiple actuations of a metered dose inhaler with large-volume spacer).
Step 5 Inhaled short acting β_2-stimulant as required with Regular high-dose inhaled corticosteroids (large-volume spacer) *and with* one or more long-acting bronchodilators (see step 4) *plus* Regular prednisolone tablets (as single daily dose).	*Note*: In addition to regular prednisolone tablets, continue high-dose inhaled corticosteroids (in exceptional cases doses exceeding 2 mg may be used).

Stepping down

Review treatment every 3–6 months; if control is achieved, stepwise reduction may be possible; in patients whose treatment was started recently at step 4 or 5 (or contained corticosteroid tablets), reduction may take place after a short interval; in chronic asthma a 3–6-month period of stability should be shown before slow stepwise reduction is undertaken.

* These recommendations are based on tables in: British Thoracic Society and others (1993) **Guidelines on the management of asthma**. *Thorax*, **48**, Supp, S1. Alternative recommendations are given for children. Reproduced by permission of BMJ Specialist Journals.

Recommendations for diagnosis, staging and surgical treatment of carcinoma of bronchus

(Deutsche Gesellschaft für Thorax-, Herz- und Gefässchirurgie, Deutsche Gesellschaft für Pneumologie und Tuberkulose (1988))

Basic diagnosis:
History, clinical examination, laboratory tests, radiology of thorax, lung function tests, sputum cytology, bronchoscopy with cytology/biopsy.

Staging investigations:
Computerized tomography, upper abdominal ultrasound, skeletal scintigraphy, CT.

Staging of carcinoma of bronchus

T – **Primary tumour**
TX   Primary tumour cannot be assessed, or demonstration of malignant cells in sputum or bronchial washings but tumour not visible radiologically or at bronchoscopy.
T0   No evidence of primary tumour.
Tis   Carcinoma *in situ*.
T1   Tumour 3 cm or less in widest diameter, surrounded by lung parenchyma or visceral pleura, no bronchoscopic evidence of infiltration proximal to a lobar bronchus (main bronchus free).
T2   Tumour with one of the following characteristics regarding size or extent:
• Tumour greater than 3 cm in largest diameter,
• Tumour with involvement of main bronchus, 2 cm or more distal to carina,
• Tumour infiltrates visceral pleura,
• Associated atelectasis or obstructive inflammation up to hilum but not of the entire lung.
T3   Tumour of any size with direct infiltration of one of the following structures: Chest wall (including tumours of the superior fissure), diaphragm, mediastinal pleura, pericardium; **or** tumour in main bronchus less than 2 cm distal to carina but carina itself not involved; **or** tumour with atelectasis or obstructive inflammation of the entire lung.
T4   Tumour of any size with infiltration of one of the following structures: mediastinum, heart, great vessels, trachea, oesophagus, vertebral body, carina; **or** tumour with malignant effusion.

N – **Regional lymph nodes**
NX   Regional lymph nodes cannot be assessed.
N0   No metastases in regional lymph nodes.
N1   Metastases in ipsilateral peribronchial lymph nodes and/or in ipsilateral hilar lymph nodes (including direct extension of the primary tumour).
N2   Metastases in ipsilateral mediastinal and/or subcarinal lymph nodes.
N3   Metastases in contralateral mediastinal, contralateral hilar, ipsi- or contralateral scalene or supraclavicular lymph nodes.

M – **Distant metastases**
MX   The presence of distant metastases cannot be assessed.
M0   No distant metastases.

TNM categories

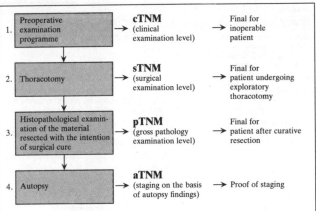

1.	Preoperative examination programme	→	**cTNM** (clinical examination level)	→ Final for inoperable patient
2.	Thoracotomy	→	**sTNM** (surgical examination level)	→ Final for patient undergoing exploratory thoracotomy
3.	Histopathological examination of the material resected with the intention of surgical cure	→	**pTNM** (gross pathology examination level)	→ Final for patient after curative resection
4.	Autopsy	→	**aTNM** (staging on the basis of autopsy findings)	→ Proof of staging

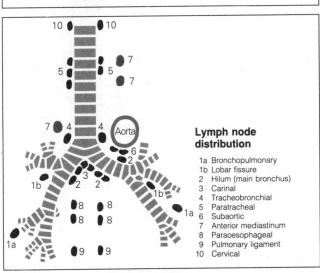

Lymph node distribution

1a Bronchopulmonary
1b Lobar fissure
2 Hilum (main bronchus)
3 Carinal
4 Tracheobronchial
5 Paratracheal
6 Subaortic
7 Anterior mediastinum
8 Paraoesophageal
9 Pulmonary ligament
10 Cervical

Carcinoma of bronchus – histology

Histology

NSCLC (non-small cell lung cancer):	SCLC (small cell lung cancer):
Squamous cell carcinoma	Small cell bronchial carcinoma
Adenocarcinoma	
Large cell, undifferentiated carcinoma	
Other, rare tumours	

Classification SCLC:

'Limited disease' (LD):
Tumour confined to one hemithorax, no major atelectases, no pleural effusion, no venous inflow obstruction, no recurrent laryngeal paresis

'Extensive disease' (ED):
Tumour extension to contralateral hemithorax, major atelectases, pleural effusion, venous obstruction, recurrent laryngeal paresis, involvement of supraclavicular nodes, distant metastases

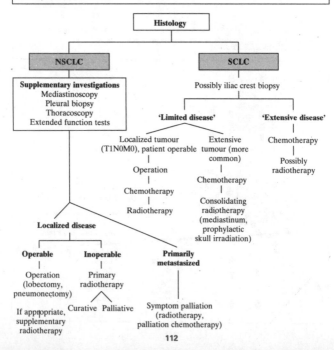

Carcinoma of bronchus – surgery

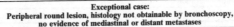

```
                        Exceptional case:
Peripheral round lesion, histology not obtainable by bronchoscopy,
        no evidence of mediastinal or distant metastases
```

Operable	Inoperable
Operation	**Percutaneous biopsy (guided by image intensifier or CT)**
Histology	
pTNM	

NSCLC	SCLC	NSCLC	SCLC
Further investigation	Chemotherapy ǀ Reinforcing radiotherapy	If appropriate, primary radiotherapy ǀǀ Follow-up; therapy only when symptomatic	Chemotherapy ǀ Reinforcing radiotherapy

Scheme for preoperative function tests

(for patients with carcinoma of bronchus) (Deutsche Gesellschaft für Thorax-, Herz- und Gafässchirurgie, Deutsche Gesellschaft für Pneumologie und Tuberkulose (1988))

Definitive measurement: FEV_1 (preoperative), if appropriate supplemented by regional analysis by means of quantitative isotope perfusion scanning

1st stage of function testing: plannd operation:

FEV_1

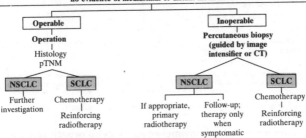

	If:	If:		
Operable	> 2.50 l ← Pneumonectomy	≤ 2.50 l	then: Isotope	Calculated
	> 1.75 l ← Lobectomy	≤ 1.75 l	perfusion scan →	postoperative
	> 1.50 l ← Segmental resection	≤ 1.50 l		FEV_1*

2nd stage of function testing: Calculated postoperative FEV_1*

	Operable	High risk	Inoperable
Pneumonectomy	> 1.5 l	1.0–1.5 l	< 1.0 l
Lobectomy	> 1.5 l	0.8–1.2 l	< 0.8 l
Segmental resection	> 1.2 l	0.8–1.2 l	< 0.8 l

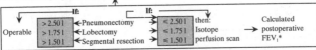

Further investigations necessary (e.g. microcatheter)

*Calculation of postoperative FEV_1:

$$FEV_{1(postop.)} = FEV_{1(preop.)} \frac{100 - A - 0.37B}{100}$$

A   Perfusion of resection
B   Perfusion of the side to be operated
0.37 Constant for the early postoperative phase

Example: Patient has tumour in right upper lobe and preop. FEV_1 of 1.4 l. Perfusion in projection of right upper lobe is completely abolished. Residual perfusion of right lung amounts to 40%.

Calculation for resection of right upper lobe:

$$FEV_{1(postop.)} = 1.4 \frac{100 - 0 - (40 \times 0.37)}{100} = 1.19\ l$$

Hence: postop. FEV_1 1.19 l:
high risk for lobectomy

Treatment of tuberculosis

Standard therapy – duration 6 months

Initial phase (2 months)	Continuation phase (4 months)[†]
Triple therapy regimen Isoniazid + rifampicin + pyrazinamide OR	Isoniazid + rifampicin
Quadruple therapy regimen (if drug resistance is thought likely) Isoniazid + rifampicin + pyrazinamide + ethambutol (or streptomycin*)	Ethambutol is added if resistance is thought likely OR Streptomycin is added if resistance to isoniazid is thought likely

* Now used only rarely

[†] Longer treatment may be necessary for bone and joint infections; for meningitis or for resistant organism

Dosage for standard unsupervised (daily) 6-month regimen

Antituberculous drug	Children Daily dose (mg/kg body weight)	Adults	
		Body weight	Daily dose
Isoniazid	10 (max 300 mg)	All weights	300 mg
Rifampicin	10	< 50 kg > 50 kg	450 mg 600 mg
Pyrazinamide (for first 2 months only)	35	< 50 kg > 50 kg	1.5 g 2.0 g
Ethambutol** first 2 months after 2 months	15 or 25 15	All weights All weights	15 or 25 mg/kg body weight 15 mg/kg body weight

** Not for children under 6 years of age

Dosage for fully supervised intermittent 6-month regimen

Antituberculous drug	Regimen	Children (mg/kg body weight)	Adults
Isoniazid	3 times a week	15	15 mg/kg body weight
Rifampicin	3 times a week	15	600–900 mg
Pyrazinamide (for first 2 months only)	3 times a week	50	2 g (if body weight < 50 kg) 2.5 g (if body weight > 50 kg)
	OR		
	Twice a week	75	3 g (if body weight < 50 kg) 3.5 g (if body weight > 50 kg)
Ethambutol**	3 times a week	30	30 mg/kg body weight
	OR		
	Twice a week	45	45 mg/kg body weight

** Not for children under 6 years of age

Tuberculin testing

Only purified tuberculin (Tuberculin PPD) is available for skin testing.

Available as 100 000 units/ml (for Heaf test (multiple puncture)), and diluted 1 in 100 (1000 units/ml), 1 in 1000 (100 units/ml) and 1 in 10 000 (10 units/ml).

1. **Heaf test (multiple puncture test)**
   The reaction produced is equivalent to that produced by 5 international units of intradermal PPD.

2. **Mantoux test (intradermal test)**

   The initial diagnostic dose in patients in whom tuberculosis is suspected (or who are known to be hypersensitive to tuberculin) is 1 unit of tuberculin PPD in 0.1 ml by intradermal injection and in subsequent tests 10 and finally 100 units in 0.1 ml may be given. For routine pre-BCG skin testing the 10-unit dose of tuberculin PPD is used.

   The tests are read after at least 72 hours and not later than 1 week.

   The reaction is positive if there is palpable induration of 6 mm or more in diameter.

   A negative result when testing with 100 international units makes the presence of tuberculosis most unlikely.

International classification of pneumoconiosis (ILO 1980)

(After Thürauf J., Erlangen. Reprinted with permission of Boehringer Ingelheim)
This classification is used for the evaluation of silicosis or asbestosis. Other interstitial lung diseases and pleural disorders can be similarly assessed and classified by analogy.

Image quality	+ = good	± = acceptable	± = inadequate	u = useless

Opacities	Profusion				
	12-step scale	0/−	1/0	2/1	3/2
	(cf. standard film)	**0/0**	**1/1**	**2/2**	**3/3**
		0/1	1/2	2/3	3/+

The first figure indicates the 'initial' classification choice, the second the possible alternative.

Transitional forms are indicated, e.g. 1/2 or 2/1.

Definition of profusion

Category 0:   Round or irregular opacities are absent, or less profuse than in category 1

Category 1:   Round or irregular opacities are clearly present, but in small numbers

Category 2:   Numerous round or irregular opacities; normal lung markings still visible

Category 3:   Very numerous round or irregular opacities; normal lung markings partly or totally obscured

Distribution (*Lung fields*)   right upper   = RU | LU = left upper
right middle = RM | LM = left middle
right lower = RL | LL = left lower

Size *small*
Shape: round   p = ● 1.5 mm   q = ● 1.5–3 mm   r = ● 3–10 mm
(diameter)
irregular   s = 1.5 mm   t = 1.5–3 mm   u = 3–10 mm
(width)
mixed   p/s
(e.g.)   q/t

large   A = 1–5 cm ∅ (+∅)   B = 5 cm - RU   C = > RU

Type   wd = ● well-defined   id = ill-defined

Pleural thickening	**Diffuse**	Spread	0 = absent; <1	1 = < 1/4 of lateral chest wall
			2 = 1/4–1/2 of lateral chest wall	3 = > 1/2 of lateral chest wall
		Thickness	a = < 5 mm b = 5–10 mm	c = > 10 mm
		Localization	R = right sided	L = left sided
	Plaques	Spread	0 = absent; < 1	1 = < 2 cm max. length
			2 = 2–10 cm max. length	3 = > 10 cm max. length
		Thickness	a = <5 mm b = 5–10 mm	c = > 10 mm
		Localization (chest wall, diaphragm)	R = right sided	L = left sided

Costophrenic angle	Obliteration R = right sided	L = left sided

Pleural	**Spread** 0 = absent; < 1 1 = < 2 cm ∅ (+∅) 2 = 2–10 cm ∅ 3 = >10cm ∅
	Localization (chest wall, diaphragm, elsewhere) R = right sided L = left sided

Abbreviations

ax confluent small opacities	em emphysema	me mesothelioma of pleura
bu bullous emphysema	es egg-shell hilus (calcification)	od other disorders/phenomena (specify)
ca cancer of lung	fr fracture of rib	pi pleural thickening
cn calcification in small opacities	hi hilar/mediastinal lymph node enlargement	(interlobar/mediastinal)
co heart, size/alteration in shape	ho honeycomb lung	px pneumothorax
cp cor pulmonale	idd indistinct diaphragm	rp rheumatoid pneumoconiosis
cv cavity	(>1/3 of hemidiaphragm)	(Caplan's syndrome)
di distortion	idh indistinct heart outline (>1/3 heart edge)	tba active tuberculosis
ef pleural effusion	kl Kerley lines (basal, perihilar)	tbu inactive tuberculosis

Cardiopulmonary resuscitation (Marsden, 1989)

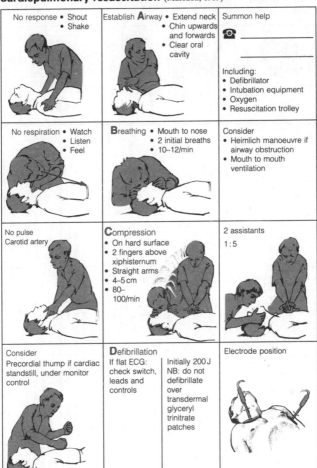

| No response | • Shout
• Shake | Establish **A**irway | • Extend neck
• Chin upwards and forwards
• Clear oral cavity | Summon help
☎ _____

_____

Including:
• Defibrillator
• Intubation equipment
• Oxygen
• Resuscitation trolley |

| No respiration | • Watch
• Listen
• Feel | **B**reathing | • Mouth to nose
• 2 initial breaths
• 10–12/min | Consider
• Heimlich manoeuvre if airway obstruction
• Mouth to mouth ventilation |

| No pulse
Carotid artery | **C**ompression | • On hard surface
• 2 fingers above xiphisternum
• Straight arms
• 4–5 cm
• 80–100/min | 2 assistants
1 : 5 |

| Consider
Precordial thump if cardiac standstill, under monitor control | **D**efibrillation
If flat ECG: check switch, leads and controls | Initially 200 J
NB: do not defibrillate over transdermal glyceryl trinitrate patches | Electrode position |

117

Cardiac arrest

(Chamberlain, 1989)

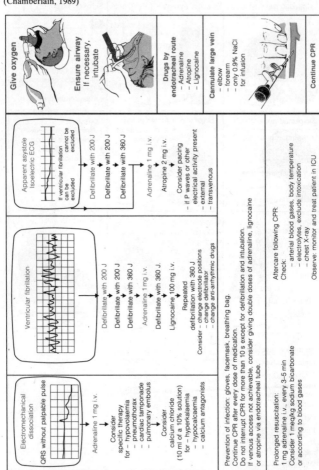

Give oxygen

Ensure airway
If necessary, intubate

Drugs by endotracheal route
- Adrenaline
- Atropine
- Lignocaine

Cannulate large vein
- elbow
- forearm
- only 0.9% NaCl for infusion

Continue CPR

Apparent asystole
Isoelectric ECG

If ventricular fibrillation cannot be excluded

Defibrillate with 200 J
Defibrillate with 200 J
Defibrillate with 360 J

→ Adrenaline 1 mg i.v.

Atropine 2 mg i.v.

Consider pacing
- if P waves or other electrical activity present
- external
- transvenous

Ventricular fibrillation

Defibrillate with 200 J
Defibrillate with 200 J
Defibrillate with 360 J

Adrenaline 1 mg i.v.

Defibrillate with 360 J.
Lignocaine 100 mg i.v.
Repeated defibrillation with 360 J
Consider – change electrode positions
– change defibrillator
– change anti-arrhythmic drugs

Electromechanical dissociation
QRS without palpable pulse

Adrenaline 1 mg i.v.

Consider specific therapy
for – hypovolaemia
– pneumothorax
– cardiac tamponade
– pulmonary embolus

Consider calcium chloride
(10 ml of a 10% solution)
for – hyperkalaemia
– hypocalcaemia
– calcium antagonists

Prevention of infection: gloves, facemask, breathing bag.
Continue CPR after every dose of medication.
Do not interrupt CPR for more than 10 s except for defibrillation and intubation.
If venous access not achievable, consider giving double doses of adrenaline, lignocaine or atropine via endotracheal tube.

Prolonged resuscitation:
1 mg adrenaline i.v., every 3–5 min
Consider 1 meq/kg sodium bicarbonate or according to blood gases

Aftercare following CPR:
Check:
– arterial blood gases, body temperature
– electrolytes, exclude intoxication
– chest X-ray
Observe: monitor and treat patient in ICU

Antidotes in poisoning

Conducting the telephone call

Caller		Name, address, telephone number
Patient	Who	Age, weight, sex, location
	What	Description of poison (package label), consumption (route)
	How much	Most exact amount possible (if necessary, estimate)
	When	Time of consumption, confirmed or only suspected
	Condition	First symptoms, measures already taken, respiration, circulation, state of consciousness
	Advice	Emergency measures before arrival of ambulance

Suspected poison	Antidote
Amphetamine	Ammonium chloride
Arsenic, organic and inorganic mercury salts	Dimercaprol (BAL) (chlorpromazine, ± beta-blockers)
Atropine, antihistamines	Pyridostigmine, neostigmine
Barium	Sodium sulphate
Benzodiazepines	Flumazenil
Carbon monoxide	Oxygen (hyperbaric if possible)
Cyanide	Amylnitrite, dicobalt edetate, sodium nitrite, sodium thiosulphate, hydroxocobalamin (vitamin B_{12})
Digoxin	Digoxin-specific antibody (Digibind)
Extrapyramidal symptoms	Biperiden
Iron	Desferrioxamine
Herbicides, paraquat	Bentonite (Fuller's earth, activated charcoal)
Hyperthermia, malignant	Dantroline
Isoniazid	Pyridoxine (vitamin B_6)
Methaemoglobinaemia (nitrites)	Methylene blue
Methanol, glycol	Ethyl alcohol
Opioids	Naloxone
Organophosphorus insecticides (acetylcholinesterase inhibitors)	Atropine (pralidoxime mesylate (P2S))
Paracetamol	Acetylcysteine, methionine
Phosgene	Hexamine
Radioisotopes, heavy metals	Sodium calcium edetate, dimercaprol (BAL), penicillamine
Warfarin	Vitamin K

Activated charcoal administration in poisoning

Simultaneous administration of activated charcoal can delay the absorption of most chemicals. Some substances are only insignificantly bound (see table). With several drugs the administration of activated charcoal is appropriate even after absorption or after parenteral administration (substances with small distribution volumes, weak plasma protein binding and/or known enterohepatic circulation and/or known secretion into the gastrointestinal tract) (see table).

Elimination accelerated even after absorption or parenteral administration	Insignificant absorption by activated charcoal
Antidepressants	Acetylcysteine
Carbamazepine	Alkali
Dapsone	Boric acid
Digitoxin	Caustic alkalis (sodium/potassium hydroxide)
Digoxin	Cyanide
Glutethimide	DDT
Meprobamate	Ethanol
Methotrexate	Malathion
Nadolol	Mercury
Phenobarbitone	Methanol
Phenylbutazone	Mineral acids
Phenytoin	Salts (lithium salts, iron salts)
Salicylate	
Theophylline	

Vesicle formation in poisoning

Amitriptyline, barbiturates, bites (snake, spider), CO, diphenoxylate, glutethimide, meprobamate, methadone, methaqualone, nitrazepam, tricyclic antidepressants.

Fetor in poisoning		Radio-opaque drugs
Drug	**Fetor**	**Regularly radio-opaque**
Amylnitrite	Fruity	Acetazolamide
Arsenic	Garlic-like	Acetylcarbromal
Chloral hydrate	Pungent	Barium
Chloroform	Acetone-like, fruity	Busulphan
Cyanide	Bitter almonds	Carbromal
Ethanol	Alcohol-like	Chloral hydrate
Ethchlorvynol	Pungent	Iodine-containing substances
Isopropanol	Acetone-like, fruity	Iron-containing substances
Malathion	Garlic-like	Potassium-containing substances
Mercaptan	Rotten eggs	
Methanol	Alcohol-like	**Inconstantly radio-opaque**
Organophosphate	Garlic-like	Antihistamines
Paraldehyde	Pungent	Phenothiazines
Parathion	Garlic-like	Tricyclic antidepressants
Phophorus	Garlic-like	
Salicylate	Acetone-like	
Hydrogen sulphide	Rotten eggs	
Tellurium	Garlic-like	
Thallium	Garlic-like	

Poisons information centres
(Consult day and night)

Belfast	01232 240503
Birmingham	0121 507 5588 *or* 0121 507 5589
Cardiff	01222 709901
Dublin	Dublin 837 9964 *or* Dublin 837 9966
Edinburgh	0131 229 2477
Leeds	0113 243 0715 *or* 0113 292 3547
London	0171 635 9191 *or* 0171 955 5095
Newcastle	0191 232 5131

Note: Some of these centres also advise on laboratory analytical services which may be of help in the diagnosis and management of a small number of cases.

Estimation of suicide risk

(Kielholz, 1971)

1. Suicide indices
   * Previous suicide attempts, direct or indirect suicide threats
   * Expression of explicit ideas concerning the preparation and performance of a suicidal act, or 'unnatural tranquillity'
   * Dreams of self-destruction, falls or disasters
   * History of suicide in family or close contact (suggestion)
2. Morbid signs
   * Onset or waning of depressive phases, confusional states
   * Agitated anxiety, inhibition of affect or aggression
   * Severe feelings of guilt or inadequacy
   * Periods of biological upheaval (puberty, pregnancy, puerperium, menopause)
   * Chronic sleep disturbances
   * Incurable illness or delusion of illness
   * Alcoholism and toxic confusional states
3. Enviromental factors
   * Disrupted family relations in childhood (broken home)
   * Loss or primary lack of human contacts (blighted love, loneliness, rejection)
   * Loss of employment, lack of job satisfaction, financial worries
   * Lack of religious affiliation

Activity profiles of antidepressants

(After Kielholz (1966))

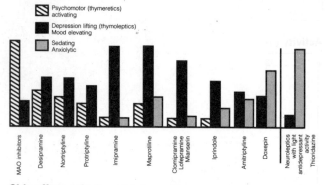

Side effects of tri- and tetracyclics

	Postural hypotension	Anticholinergic	Quinine-like	Adrenergic
Amitriptyline	+ + + + +	+ + + + +	+	+
Doxepin	+ + +	+ + +	±	0
Imipramine	+ + + +	+ + + +	+	+ + +
Nortriptyline	+ +	+ +	+	+ + +
Desipramine	+ +	+ +	+	+ + + + +
Maprotiline	+	+	+	+ + + + +
Trazodone	+	+	−	0
Trimipramine	+	+ +		+
Amoxapine	+	+		+ + +
Protriptyline	+	+ + +		+ + +

Review of psychotropic drugs

Classification	Main action	Principal agent
Minor tranquillizer	Non-hypnotic sedative **without** antipsychotic effect	Benzodiazepine Meprobamate
Major tranquillizer (neuroleptics)	Non-hypnotic sedative **with** antipsychotic effect	Phenothiazine Butyrophenone Thioxanthene
Thymoleptics	Mood-lightening antidepressants	Tricyclic antidepressants
Thymeretics	Disinhibiting antidepressants	MAO inhibitors
Lithium	Stabilization of cyclic depression	Various salts
Stimulants	Motivation enhancing	Amphetamine

Activity profile of neuroleptic drugs

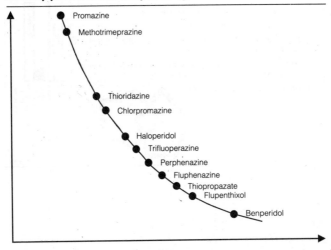

Promazine
Methotrimeprazine
Thioridazine
Chlorpromazine
Haloperidol
Trifluoperazine
Perphenazine
Fluphenazine
Thiopropazate
Flupenthixol
Benperidol

Short test of cerebral function

Questions	Points
Orientation	
1. What is today's date? Day of week? Month? Year? Season?	5
2. Where are you now? Hospital? Ward? Town? Country?	5
Memory	
3. Memorize: lemon, key, ball* (Dictate ca. every 1 s, have patient repeat until he or she can remember the words)	3
Attention	
4. Subtract 7s from 100 (93, 86, 79, 65) or spell **nature** backwards (erutan)	5
Short-term memory	
5. Repeat the words memorized at (3) above	3
Speech	
6. Name: pencil (ballpoint), show patient a watch	2
7. Repeat: none and, when or but	1
8. Three-step command: take the paper in the left hand, fold it in half, lay it on the floor	3
9. Write a sentence (must contain subject and object and make sense; spelling mistakes do not count)	1
10. Draw the following figure with closed eyes:	1

*Choose other words when repeating test

Total

0–23: Suspicion of organic lesion

Substance abuse

	Opiates	Hypnotics	Tranquillizers	Alcohol	Stimulants	Hallucinogens	Cannabis
Examples	Heroin Cocaine Morphine Opium Methadone	Barbiturate Glutethimide	Benzodiazepine Meprobamate	Ethanol C_2H_5OH	Amphetamine Sympathico- mimetics Appetite suppressants	LSD* PCP* Mescalin Psilocybin	δ-9- tetrahydro- cannabinol (THC)
Respiration	↓ Hypoxia Toxic pulmonary oedema	↓ Hypoxia, possibly respiratory acidosis		Alcoholic fetor Aspiration pneumonia		↓	↓ Dry mouth
Consciousness	↓ to coma				Possibly delirium	Possibly delirium, coma	
Pupils	Contraction Note: Pethidine→ Dilatation	Contraction		Dilatation Nystagmus	Dilatation	Dilatation Nystagmus	Dilatation Conjunctival irritation
Circulation	↓ Cocaine→ Cardiovascular complications	↓ Hypothermia	↓	↓↑ Facial flushing	↑ Fever	↑ Palpitation	↑
Psychological symptoms	Euphoria Hallucinations	Hallucination Agitation		Slurred speech Incoordination	Flight of ideas Anxiety Paranoia	Hallucinations Anxiety Confusion Delusions Violence (PCP)	Hallucinations Euphoria
Therapy of intoxication	**Preservation and protection of vital functions** Airway, circulatory support, oxygen, gastric lavage, dialysis, haemoperfusion, hypothermia protection, rhabdomyolysis						
	Naloxone		Flumazenil	Thiamine			
Withdrawal symptoms	Mydriasis Myalgia Abdominal cramps Nausea Vomiting Yawning Sweating Tears Insomnia	Autonomic hyperactivity Nausea, vomiting, anxiety Sleep disturbances, tremor Grand mal seizures		Autonomic hyperactivity Sweating Vomiting Epilepsy Liver failure Hallucinations Restlessness	Restlessness Exhaustion Psychomotor agitation	Agitation 'Bad trip'	Anxiety Tremor Nystagmus (and others, cf. opiates)
Therapy withdrawal	Autonomic hyperactivity is an important pathophysiological mechanism in the acute withdrawal phase; hence administration of alpha- and/or beta-blockers must be considered						
	Clonidine Baclofen Methotri- meprazine			Chlormethiazole Anticonvulsants			Diazepam 'Talk down' Anxiolytics PCP: Haloperidol
Warning	In emergency treatment of patients with substance abuse note danger of infection with HIV and hepatitis viruses						
	*LSD, lysergic acid diethylamide; PCP, Phenycyclidine						
Literature	American Psychiatric Association (1987)						

Acid–base disturbances

Respiratory alkalosis (hyperventilation)	
1. Central	Stimulation of respiratory centre (anxiety, fever, hypoxaemia, salicylate, exertion)
2. Thoracic	Reflex stimulation of respiratory centre (pulmonary embolus, pneumonia, atelectasis, pulmonary oedema, asthma)
3. Various	Sepsis, overbreathing, pregnancy, hepatic cirrhosis

Respiratory acidosis (Hypoventilation)	
1. Central	Disturbed function of respiratory centre (trauma, drugs/poisoning)
2. Thoracic	Disturbed mechanics of breathing (poliomyelitis, myasthenia gravis, trauma)
	Disturbed lung structure (emphysema)

Metabolic alkalosis	
1. ↑ Acid loss	Loss of gastric juice, diuretic therapy, severe potassium depletion, Cushing's syndrome, Conn's syndrome
2. ↑ HCO_3^- supply	Iatrogenic HCO_3^- administration, milk-alkali syndrome, overventilation of chronically hypocapnic patients, metabolism of ketone bodies and lactate to HCO_3^-

Metabolic acidosis (Kussmaul respiration)		
1. ↑ Acid supply (↑ anion gap, normochloraemia)	Ketoacidosis	(Diabetes, starvation, alcohol)
	Lactic acidosis	(Shock, biguanide poisoning, CO poisoning, terminal hepatic cirrhosis, leukaemia)
	Drugs/poisoning	(Methyl alcohol, ethylene glycol, salicylate, isoniazid, cyanide, nitroprusside)
2. ↑ HCO_3^- loss (normal anion gap, hyperchloraemia)	HCO_3^- loss	(Diarrhoea, intestinal fistulae, pancreatic fistulae, ileostomy, carbonic anhydrase inhibitor administration, ureterosigmoidostomy)
	Chloride retention	(Renal tubular acidosis, administration of arginine, lysine, NH_4Cl)
3. ↓ Acid excretion	Renal failure, hypoaldosteronism, congenital enzyme deficiencies	

Anion gap:

· Normal value: 8–12 mmol/l

$$\text{Anion gap} = Na^+ - (Cl^- + HCO_3^-)$$

Acid–base nomogram
(After Siggaard–Andersen (1963))

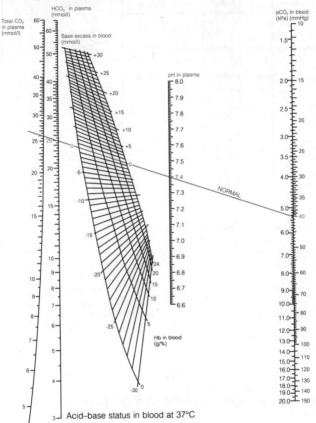

Acid–base status in blood at 37°C

To use:
1. Connect pCO_2 and pH, read off on left HCO_3^- or total CO_2.
2. Measure Hb concentration, read off base excess on appropriate Hb line.

Blood gas analysis (normal values)

Estimation	Units	Arterial	Venous	Capillary
pH		7.38–7.42	7.36–7.40	7.38–7.42
pO₂	mmHg	90–100	35–45	>80
	kPa	12–13.3	4.6–6.0	>10.6
pCO₂	mmHg	35–45	40–50	38–45
	kPa	4.6–6.0	5.3–6.6	5.1–6.0
Oxygen saturation (SO₂)	%	95–97	55–70	95–97
Standard bicarbonate (HCO₃⁻)	mmol/l	21–29	24–30	21–29
Base excess (BE)	mmol/l	−2 to +2	−2 to +2	−2 to +2

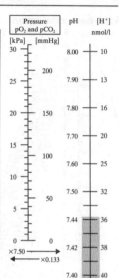

Estimation of acid–base disturbances

Required: pH, pCO₂ and HCO₃⁻

Definitions of acid–base disturbances

Acidosis: pH below 7.36
Respiratory acidosis: p_aCO_2 above 45 mmHg (≈6 kPa)
Respiratory alkalosis: p_aCO_2 below 35 mmHg (≈4.5 kPa)

Alkalosis: pH above 7.44
Metabolic acidosis: Bicarbonate below 21 mmol/l
Metabolic alkalosis: Bicarbonate above 29 mmol/l

pCO₂ \ HCO₃⁻	Under 21 mmol	21–29 mmol/l	Above 29 mmol/l
Above 6 kPa 45 mmHg	Combined metabolic and respiratory acidosis	Respiratory acidosis	Metabolic alkalosis and respiratory acidosis
4.5–6.0 kPa 35–45 mmHg	Metabolic acidosis	Normal	Metabolic alkalosis
Below 4.5 kPa 35 mmHg	Metabolic acidosis and respiratory alkalosis	Respiratory alkalosis	Combined metabolic and respiratory alkalosis

Calculation of the bicarbonate required to correct pH

Bicarbonate required = negative base excess (base deficit) × 0.3 × body weight in kg

The formula permits the direct calculation of the required amount of sodium bicarbonate in millilitres, if 8.4% sodium bicarbonate is used (1 ml = 1 mmol)

Approximate relationship between pH and H⁺ ion concentration

$$[H^+] = \frac{24 \times pCO_2}{HCO_3^-} \qquad pH = 6.1 + \frac{HCO_3^-}{pCO_2}$$

nmol/l

Sodium and potassium

Hypernatraemia	Hyponatraemia

1. ↑ **Intake**
   Salt consumption
   Sodium bicarbonate
   Sodium penicillin
2. ↓ **Renal excretion**
   Diabetes insipidus
   (renal, posterior pituitary)
   Osmotic
3. **Endocrine**
   Cushing's syndrome
   Primary hyperaldosteronism
   Hyperosmolar diabetic coma
4. **Others**
   Laboratory error
	1. ↓ **Intake**
	   Polydipsia
	2. ↑ **Gastrointestinal losses**
	   Vomiting, diarrhoea
	   Aspiration of gastric juice
	   Fistulae
	3. ↑ **Renal losses**
	   Polyuric phase of acute renal failure
	   Salt-losing nephritis
	   Diuretics
	   Osmotic
	4. **Endocrine**
	   Addison's disease
	   Inappropriate ADH secretion (see p. 130)
	   Ketoacidotic diabetic coma
	5. **With water balance disturbances**
	   (cf table p. 130)
	6. **Others**
	   Laboratory error
	   Dilutional
	   False, in hyperlipidaemia, hyperproteinaemia

Sodium deficit in mmol/l
$$\frac{(142 - \text{measured Na}^+) \times \text{body weight}}{5}$$

Hyperkalaemia	Hypokalaemia

1. ↑ **Intake**
   Potassium infusion
   Stored blood transfusion
2. ↓ **Renal excretion**
   Acute renal failure
   Chronic renal failure
   Addison's disease
   Hypoaldosteronism
   Potassium-sparing diuretics
   ACE inhibitors
3. **Displacement from cells**
   Acidosis
   Crush syndrome
   Haemolysis, rhabdomyolysis
   Burns
   Digitalis intoxication
   Succinyl choline
   Hyperkalaemic periodic paralysis
4. **Others**
   Poor phlebotomy technique
   in vitro haemolysis
   Laboratory error
   Thrombocytosis, leucocytosis
	1. ↓ **Intake**
	   Malnutrition
	2. ↑ **Gastrointestinal losses**
	   Vomiting, diarrhoea, fistulae
	   Laxative abuse
	3. ↑ **Renal losses**
	   Osmotic diuresis
	   Diuretics (saliuretics, carbonic anhydrase inhibitors)
	   Cushing's syndrome
	   Hyperaldosteronism (primary and secondary)
	   Renal tubular acidosis
	   Metabolic alkalosis
	4. **Displacement into cells**
	   Alkalosis
	   Insulin therapy
	   Hypokalaemic periodic paralysis
	5. **Others**
	   Magnesium deficiency
	   Laboratory error
	   Diabetic ketoacidosis

Potassium replacement and pH

Calculation:

1. Determine body potassium

mmol/kg	Male	Female
Normal	45	40
Moderate weight loss	38	33
Severe weight loss	30	26

2. Read off arterial pH and K$^+$ from nomogram and assess body weight condition.
3. Calculate K$^+$ requirement/excess by multiplying body potassium by weight and read off on the nomogram the percentage adjustment.

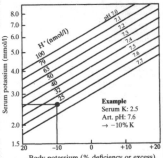

Example
Serum K: 2.5
Art. pH: 7.6
→ −10% K

Calcium and phosphorus

Hypercalcaemia	Hypocalcaemia
↑ Intake	↓ Intake
Hypervitaminosis A/D	Malabsorption
Milk-alkali syndrome	
	Endocrine
Endocrine	Hypoparathyroidism
Primary hyperparathyroidism	Secondary hyperparathyroidism
Tertiary hyperparathyroidism	Vitamin D deficiency (rickets, osteomalacia)
Hyperthyroidism	
Acromegaly	**Electrolyte disturbances**
Adrenal cortical insufficiency	Hypomagnesaemia
Ectopic ADH production	Hyperphosphataemia
Drugs	**Drugs**
Thiazide diuretics	Anticonvulsants
Lithium	
	Others
Others	Hypoalbuminaemia
Bone metastases	Pancreatitis
Therapy of tumours with metastases	Distal renal tubular acidosis
Multiple myeloma	Laboratory error
Immobilization	
Sarcoidosis	
Recovery phase of acute renal failure	
Laboratory error	

Correction for serum albumin
Add 0.02 mmol/l Ca for each g/l of serum albumin below 40 g/l, subtract 0.02 mmol/l Ca for each g/l of serum albumin above 40 g/l.

Hyperphosphataemia	Hypophosphataemia
↑ Intake	↓ Intake
	Malnutrition
Endocrine	Malabsorption
Hypoparathyroidism	Chronic alcoholism
Secondary and tertiary hyperparathyroidism	Parenteral nutrition without P supplement
Diabetic coma	
Hyperthyroidism	↑ Renal losses
Acromegaly	Renal tubular acidosis
	Fanconi syndrome
Drugs	
Diphosphonate	**Endocrine**
Cytostatic agents	Primary hyperparathyroidism
	Vitamin D-resistant rickets
Others	
Acidosis	**Electrolyte disturbances**
Renal failure	Hypercalcaemia
Burns	Hypomagnesaemia
Laboratory error	
	Drugs
	Diuretics
	Phosphate binders
	Antacids, salicylate poisoning
	Others
	Alkalosis
	Gram-negative septicaemia
	Laboratory error

Magnesium

Hypermagnesaemia	Hypomagnesaemia
↑ **Intake** Mg^{2+}-containing antacids and laxatives Mg^{2+} infusions	↓ **Intake** Malnutrition Malabsorption Chronic alcoholism Parenteral nutrition without Mg^{2+}-supplements
↓ **Renal excretion** Renal failure	↑ **Renal losses** Diuretics (apart from potassium sparers) Diabetic ketoacidosis Renal tubular defects
	↑ **Gastrointestinal losses** Vomiting, diarrhoea Aspiration of gastric juice Small intestine bypass
	Endocrine Hyperaldosteronism Hyperthyroidism Vitamin D therapy
Others Rhabdomyolysis Burns Laboratory error	**Others** Pancreatitis With hypercalcaemia After aminoglycoside antibiotics After cisplatin treatment Laboratory error

Syndrome of inappropriate ADH secretion (SIADH)

Criteria:
- Hyponatraemia and low serum osmolality
- No dehydration
- Urine osmolality higher than serum osmolality
- Increase of sodium and serum osmolality with water restriction
- Normal function of kidneys, pituitary, thyroid and adrenals

Causes	
CNS disorders	Encephalitis, meningitis, brain abscess, cerebral tumour, skull/cerebral trauma, subarachnoid haemorrhage, subdural haematoma, venous sinus thrombosis, Guillain-Barré syndrome, cerebral lupus erythematosus
Lung disorders	Pneumonia (bacterial and viral), tuberculosis, lung abscess, empyema, chronic obstructive airways disease, PEEP ventilation
Ectopic ADH production (paraneoplastic)	Small cell carcinoma of bronchus, carcinoma of pancreas, carcinoma of duodenum, leukaemia, Hodgkin's lymphoma, thymoma
Drug induced	Carbamazepine, chlorpropamide, clofibrate, cyclophosphamide, lithium, narcotics, nicotine, oxytocin, thiazides, tricyclics, vasopressin, vinblastine, vincristine
Others	Hypothyroidism, Addison's disease, hypopituitarism, emotional stress

Water excess in litres $= \dfrac{(142 - \text{measured Na}^+) \times \text{body weight}}{700}$

Anatomy of the digestive organs

Oesophagus

1 Mouth of oesophagus (Zenker's diverticulum)
2 Aortic impression (traction diverticulum)
2a Aorta
3 Diaphragmatic impression

Stomach

3a Cardia
4 Fundus (with air bubble)
5 Lesser curvature
5a Angular notch (incisura angularis)
6 Greater curvature
7 Body
8 Antrum
9 Pylorus

Small bowel (2.5–4.5 m)

Duodenum (25–30 cm)

9a Duodenal bulb
10 First (superior) part
11 Second (descending) part
11a Third (horizontal, inferior) part
12 Fourth (ascending) part
13 Duodenojejunal flexure

14 **Jejunum**
15 **Ileum**
(Meckel's diverticulum)
30–100 cm
prox. of 15a

Large bowel (~1.5 m)

15a Ileocaecal valve
16 Appendix
17 Caecum
18 Ascending colon
19 Hepatic (right) flexure
20 Transverse colon
21 Splenic (left) flexure
22 Descending colon
23 Sigmoid colon
24 Rectum
25 Rectal ampulla

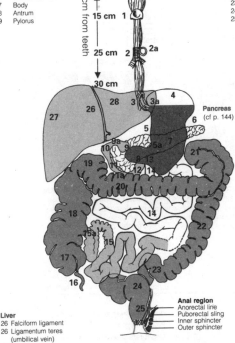

cm from teeth
15 cm 1
25 cm 2 2a
30 cm

Pancreas (cf p. 144)

Anal region
Anorectal line
Puborectal sling
Inner sphincter
Outer sphincter

Liver

26 Falciform ligament
26 Ligamentum teres (umbilical vein)
27 Right lobe
28 Left lobe

Typical radiological wall appearances

Jejunum:

Ileum:

Circular folds

Colon:

Haustrations
Semicircular folds

Abdominal ultrasound – anatomy and technique

Longitudinal section – anatomy

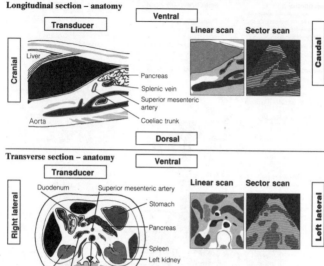

Ventral

Transducer

Linear scan   Sector scan

Cranial | Caudal

Liver
Pancreas
Splenic vein
Superior mesenteric artery
Coeliac trunk
Aorta

Dorsal

Transverse section – anatomy

Ventral

Transducer

Linear scan   Sector scan

Right lateral | Left lateral

Duodenum   Superior mesenteric artery
Stomach
Pancreas
Spleen
Left kidney
Right kidney
Aorta
Vena cava

Dorsal

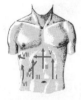

Schematic examination sequence (I–VII) of liver and gall bladder with the required planes of cut in ultrasound

Systematic method of ultrasound nomenclature:
1. Description of the echoes: strength (strong/weak), size (fine/coarse), interval between echoes (dense/isolated).
2. Assessment of the echo pattern: distribution of the echoes (homogeneous/patchy).
3. Assessment of the sound distribution: sound reduction (shadow), 'relative sound enhancement' (behind fluids).
4. Circumscribed changes (weak echo).

Glossary of ultrasound morphology:

Echo-free with distal 'sound enhancement'

Echo-poor/poor reflection

Echo-dense/echogenic/reflective/rich reflections

Homogeneous/regular

Patchy/irregular

Bright reflections/with distal sound shadow

Ultrasound of the liver

Characteristics of diffuse and circumscribed changes of hepatic parenchyma

Hepatic parenchymatous diseases		Normal liver	Acute hepatitis, acute congestion	Fatty liver	Cirrhosis
	Size (cm) midclavicular line	12 cm (±2)	>12 cm	>12 cm	>12 cm or <12 cm
	Contour ventral	Flat	Convex	Convex	Convex
	dorsal	Concave	Convex	Convex	Convex
	Caudal liver edge	Acute-angled	Rounded	Blunt-angled	Swollen
	Inner structure	Fine Regular	Fine Regular	Coarse Dense Regular	Coarse Dense Irregular
	Sound conduction	Normal	Mildly reducing	Moderately reducing	Moderately reducing

		Margin	Shape	Size	Echo pattern	Distal reflections	Localization
Echogenic (echo-dense) circumscribed liver lesions	Metastases ca. 30%	Smooth	Irregular	Variable	Irregular, often less echogenic rim – 'bull's eye'	Reduced	Multiple/ overlapping
	Liver cell neoplasms	Irregular	Irregular	Variable	Irregular	Reduced	Solitary/ overlapping
	Cholangio-carcinoma	Smooth	Irregular	Variable	Irregular	Reduced	Solitary/ portal
	Haemangioma	Smooth	Regular	Variable	Regular	Slightly enhanced	Solitary/ multiple
	Organized haematoma	Anatom. determined	Variable	Variable	Regular	Reduced	Solitary
	Localized fatty infiltration	Irregular	Determined	Variable	Regular	Reduced	Solitary/ multiple
Weaker echogenic circumscribed liver lesions	Metastases ca. 60%	Irregular	Round, oval	Variable	Irregular	Enhanced/ reduced	Multiple/ overlapping
	Adenoma	Regular	Round, oval	Variable	Regular	Reduced	Often solitary
	Focal nodular hyperplasia	Irregular	Round, oval	Variable	Regular	Reduced	Often solitary
	Fresh abscess	Irregular	Round, oval	Variable	Irregular	Reduced	Mostly solitary
	Liver cell neoplasm	Irregular	Round, oval	Variable	Irregular	Reduced	Mostly solitary/ overlapping
	Lymphoma	Regular	Round, oval	Variable	Regular	Reduced/ enhanced	Multiple
Non-echogenic circumscribed liver lesions	Congenital cyst	Regular	Round	Variable	Free	Increased	Ubiquitous
	Post-traumatic cyst	Regular	Irregular	Variable	Free	Increased	Mostly solitary
	Hydatid	Regular	Round	Variable	Daughter cysts	Increased	Solitary/ multiple
	Fresh haematoma	Anatom. determined	Irregular	Variable	Possibly	Increased	Solitary
	Chronic abscess	Irregular	Irregular	Variable	Possibly	Increased	Solitary/ multiple
	Metastases	Irregular	Irregular	Variable	In region of rim	Increased	Often multiple

Ultrasound of gall bladder, pancreas and kidney

Normal findings	Sonographic criteria in pathological findings

Gall bladder normal	Gallstone	Cholesterol-polyps	Acute cholecystitis	Adeno-myomatosis	Carcinoma
Length 8–11 cm Thickness 3–4 cm Capacity 30–55 ml Wall ≤ 3 mm **Extrahepatic bile duct** normal 4–6 mm pathological >7 mm (After cholecystectomy 9–11 mm normal)	• Echogenic reflections, often bowed • Distal sound shadow (>3 mm) • Mobile on change of posture	• Wall-associated echogenic structures • Immobile • No sound shadow	• Wall thickness >3 mm, several layers • Tenderness on palpation • Pericholecystitis	• Irregular moderate wall thickening up to filling of lumen	• Wall thickening • Irregular borders, often beyond gall bladder • Usually evidence of stones

Pancreas normal A = 3 cm B = 2 cm C = 3 cm	Acute pancreatitis	Chronic pancreatitis	Carcinoma
Pancreatic duct ≤ 3–4 mm	• Pancreas enlarged • Poorly demarcated from surroundings • Homogeneous/non-homogeneous, faint echo	• Pancreas reduced • Sometimes circumscribed enlargement, 'pseudo-tumorous pancreatitis' • Pseudocysts • Calcification • Pancreatic duct dilated	• Circumscribed enlargement • Non-homogeneous • Pancreatic duct widened • Vascular displacement

Pancreatic duct ≤ 3–4 mm

Superior mesenteric artery

Confluent part of superior mesenteric and portal veins

Vena cava   Aorta   Splenic vein

Kidney normal	Atrophic kidney	Obstructed kidney	Carcinoma
6–12 cm Cortical width >1.5 cm, age dependent Difference between sides >1.5 cm, pathological	• Kidney small • Poorly demarcated • Ill-defined	• Dilatation of renal pelvicalyceal system	• Circumscribed organ border, overlapping echos

Ultrasound of adrenals and spleen

Normal findings	Sonographic criteria in pathological findings	

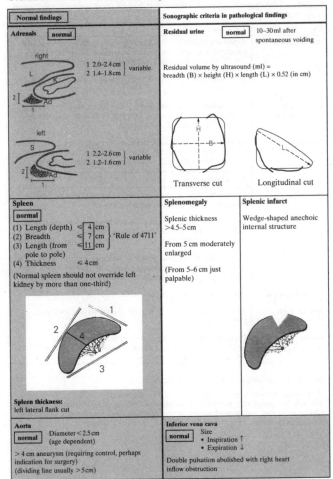

Adrenals | normal |

right

1 2.0–2.4 cm
2 1.4–1.8 cm } variable

L
K
Ad
2
1

left

1 2.2–2.6 cm
2 1.2–1.6 cm } variable

S
Ad
2
1

Residual urine | normal | 10–30 ml after spontaneous voiding

Residual volume by ultrasound (ml) =
breadth (B) × height (H) × length (L) × 0.52 (in cm)

Transverse cut   Longitudinal cut

Spleen

| normal |

(1) Length (depth) ≤ 4 cm
(2) Breadth ≤ 7 cm } 'Rule of 4711'
(3) Length (from ≤ 11 cm
    pole to pole)
(4) Thickness ≤ 4 cm

(Normal spleen should not override left kidney by more than one-third)

Splenomegaly

Splenic thickness >4.5–5 cm

From 5 cm moderately enlarged

(From 5–6 cm just palpable)

Splenic infarct

Wedge-shaped anechoic internal structure

Spleen thickness:
left lateral flank cut

Aorta

| normal | Diameter < 2.5 cm
         (age dependent)

> 4 cm aneurysm (requiring control, perhaps indication for surgery)
(dividing line usually > 5 cm)

Inferior vena cava

| normal | Size
• Inspiration ↑
• Expiration ↓

Double pulsation abolished with right heart inflow obstruction

Acute abdomen

Definition: Undiagnosed abdominal pains which demand rapid diagnosis and surgical or medical treatment.

Causes	Intra-abdominal
Inflammation	**Acute appendicitis** (~54%), **acute cholecystitis** (~14%), **acute pancreatitis** (~5%), peritonitis of unknown origin (~1%), diverticulitis, ileitis, colitis, subphrenic abscess, salpingitis, pyelonephritis Infectious diseases: malaria, tuberculosis, typhoid fever, viral hepatitis
Perforation/ haemorrhage	**Gastric/duodenal perforation** (~7%) (ulcer, carcinoma), gall bladder perforation, ectopic pregnancy, rupture of spleen or liver, aortic dissection
Occlusion of organ/vessel	**Ileus** (~11%), **acute mesenteric artery occlusion** (~3%), **biliary colic**, hernia, renal calculi, torsion, volvulus (ovarian tumour/ cyst), acute hepatic vein occlusion (Budd–Chiari syndrome)
	Extra-abdominal
Poisoning	**Foodstuffs**, lead, alcohol, arsenic, thallium, vegetable poisons, mushrooms, mercury, carbon tetrachloride
Metabolic	Diabetic precoma, familial hyperlipidaemia, acute intermittent porphyria, Addison's disease, periodic peritonitis (familial Mediterranean fever), hypercalaemia, hyponatraemia
Cardiovascular	**Myocardial infarct (esp. posterior wall)**, acute right heart failure (hepatic congestion), pulmonary embolus, thrombosis of mesenteric artery/vein, periarteritis nodosa, lupus erythematosus
Haematological	Haemolytic anaemia, acute/chronic leucosis, polycythaemia
Neurological	Tabes dorsalis, herpes zoster, intervertebral disc prolapse, vertebral fracture
Others	Psychoses, acute urinary retention, basal pneumonia, pneumothorax; acute glaucoma; haematoma of rectus abdominis, Bornholm disease (Coxsackie)

In pregnancy, arising from reproductive organs:

(Note: also consider the above listed differential diagnoses)
Extrauterine pregnancy, premature separation of the placenta, rupture/perforation/ torsion of uterus, inversion of uterus, fibroid complications, hydramnios, postpartum pneumoperitoneum, torsion of stalk or rupture of adnexal tumour

Principal symptoms	
General condition:	Shock, restlessness, shallow respiration, air hunger
Pain:	Localization, time course and manner of onset, pain-relieving/accentuating factors
Peritonitis	Diffuse or local; rebound tenderness (visceral peritoneum), guarding (visceral and parietal peritoneum); **nausea, vomiting, retention of faeces and flatus, urinary retention, fever**

Examination	
Inspection:	Operation scars, visible peristalsis; **lips/buccal mucosa:** abnormal pigmentation (Addison's disease, Peutz–Jeghers syndrome); **gums:** lead line; **skin:** pigmentation, petechial haemorrhages, collagenoses
Palpation:	Rebound tenderness, guarding, liver/spleen, tumour, rectal, femoral pulses, hernial orifices, supraclavicular lymph nodes (carcinoma of stomach), genitalia
Auscultation:	Bowel sounds (normal/increased/absent); heart (persistent arrhythmia, cardiac abnormality); lungs (pneumonia, effusion, pneumothorax)
Percussion:	Dullness in flanks
Others:	Pupil reactions (tabes dorsalis), ocular pressure (glaucoma), meningism

X-ray

Plain erect abdominal film
- **Free air under diaphragm** (Note: exclude previous laparotomy/laparoscopy, tubal isufflation) → perforation gastrointestinal tract; differential diagnosis: subphrenic abscess, loop of colon between liver or spleen and diaphragm, rarely gas-forming peritonitis; perhaps repeat film in left lateral position (air more readily demonstrable), perhaps repeat after 1 hour
- Free air subhepatic, pericaecal, retroperitoneal
- Free air in bile ducts (→ perforation)
- Gas and **fluid level** in stomach, small bowel, large bowel (indicative of ileus)
- Calculi/calcification: pancreas, gall bladder, kidney, urinary tract, vessels, hydatid cyst
- Size of kidneys, liver, spleen; psoas shadow

Chest X-ray: (Air under diaphragm, pleural effusion, infiltration, cardiac outline)

Abdominal ultrasound	

Laboratory	(Also preliminary for possible operation) Red/white cells, platelets, prothrombin time, electrolytes, creatinine, glucose, SGOT, SGPT, CPK, amylase (blood gases)

ECG

Ileus

Localization of Gas collection and **fluid level** (above the obstruction) →		Localization of the suspected stenosis/obstruction
Fluid level in: distended stomach		Pyloric stenosis
stomach and duodenum	No fluid levels in large bowel	Duodenum
standing loops of bowel in **middle** and **left** upper abdomen		**High** small bowel ileus
middle and **right** lower abdomen		**Low** small bowel ileus
Colon and possibly small bowel considerably distended (typical parietally placed gas-filled loops of bowel), with fluid levels	Fluid levels in large bowel	Large bowel ileus

Fluid level development

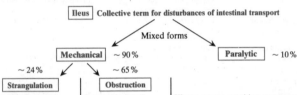

Ileus | Collective term for disturbances of intestinal transport

Mixed forms

Mechanical ~ 90%   **Paralytic** ~ 10%

~ 24%   ~ 65%

Strangulation

Lumen blockage and disturbance of circulation (usually history of operation, scar!), acute dramatic onset, colicky **pains**, typically metallic, tinkling, gurgling bowel sounds, later silence, retention of faeces and flatus, vomiting, shock

Causes: Adhesions, wedging of bowel in mesenteric lacunae, incarcerated hernia, intussusception, volvulus, malrotation

Obstruction

Lumen blockage/compression

Gradual onset, **pains**, increasing retention of stool and flatus, hyperperistalsis, increased bowel sounds

Causes: Adhesions, stenoses, strictures, tumours, atresia, reduplications, Crohn's disease, megacolon, peritoneal carcinomatosis, irradiation damage, foreign bodies (gallstones, bezoars, constipation), ascarides

Hiccup, nausea, vomiting, stoppage of stool and flatus, absent bowel sounds, **'deathly silence'**, succussion splash, meterorism, **pains** usually absent

Causes:
- **Peritoneal irritation**
  Peritonitis, pancreatitis, perforation, haemorrhage, trauma, carcinomatosis
- **Reflex**
  Renal colic, after laparotomy, cholelithiasis, mesenteric vascular thromboses
- **Toxic**
  Sepsis, pneumonia, uraemia, diabetic coma
- **Neurogenic**
  Cerebral (stroke, tumour), vagal excitation, spinal cord affections (injury, tumour, infections), disturbances of neuromuscular transmission (hypokalemia, anticholinergics)

Gastrointestinal bleeding

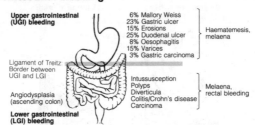

Upper gastrointestinal (UGI) bleeding

6% Mallory Weiss
23% Gastric ulcer
15% Erosions
25% Duodenal ulcer
8% Oesophagitis
15% Varices
3% Gastric carcinoma

} Haematemesis, melaena

Ligament of Treitz: Border between UGI and LGI

Angiodysplasia (ascending colon)

Lower gastrointestinal (LGI) bleeding

Intussusception
Polyps
Diverticula
Colitis/Crohn's disease
Carcinoma

} Melaena, rectal bleeding

Melaena:
Arises when blood remains in the gut for at least 8 h (Check: Tarry stool on finger stall?). Cause 70–80% UGI; <60 ml blood: solitary tarry stool, >60 ml blood: ca. 3 day tarry stool.

Rectal bleeding:
Rectal blood loss (light- or dark-coloured blood) → LGI, but be aware of profuse UGI with rapid intestinal passage, e.g. bleeding duodenal ulcer (p. 157).

Grade I! → with cardiovascular stability: primary exclusion of UGI by gastroduodenoscopy.

Diagnosis of UGI:
90% of all GI bleeds are UGI! → nasogastric intubation (altered blood: 'coffee grounds'?), → digital rectal examination (tarry stool on finger stall?) → oesophagogastroduodenoscopy, later proctosigmoidoscopy, colonoscopy.

Diagnostic sequence of upper GI bleeding

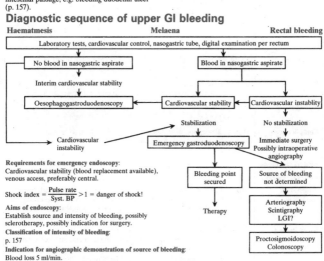

Haematmesis   Melaena   Rectal bleeding

Laboratory tests, cardiovascular control, nasogastric tube, digital examination per rectum

No blood in nasogastric aspirate → Interim cardiovascular stability → Oesophagogastroduodenoscopy

Blood in nasogastric aspirate → Cardiovascular stability / Cardiovascular instablity

Cardiovascular stability → Stabilization → Emergency gastroduodenoscopy

Cardiovascular instability →

Cardiovascular instablity → No stabilization → Immediate surgery Possibly intraoperative angiography

Emergency gastroduodenoscopy → Bleeding point secured → Therapy

Source of bleeding not determined → Arteriography Scintigraphy LGI? → Proctosigmoidoscopy Colonoscopy

Requirements for emergency endoscopy:
Cardiovascular stability (blood replacement available), venous access, preferably central.

$$\text{Shock index} = \frac{\text{Pulse rate}}{\text{Syst. BP}} > 1 = \text{danger of shock!}$$

Aims of endoscopy:
Establish source and intensity of bleeding, possibly sclerotherapy, possibly indication for surgery.

Classification of intensity of bleeding:
p. 157

Indication for angiographic demonstration of source of bleeding:
Blood loss 5 ml/min.

Indication for scintigraphic demonstration of source of bleeding:
Blood loss 0.1 ml/min. Localization of blood loss less specific!

Crohn's disease/ulcerative colitis

	Regional enteritis (Crohn's Disease)	Ulcerative colitis

Localization:

Oesophagus, Stomach, Duodenum 3–5%

Only small bowel 25–30%

Total colitis 15–20%

Small and large bowel 45%

Partial colitis 30–50%

Terminal ileum 80%

Backwash ileitis

Rectum 11–20%

Anorectal disorders (anal fistulae, anal fissures, perianal abscesses) 30–40%

Proctitis 30–50%

	Regional enteritis (Crohn's Disease)	Ulcerative colitis
Onset	Gradual	Gradual, sometimes acute
Symptoms	Diarrhoea, rarely rectal bleeding	Rectal bleeding, blood and mucus in stool
Pain	Tenesmus rarely, cramping colicky pains right lower abdomen	Tenesmus, cramping pains, frequently left lower abdomen
Age of onset	20–40 years (5% > 50 years)	20–40 years (10% > 50 years)
Complications	Abscess, absorption of B_{12} and folic acid ↓, stenoses, perforation, peritonitis	Anal bleeding, toxic megacolon (2–13%)
Risk of carcinoma	?	Substantially increased
Perianal lesions	15–50% fistulae, fissures, abscesses	Rarely
Associated conditions	Iritis, arthritis, cholecystitis, gallstones, pyoderma gangrenosum, erythema nodosum	Iritis, arthritis, primary sclerosing cholangitis, erythema nodosum, ankylosing spondylitis, pyoderma gangrenosum
X-ray findings	Fissures, strictures, especially right-sided, distance phenomenon, wall thickening, cobblestoning, skip lesions; demonstration by small bowel enema	Superficial ulcers, distal, continuous segmental, collar stud ulcers, pseudopolyps, loss of haustrations, hose-pipe appearance

	Regional ileitis (Crohn's disease)	Ulcerative colitis
Endoscopy	Aphthoid lesions, confluent ulcers	Initially only discrete mucosal changes, often rectal involvement, superficial and deep ulcers, pseudopolyps, mucosal bridging; end stage: shortening of the bowel and stenoses
Histology	Granulomata, transmural inflammation	Crypt abscesses
Therapy	Vitamin and mineral supplements	
Mild/moderately severe inflammation	Prednisolone 1st week 60 mg/day orally* 2nd week 40 mg/day orally 3rd week 40 mg/day orally 4th week 30 mg/day orally 5th week 20 mg/day orally 6th week 20 mg/day orally Possibly longer Maintenance dose: 10 mg/day	Left-sided colitis Rectal: mesalazine 1–4 g/day, possibly steroid enemas • Left-sided involvement: topical 1 g mesalazine + oral sulphasalazine 2–4 g/day or mesalazine 3–4 g/day
Severe inflammation	Prednisolone 60–100 mg/day orally; weekly reduction by 5–10 mg	Prednisolone 60–100 mg/day orally*
Refractory to therapy	Bacterial superinfection? Azathioprine 50 mg b.d. (2 mg/kg body weight daily)	Bacterial superinfection? Colectomy, ileoanal pouch
Fistulae	Metronidazole 400 mg t.d.s. (10 mg/kg body weight) (8–10 weeks) or azathioprine 50 mg b.d. (at least 3–4 months, as no effect earlier!)	

* In 2 divided doses.

Classification of degree of severity

Mild attack: ≤ 5 stools/day, little blood, temp. $< 37°C$, little malaise

Moderately severe attack: 5–8 stools/day, mucus and blood, temp. $> 38°C$, definite malaise

Severe attack: > 8 stools/day, bloody, temp. $> 38°C$, pulse rate > 100/min, anaemia, severe malaise

Differential diagnosis: Infective inflammations (*Yersinia enterocolitica*, Shigellae, Salmonellae, Chlamidiae), drug-induced, pseudomembranous colitis (*Clostridium difficile*), ischaemic, post-irradiation colitis, collagenoses

Estimation of severity of the inflammatory changes, examination, laboratory parameters after the classification of

- Best index (*Gastroenterology*, **70**, 439–444 (1976))

  or

- van Hees index (*Gut*, **21**, 269–286 (1980))

Pancreas and pancreatitis

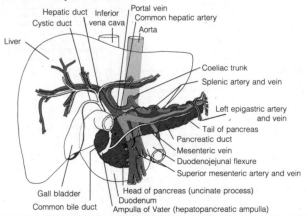

Hepatic duct Inferior Portal vein
Cystic duct vena cava Common hepatic artery
Aorta
Liver

Coeliac trunk
Splenic artery and vein

Left epigastric artery
and vein
Tail of pancreas
Pancreatic duct
Mesenteric vein
Duodenojejunal flexure
Superior mesenteric artery and vein

Gall bladder Head of pancreas (uncinate process)
Common bile duct Duodenum
Ampulla of Vater (hepatopancreatic ampulla)

Clinical:	Acute spontaneous pain in upper abdomen or back.	**Acute pancreatitis**
Morphology:	**Oedematous:** 85%, mortality <1%; interstitial oedema; mild forms recovering spontaneously in 5–7 days in 85–90% of cases. **Necrotizing:** 15%, mortality up to 100%. Severe forms with fat and parenchymal necrosis, haemorrhages, shock, renal failure, encephalopathy, cardiovascular and pulmonary disturbances; skin signs: **Cullen's sign:** periumbilical dusky skin discoloration; **Turner's sign:** blue-red to brownish discoloration of the skin in the flanks. Both signs are an expression of a severe necrotizing pancreatitis. Clinical and morphological severity do not always correlate.	
Basic diagnosis:	**1. Laboratory:** Amylase ↑ in serum and urine, lipase ↑, leucocytes ↑, LDH ↑, electrolytes (calcium ↓, arterial blood gases, pH ↓, pO_2 <8kPa), blood glucose ↑, albumin ↓, serum urea, creatinine. **2. Chest X-ray:** left-sided atelectasis, pleural effusion? **3. Plain X-ray abdomen:** Pancreatic calcification? **4. Ultrasound:** Pancreatic oedema, calcification, pseudocysts, retrocolic or intra-abdominal fluid, ascites, gallstones. **5. CT** with i.v. contrast: necrotizing pancreatitis demonstrable in 100%! **6. ERCP:** Outflow obstruction in common bile or pancreatic ducts?	
Therapy:	**Nil by mouth,** nasogastric tube, i.v. fluids (3–4 l/day), electrolyte replacement, morphine derivatives contraindicated (spasm of papilla!), H_2-blockers, if necessary antibiotics (against aerobes and anaerobes), if necessary early PEEP ventilation (pO_2 <9.5kPa), insulin supplements.	

Clinical:	Recurrent persistent non-colicky girdle pains, in later stages usually painless, weight loss, indigestion, diabetes.	**Chronic pancreatitis**
Diagnosis:	Pancreatic calcification (confirming): CT/abdominal film/ultrasound/ERCP. Pancreatic pseudocysts, steatorrhoea, diabetes mellitus.	
Morphology:	p. 157	
Exocrine disturbances:	Only if >70% of pancreatic tissue is destroyed → abnormal pancreozymin-secretin test, faecal chymotrypsin <3 U/g, abnormal B_{12} absorption in 40%, faecal fat >9.5%.	
Therapy:	In acute attack treat as for acute pancreatitis. Alcohol restriction, enzyme supplements, at least 60 000 FIP units lipase, enzymes at meal times, low-fat diet, if necessary insulin.	

Oesophageal varices haemorrhage

Classification of hepatic cirrhosis
(After Child and Turcotte (1964))

	A	B	C
Serum bilirubin μmol/l (mg/dl)	<40 (<2)	40–50 (2–3)	>50 (>3)
Serum albumin g/l (mg/dl)	>35 (>3.5)	30–35 (3–3.5)	<30 (<3)
Ascites	None present	Easily controllable with drug therapy	Barely controllable with drug therapy
Nutritional state	Very good	Good	Poor, cachexia
Neurological symptoms	None	Minimal	Advanced coma

Staging of oesophageal varices: see endoscopic staging, p. 157.

Treatment of haemorrhagic shock in hepatic cirrhosis

a) General measures

- Central venous access, or at least two peripheral lines of large calibre.

- Fresh blood, not older than 48 hours, ammonia ↑, transfused under pressure, fresh plasma. Note: calcium supplements with citrated blood, ca. 10 ml 10% calcium gluconate/1 l blood.

- Empty stomach, rinse with water at normal temperature, exact balance.

- Vasopressin, 2 mg bolus initially (slowly over 2 min, 1 mg 4–6 times/day i.v.). Attention: cardiovascular side effects!

- Somatostatin 500 μg/hour, effectiveness 0–100%!

- Control: blood count, acid–base status, electrolytes, urea, creatinine (target: Hb 9 g/dl, potassium 4 mmol/l, pH 7.4)

- Emergency endoscopy: aim sclerotherapy, localization of bleeding source

- Emergency endoscopy not possible → see p. 146.

b) Balloon tamponade with Sengstaken–Blakemore tube

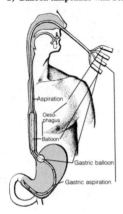

Use the SB tube judiciously as many complications may occur. The procedure is very unpleasant for the patient.

Do not use if patient:
- has severe encephalopathy with no pharyngeal reflex;
- has had recent oesophageal surgery;
- has known oesophageal stricture.

1. Check tube and balloons for patency. Cool in refrigerator. (Makes insertion easier)
2. Turn patient on side, with head tilted slightly down.
3. Insert gag in patient's jaws to keep mouth open throughout procedure.
4. Lubricate cooled tube and insert via mouth or nose. (Nasal ulceration and trauma more common with nasal route.)
5. Insert to at least 60 cm, and check tube is not coiled in pharynx. (Suction on gastric aspiration port should produce large volumes of blood.)
6. Inflate gastric balloon with about 300 ml air. Use e.g. bladder irrigation syringe. Secure with clamp.
7. Withdraw tube until firm resistance is felt (at the oesophagogastric junction).
8. Inflate oesophageal balloon with sphygmomanometer cuff to a pressure of 40 mmHg. Secure with clamp.
9. Secure tube with adhesive plaster to prevent displacement.
10. Check tube and balloon positions with chest X-ray.
11. Monitor pressure in oesophageal balloon hourly. Use low-pressure suction on oesophageal aspiration port to prevent blocking.

Keep tube *in situ* and balloons inflated for maximum 24 h, preferable 12 h. (To avoid oesophageal ulceration.) When bleeding controlled: deflate (first oesophageal balloon, then gastric balloon); keep deflated tube *in situ* without fixation at least for 6–12 h; if bleeding remains controlled, check if balloons are really empty, and then withdraw.

Note: Bleeding may not be arrested in up to 10% of patients.

Complications include oesophageal rupture, aspiration-pneumonia (occurs in 10% of patients), oesophageal ulceration, migration of oesophageal balloon with upper airway obstruction.

Continuous supervision of patient is essential

(After McCormick, Burroughs and McIntyre (1990))

c) Prophylaxis of hepatic coma

Clearance of blood from intestinal tract, alteration of bacterial flora, correct acid–base balance and electrolytes.
- High enema with 750 ml water and 250 ml lactulose
- 20 ml lactulose via gastric tube, at first 2-hourly, up to 150 ml/day, stool pH < 5
- Parenteral nutrition, high-calorie **glucose solution**, potassium supplements, special amino acid infusion, no protein intake. Beware: sedatives and diuretics!

Prophylaxis of recurrent bleeding and indication for surgical intervention

Precondition: endoscopically confirmed variceal haemorrhage.

Therapy
1. **Sclerotherapy**: Obliteration of the varices or regression to Stages I–II.
   Discontinuation of therapy: if no reduction in size of the varices, sclerotherapy ulcers, appearance of fundal varices, mediastinitis.
2. **Portosystemic shunt** (always after medical/surgical consultation), emergency shunt obsolete.
   - Portocaval shunt: patient < 62 years, Child–Turotte class A/B (end-to-side)
   - Distal-splenorenal shunt (Warren)
   - Mesocaval shunt (H-shunt (Drapanas))
3. Perhaps transjugular intrahepatic stent (TIPS), Child–Turotte class C
4. Perhaps liver transplant

Disgnosis of ascites

Standard programme	Portal ascites	Malignant/inflammatory
Colour of ascitic fluid	Clear	Clear/haemorrhagic/chylous
Protein concentration	$<3.0\,$g/dl	$>3.0\,$g/dl
Leucocytes	<200/mm^3	>500/mm^3 (or >200 neutrophil granulocytes/mm^3)
pH	$\geqslant7.45$	<7.35
Cholesterol	$\leqslant48\,$mg%	$>48\,$mg%
Cytology	Negative	Positive (carcinoembryonic antigen, alpha-fetoprotein)
Blood cultures (aerobic/anaerobic)	Negative	Negative/positive

Optional
- Supicion of spontaneous bacterial peritonitis (SBP): >200 neutrophil granulocytes/mm^3, direct slide preparation, centrifuge 250 ml ascitic fluid, sediment in aerobic/anaerobic blood cultures
- Suspicion of TB: glucose quotient serum/ascites >1, Ziehl–Neélsen stain
- Suspicion of pancreatogenic ascites: amylase quotient serum/ascites >1

Treatment of portal ascites

Target: weight reduction of ca. 0.5–1.5 kg/day

Basic therapy
Salt restriction, max. 3 g daily, normalization of albumin concentration, if necessary supplementation with 25% (salt-free!) human albumin; serum sodium $<130\,$mmol/l, additional fluid restriction (e.g. max. 800–1000 ml/day); spontaneous diuresis sodium $<10\,$mmol/l, diuretics (spironolactone 100 mg/day). If no satisfactory weight reduction after 4 days ($<1.5\,$kg), $\rightarrow$ gradual increase of diuretic dose (spironolactone) by 100 mg daily over 3–4 days to max. 400 mg/day, additionally small amounts of a loop diuretic to max. 80 mg/day!

Causes of treatment failure
Sodium intake too high (through drugs dissolved in NaCl, e.g. antibiotics), cause of ascites undetermined, SBP, worsening of liver function, impairment of renal function (e.g. nephrotoxic substances, antibiotics, anti-inflammatory agents).

Paracentesis
Indication, e.g. excessive feeling of distension, dyspnoea. Substitution required: 6–8 g albumin/1 l ascites.

Ascites refractory to treatment
Only $<5\%$ unresponsive to conservative therapy. Palliative measure: peritoneal–venous shunt (Denver/LeVeen shunt).

Treatment of malignant ascites
Paracentesis, Denver shunt as palliative measure. At present still experimental: trial of tumour necrosis factor (TNFα): first paracentesis as complete as possible slowly over 24 h, then instillation of 50 µg TNFα dissolved in 500 ml NaCl into the ascites once a week, repeated up to 3 times, side effect: temp. 38°C.

Portal hypertension

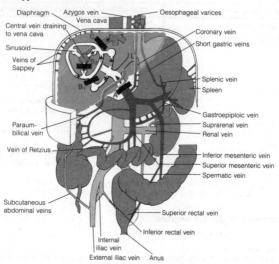

Localization of the obstruction to flow	Frequent	Rarely	Oesophageal varices	Ascites	Splenomegaly
A Prehepatic	Portal vein thrombosis	Arteriovenous fistulae	Marked	Rarely	Marked
B Intrahepatic					
B₁ Presinusoidal	Primary biliary cirrhosis	Schistosomiasis*	Marked	Marked	Rarely
		Sarcoidosis	Marked	Rarely	Marked
		Haemochromatosis	Marked	Rarely	Marked
		Lymphatic system disease	Marked	Marked	Marked
Sinusoidal	Cirrhosis of liver Alcoholic cirrhosis	Nodular hyperplasia	Marked	Marked	Marked
B₂ Postsinusoidal	Alcoholic cirrhosis	Veno-occlusive syndrome	Marked	Marked	Marked
		Budd–Chiari syndrome	Marked	Marked	Marked
C Posthepatic	Right heart failure	Budd–Chiari syndrome	Marked	Very marked	Very marked
	Constrictive pericarditis	Thrombosis of inferior vena cava	Marked	Marked	Marked

* Commonest cause of portal hypertension worldwide.

Jaundice

Differential diagnosis	Prehepatic jaundice, haemolysis, bilirubin transport defect	Intrahepatic jaundice (parenchymatous)	Extrahepatic jaundice (obstructive)
Serum Bilirubin			
• **indirect** (unconjugated)	↑	– (↑)	–
• **direct** (conjugated, glucuronidated)	–	↑ (↑)	↑ (↑)
SGOT	(↑)	↑↑↑	↑/↑↑
SGPT	–	↑↑↑	↑/↑↑
AP	–	(↑)/↑↑	↑↑↑
LAP	–	(↑)/↑↑	↑/↑↑↑
Gamma-GT	–	↑/↑↑	↑↑/↑↑↑
LDH	↑↑/↑↑↑	↑/↑↑	↑
Urine Bilirubin	–	↑	↑
Urobilinogen	↑	↑/↓	↓/–
Urine colour	Light	Dark	Dark
Stool colour	Normal	Normal/pale	Pale (putty coloured)
Pruritus	–	(+)	+
Clinical	Spleen ↑ Signs of anaemia	Liver values ↑ Cirrhosis, skin signs	Colic Tumour, lymphoma Weight ↓
Special serological tests	Reticulocytes ↑ Haptoglobin ↓ Triglycerides ↑ (Zieve's syndrome) Blood film	Hepatitis serology, CMV, EBV, malaria leptospirosis, bacterial causes, antinuclear antibodies, antimitochondrial antibodies, caeruloplasmin	Carcinoembryonic antigen CA 19-9 tumour marker
Ultrasound/CT	Bile passages normal	Bile passages normal	Bile passages dilated Proximal obstruction/PTC Distal obstruction/ERCP
Without haemolysis	Haemoglobinopathy, spherocytosis, thalassaemia, sickle cell anaemia, Gilbert's syndrome*		

*Gilbert's syndrome: 5–7% of population, men four times more frequently, young persons, autosomal dominant. Diagnosis: intermittent jaundice, indirect bilirubin up to 80µmol/l **Starvation test**: 400 cal/day → doubling of bilirubin; **nicotinic acid**: 50mg i.v. → bilirubin ↑; phenobarbitone 60mg t.d.s. → fall in bilirubin; treatment: none, prognosis excellent. PTC, percutaneous transhepatic cholangiography; ERCP, endoscopic retrograde cholangiopancreatography.

Drug induced jaundice

(Biour *et al.* (1987))

Displacement of bilirubin from albumin binding	Directly hepatotoxic
Sulphonamides, ampicillin, salicylate, indomethacin, phenylbutazone, heparin (releases bilirubin by the release of long-chain fatty acids), etc.	Diclofenac, indomethacin, ketoconazole, methotrexate, mexilitine, oestrogens, phenytoin, tolbutamide, etc.

Gallstones

Cause of 80–90% of all colicky abdominal pains, ca. 12% of the population carry gallstones; male:female ratio 1:3; prevalence 30–40% at 70 years of age.

Groups at risk:
Overweight, hyperlipoproteinaemia, infections and inflammations, vagotomy/gastrectomy, disorders of the terminal ileum (resection, Crohn's disease), diabetes mellitus, hepatic cirrhosis, chronic hepatitis, haemolytic anaemia, immunodeficiency syndrome, hyperparathyroidism, pancreatitis, oestrogen/progestogen therapy, clofibrate, cholestyramine.

Pathophysiology: lithogenic index $= \dfrac{\text{Cholesterol}}{\text{Bile salts} + \text{phospholipids}}$

Symptoms: colicky pains, right upper to mid-abdomen, right shoulder, vomiting.

Stone composition:
25% cholesterol stones (>70% cholesterol), 67% cholesterol-pigment-calcium stones, 8% pigment stones.

Diagnosis:
Ultrasound sensitivity above 95%.

Complications of cholelithiasis:
Acute cholecystitis (**Charcot's triad:** colic, jaundice, intermittent fever); **Murphy's sign: pain** on palpation of gall bladder region. Chronic cholecystitis, choledocholithiasis, strangulation of gall bladder, cholangitis, biliary pancreatitis, hydrocele, empyema, gangrene, perforation, gallstone ileus. **Mirizzi syndrome:** obstructive jaundice, stone in neck of gall bladder with compression of hepatic duct, painful gall bladder region.

Incidence of carcinoma:
Increased; 70–100% of malignant gall bladders contain stones, but only 7% of all carcinomas of the gastrointestinal tract are gall bladder carcinomas. (**Courvoisier' sign: painless** enlarged gall bladder – strongly suggestive of carcinoma.)

Treatment:
Asymptomatic (no colic): no interference!
Symptomatic (colic 1–2 times per week): → op. Acute cholelithiasis, biliary pancreatitis → op.; operative mortality for **elective** surgery ca. 1.6%, over 50 years 2.8%.

Requirements for oral litholysis and MTBE treatment:
Gall bladder disease without complications, cholesterol stone up to 1.5 cm (X-ray translucent stone), gall bladder motility preserved, cystic duct patent (ultrasound: gall bladder contraction after test meal or positive cholecystogram).

Litholysis:
Ursodesoxycholic acid (UDCA) 7–10 mg/kg body weight, side effects: 10% stone calcification. Chenodeoxycholic acid (CDCA), side effects: diarrhoea, SGOT ↑, SGPT ↑. Therapy for several months; relapse ↑ after stopping treatment. Success rate ca. 90% stone dissolution after 2 years.

Local lysis with MTBE (methyl-tert-butyl ether): long-term catheter in gall bladder, irrigation 1–3 days, >90% success rate. Side effect: biliary peritonitis.

ESWL (extracorporeal shock wave lithotripsy): requirements as for oral litholysis, stone size up to 2.5 cm, if more than five stones success doubtful, after-treatment with bile acids required, recurrence after 5 years over 50%.

Choledocholithiasis:
Incidence ca. 1.3%; in 20% simultaneous stones in gall bladder and hepatic duct; this coincidence increases with age.

Diagnosis:
Ultrasound: cystic duct >0.7–0.9 cm normal, after cholecystectomy >1.0–1.2 cm; ERCP most reliable method of demonstration. In patient with gastrectomy or duodenal diverticulum → i.v. cholangiography or percutaneous transhepatic cholangiography (PTC).

Treatment:
Endoscopic stone extraction, combined with ESWL, mechanical lithotripsy, local lysis (nasobiliary tube), endoscopic papillotomy (EPT), patient >40 years mortality 1.1%; complications of EPT: haemorrhage, cholangitis, pancreatitis. Complication rate 7.5%.

Complications:
Purulent cholangitis, sepsis, biliary pancreatitis.

Complication rate: 90–95%.

Types of hepatitis

Hepatitis type Synonym	A Infectious 'short incubation hepatitis'	B 'Long incubation hepatitis'	C 'Non-A-non-B' (NANB) post-transfusion hepatitis	D 'Delta' hepatitis, only associated with HBV	E 'Enteral NAND'
Abbreviation	HAV	HBV	HCV	HDV	HEV
Incubation time	15–45 days	90–180 days	6–12 weeks	3–15 weeks	~6 weeks
Virus	RNA virus, picornavirus	Hepadna virus, DNA virus	RNA virus, C virus	Defective RNA virus, Delta virus	E virus, RNA virus
Mode of transmission	Faecal–oral	Parenteral, sexual, perinatal	Parenteral	Parenteral, sexual, perinatal	Faecal–oral
Serology	anti-HAV-IgM anti-HAV-IgG	HBs-Ag/AB HBc-Ag/AB HBe-Ag/AB HBV-DNA HBV-DNA-polymerase	Anti-HCV HCV-RNA	Anti-HDV-IgM HBs-Ag/AB HD-Ag HDV-RNA	Anti-HDV in development
Course	Recovery	HBV carrier	HCV carrier		
Fulminant	0.1–0.2%	1–3%	2%	HBV + HDV >2%	In pregnancy ↑
Chronic state	No	Yes, ~6%	Yes, ~50%	Yes	No

Hepatitis immunization

Hepatitis A: passive immunization with 5 ml gammaglobulin i.m., up to 14 days after presumed exposure; ca. 80% protection for 3 months.

Hepatitis B: passive immunization (anti-B hyperimmune serum) abandoned!

Active-passive (simultaneous) immunization: needle prick injury with HBV positive blood.

'Needle prick hepatitis': confirmed needle prick with HBs-Ag-containing blood → ≤6 hours after exposure anti-B hyperimmune serum 5 ml gluteal and simultaneously one dose active vaccine into upper arm.

Active immunization: (i.m. upper arm)
(Engerix-B, H-B-Vax) immunization at intervals of 4 weeks (2nd dose) and 6 months (3rd dose), anti-HBs assay 1 month after last immunization dose.

Indicaton: Dialysis patients, frequent contact with blood, neonates of HBs-Ag-positive mothers, spouse/contacts of HBs-Ag carriers, homosexuals, prostitutes, drug addicts, prisoners, carers of mentally handicapped.

Booster dose: Dependent on anti-HBs titre: ≤10 mU/l immediate reimmunization; over 10000 mU/ml check titre after 3–6 years.

HBV immunization also protects against simultaneous or superinfection with HDV virus.

Serological course of hepatitis

HAV

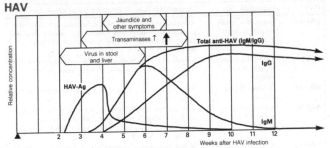

HBV

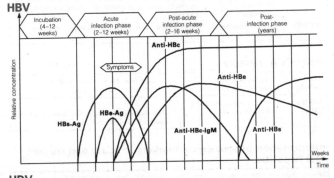

HDV

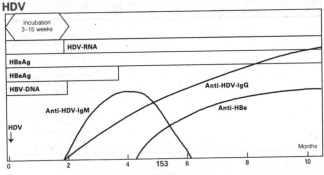

Hepatitis B markers

HBV	Hepatitis B virus	Demonstrable in blood and serum (rarely necessary)
HBs-Ag	Hepatitis B surface antigen (formerly: 'Australia antigen'	Already demonstrable ca. 14 days before clinical symptoms; generally no longer present 6 weeks after onset of illness; if longer than 6 months: chronic hepatitis, carrier often asymptomatic
Anti-HBs	Antibodies against hepatitis B surface antigen	Indicate of reactive immunity; appear relatively late (4–5 months after onset of illness) in convalescent patients
HBc-Ag	Hepatitis B core antigen	Bound to the liver cell (liver biopsy); not demonstrable in blood
Anti-HBc	Antibodies against hepatitis B core antigen	Very sensitive marker for recovered or active hepatitis B; carriers of anti-HBc without anti-HBs are potentially infectious; anti-HBc without HBs-Ag and anti-HBs can indicate fresh hepatitis B
HBe-Ag	Hepatitis B e-antigen e: virus core components	Indicates presence of Dane particles in blood; best indicator for infectiousness; if persistent, sign of chronic active hepatitis
Anti-HBe	Antibodies against hepatitis B e-antigen	When present, patient probabaly no longer infectious

Hepatitis A markers

HAV HAV-Ag	Hepatitis A virus Hepatitis A virus antigen	Already in stool before onset of illness (Determination rarely necessary)
Anti-HAV IgM	Antibodies against HAV Anti-HAV-IgM	Already present at time of first clinical symptoms (jaundice). Sign of acute phase

Interpretation of serological markers in acute and chronic viral hepatitis

HBs-Ag	HBe-Ag	HBV-DNA	Anti-HBc IgM/IgG	Anti-HBs	Anti-HBe	Anti-HAV IgM/IgG	Anti-HD-Ag	Interpretation
+	+	+	−	−	−	−	−	Early phase of acute hepatitis B
+	+	+	+ +	−	−	−	−	Acute hepatitis B, chronic hepatitis B, HBV carrier
+	−	−	+ +	+	−	−	−	Chronic hepatitis B, HBV carrier
−	−	−	+	+	+	−	−	Recent hepatitis B
−	−	−	−	+	−	−	−	Primary immune response without HBV infection. Immune response to HBV vaccination
+	+	+	+ +	−	−	−	+	Acute HBV/HDV co-infection
+	−	−	+ +	+	−	−	+	Chronic HBV infection with HDV superinfection
−	−	−	−	−	−	+ +	−	Acute/recently recovered hepatitis A
−	−	−	−	−	−	+	−	Recovered hepatitis A

Chronic active hepatitis

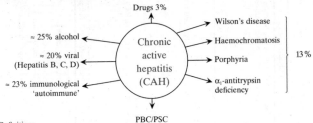

Definition:
persistent transaminases over 6 months; histology: 'piecemeal' necroses.

Specific diagnosis	Treatment
Alcoholic hepatitis SGOT/SGPT >2, gamma-GT ↑, histology 'wire mesh fibrosis' Zieve syndrome: haemolysis, cholesterol ↑, jaundice	Alcohol restriction
Immunological-autoimmune hepatitis 90% women; ANA type (ANA/SMA positive) (anti-nuclear antibody (Ab), smooth muscle Ab) LKM type (Ab against liver and kidney microsomes) SLA type (Ab against liver soluble cytoplasmic antigens)	Initially: 60 mg prednisolone daily (1st week) 40 mg prednisolone/day (2nd week) 30 mg prednisolone/day (3rd and 4th weeks) 25 mg prednisolone/day (5th and 6th weeks) Maintenance dose: 20 mg prednisolone/day Alternative: combination with 50 mg azathioprine/day; initially 30 mg prednisolone/day (2 weeks); maintenance dose 10 mg prednisolone/day, 10 mg azathioprine
Primary biliary cirrhosis (PBC) 90% women, peak >50 years, jaundice, pruritus, anti-M_2 >95% positive (antimitochondrial Ab, subtype M_2), IgM ↑ **Primary sclerosing cholangitis (PSC)** Endoscopic retrograde cholangiography; typical diagnostic appearance, staging	Symptomatic: Cholestyramine 4–16 g/day Mid-chain fatty acid diet, vitamins i.m. (A, D, E, K) once a month. Minimally life-prolonging: azathioprine 50 mg/day; ursodeoxycholic acid 13–15 mg/kg body weight/day; effect on prognosis still unclear; possibly liver transplant
Haemochromatosis idiopathic (IHC) Serum Fe >180 µg%, transferrin saturation >60%, serum ferritin >300 mg/dl, liver tissue Fe 80–1000 µg/100 mg dry weight (note: false high serum ferritin in acute inflammation, HLA-A3, B7, B14 no diagnostic significance)	Venesection, 500 ml 1–2 times a week; 500 ml blood ≡ 200 µg, → therapy at least 2–3 years, then venesection less frequently, but lifelong
Wilson's disease Serum copper <70 µg%, ceruloplasmin <10 mg%, urine copper above 400 µg/24 hours, liver tissue over 250 µg copper/g dry weight Kayser-Fleischer corneal ring	Penicillamine 20–30 mg/kg/day in three doses, $\frac{1}{2}$ hour before food, lifelong therapy. Also during pregnancy. If intolerance, restart, slow introduction of penicillamine, if necessary prednisolone 20 mg/day for 2 weeks in addition

Liver transplantation

1. Indications

Benign liver conditions	Malignant liver conditions	Metabolic disorders of hepatic origin
Posthepatitic cirrhosis Primary/secondary biliary cirrhosis Primary/secondary sclerosing cholangitis Alcoholic cirrhosis (positive compliance for at least 6 months), Budd–Chiari syndrome, cirrhosis in hepatitis B and C	Hepatic cell carcinoma (HCC), not resectable. HCC in cirrhosis, cholangiocellular carcinoma, secondary liver tumours (colorectal carcinoma, melanoma, teratoma)	Wilson's disease, α_1-antitrypsin deficiency, haemochromatosis, Crigler–Najjar syndrome

2. Contraindications. cf. also p. 173

(a) Absolute: florid sepsis, AIDS, advanced cardiopulmonary conditions, metastasizing conditions
(b) Relative: age > 55 years, portal vein thrombosis, condition after portocaval shunt, drug and alcohol abuse, advanced renal disease, hepatitis B virus complications

3. Preconditions

(a) Age 5–55 years
(b) Confirmed diagnosis of the liver condition (histology, viral serology, Child criteria)
(c) Exclusion of serious secondary disorder (heart, lung, kidney function, diabetes mellitus, infections)
(d) Demonstration of the liver vasculature (angiography, Doppler ultrasound), demonstration of the biliary passages (ERC)
(e) Exclusion of distant metastases in malignant liver tumours

Indication categories for liver transplantation in cirrhosis
(After Pichlmayer (1987))

Indication category	General condition	Liver function	Other organ systems	Independent risk factors
I Elective	Good/satisfactory Ambulant	Adequate without substitution	No serious complications	Age Previous surgery
II Complicated ('late')	Diminished/poor Mainly hospitalized	Marked and progressive intermittent deterioration	Marked repeated complications	Infective status (Duration of illness)
III Emergency	Poor Requirement for intensive care	Failure of function	Severe, untreatable complications	Accompanying illness

Endoscopic staging of abdominal disorders

Reflux oesophagitis

Ia	Mucosal erythema, solitary, multiple 'red patches'
Ib	Mucosal lesions with fibrin deposits
IIa	Longitudinal or confluent streaky lesions
IIb	Longitudinal or confluent streaky lesions with fibrin deposits
III	Entire oesophageal circumference involved, no ulceration
IV	Ulceration, scarred stenoses, bleeding

(After Spech *et al.* (1982))

Oesophageal varices

I	Straight, pink-blue veins within level of the mucosa, $\varnothing < 2\,mm$
II	More tortuous blue venous dilatations, nodular calibre variations, projecting into the lumen, $\varnothing \leqslant 2$–$3\,mm$
III	Knotted convoluted blue varices, lumen constricted to one-half, $\varnothing \leqslant 3$–$4\,mm$
IV	Grape-like livid vascular convolutions reaching to the centre of the oesophagus, with circumscribed blue-red fine telangiectases on their surface, 'varices on varices'

Gastric bleeding activity

Ia	Arterial, 'spurting' bleeding
Ib	Oozing
II	Bleeding ceased, haematin or clot on lesion, visible vessel stump
III	Lesion without above criteria

(After Forrest (1974))

Carcinoma of stomach

'Early cancer'	Infiltrating mucosa and submucosa only
'Advanced cancer'	Submucosa penetrated, polypoid, no ulceration
Linitis plastica	Diffuse infiltrating

Chronic pancreatitis

		Normal
I		Calibre variations of side arms of pancreatic duct
II		Additionally, calibre variations of main duct
III		Marked calibre variations of pancreatic duct, cystic dilatations of side arms, duct calculi, calcification of parenchyma, pseudocysts

(After Anacker and Löffler (1989))

Gastrointestinal tumours

Early gastric carcinoma

(confined to mucosa and
submucosa)
Classification according to the
Japanese Society for
Gastroenterological Endoscopy
(1962)

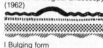

I Bulging form

II Superficial forms

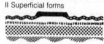

IIa Elevated

IIb Level

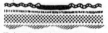

IIc Depressed

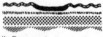

III Excavated form

Mucosa
Submucosa
Muscular layer
Serosa

Advanced gastric carcinoma

Macroscopic classification after Borrmann (1926)

I Circumscribed solitary,
polyploid carcinoma
without significant ulceration

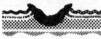

II Ulcerated carcinoma
with rampart-like edges
and sharp borders

III Ulcerated carcinoma,
which in contrast to type II
is only partly or not at all
sharply demarcated from
its surroundings. The tumour is spreading by diffuse
infiltration

IV Diffusely infiltrating
carcinoma, which often
progresses without mucosal lesions

Colorectal carcinoma Staging after Dukes (1935)

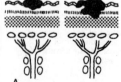

A
Tumour confined to bowel wall
(movable)

B
Tumour penetrates
bowel wall, (not
movable), lymph
nodes clear

CI
Lymph nodes
involved

CII
Metastases,
liver, lung, bones

O Tumour-free lymph nodes
● Metastases in lymph nodes

Function tests

Function test	Disorder
D-xylose absorption test: 25 g xylose orally, excretion of <3 g in 5 h abnormal	Malabsorption in proximal jejunum
Lactose tolerance test: 50 g lactose orally, rise in blood glucose <20 mg% (<11 mmol/l) after 30 min abnormal	Lactase deficiency
H₂-exhalation test: 50 g lactose orally, after 2 h H₂ exhalation (>20 ppm)	Lactase deficiency, intestinal hurry, altered small bowel bacterial flora, e.g. in Billroth-II gastrectomy
Schilling test: 1 µg cyanocobalamin (^{57}Co) orally, excretion of <7% in 24-hour urine. Note: intrinsic factor deficiency in megaloblastic anaemia	Disturbed B_{12} absorption in terminal ileum
Iodine-125-polyvinylpyrollidine: Iodine-125-PVP i.v., 4-day stool collection, radioactivity above 1.8% of the total activity pathological	Exudative enteropathy
α₁-antitrypsin clearance: <3 mg/g stool	Exudative enteropathy
Chymotrypsin: Screening test in stool, pancreas enzymes 5 days or discontinue	Exocrine pancreatic insufficiency after Billroth-II operation and diarrhoea
Secretin test: Fractionated duodenal juice analysis after secretin stimulation	Exocrine pancreatic insufficiency

Ulcer Therapy

a) **Conservative Treatment**
Avoidance of provocative factors (NSAIDs, glucocorticoids, salicylates, smoking, etc.). H₂-receptor antagonists: cimetidine, ranitidine, famotidine, nizatidine; administration at night. H⁺/K⁺-ATPase blocker: omeprazole. Antacids. Mucosa protection: sucralfate; prostaglandins – misoprostol as prophylaxis during NSAID administration.

b) **Surgical Treatment**
Gastric ulcer: Two-thirds gastrectomy – Billroth-I (gastroduodenostomy).
Duodenal ulcer: Selective proximal vagotomy (SPV). Combined gastric and duodenal ulcers: SPV with pyloroplasty, possibly two-thirds gastrectomy.
Indication for surgery: ulcer refractory to medical treatment, arterial bleeding, perforation, pyloric stenosis.

Chronic gastritis

Type A: 'Body gastritis', autoimmune, autoantibodies in 90% against parietal cells, 50% against intrinsic factor. Achlorhydria, B_{12} deficiency, pernicious anaemia.
Type B: 'Antrum gastritis', bacterial, associated with *Helicobacter pylori* (Gram-negative bacterium).
Type C: 'Fundus gastritis', chemical, drug induced.

Renal anatomy

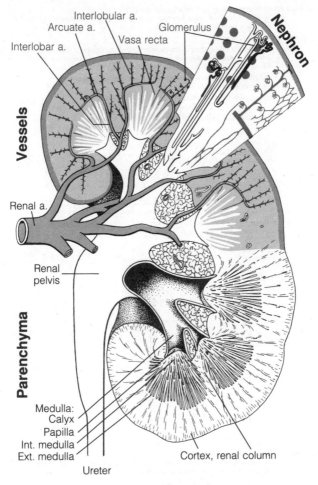

Interlobular a.
Arcuate a.
Vasa recta
Interlobar a.
Glomerulus
Nephron

Vessels

Renal a.

Renal pelvis

Parenchyma

Medulla:
Calyx
Papilla
Int. medulla
Ext. medulla
Ureter

Cortex, renal column

Nephrological formulae

Inulin (and PAH) clearance/body surface area (ml/min/m²)

'gold standard' of renal function tests, but is too inconvenient for practical purposes, therefore:

Endogenous creatinine clearance

gives higher values than inulin clearance, since creatinine is also excreted by the tubules; in practice relatively uncomplicated. Beware of collection error! Check for correct collection (i.e. collection time):

Measurement of total creatinine excretion in urine collection.
Dependent on muscle mass.

Standard values: Male: 150–200 μmol/kg/day
                 Female: 100–150 μmol/kg/day

Measured value/calculated value = 1: correct collection
                                           <1: collection too short
                                           >1: collection too long

For practical purposes and with constant renal function:

Creatinine clearance

Normal value: 90–125 ml/min

Calculation:
$$\frac{(150 - age) \times body\ weight\ (kg)}{plasma\ creatinine\ (\mu mol/l)} \qquad \text{Men: } +10\% \quad \text{Women: } -10\%$$

or
$$\frac{Urine\ volume\ (ml) \times Urine\ creatinine\ (\mu mol/l)}{Plasma\ creatinine\ (\mu mol/l) \times time\ (min)}$$

Times: 24 h = 1440 min, 12 h = 720 min, 8 h = 480 min, 6 h = 360 min, 4 h = 240 min

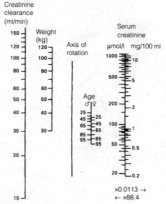

Application: 1. Connect age and weight.
                2. Rotate ruler around crossing point on axis of rotation to lie on serum creatinine value.
                3. Read off the creatinine clearance on left scale.

Urine normal values

Dip stick chemical test and examination of sediment – preferably to be performed immediately (max. 1 h) after sample is voided. HPF = high-power field

Determination	Normal values	Determination	Normal values
Dip stick test (semiquantitative)		**Quantitative estimations** (in 24 h)	
pH	4.5–8	Volume	Variable (according to fluid and NaCl intake)
Albumen	–		
Glucose	–	Specific gravity	1003–1030
Ketones	– (positive if fasting)	Osmolality	350–1400 mosmol/l
Urobilinogen	–	Residual urine	A few ml (if more than 100–150 ml needs urological investigation)
Bilirubin	–		
Blood	–		
Hb from erythrocytes	–		
Sediment examination		Sodium	100–250 mmol
Casts: hyaline	Normal (not significant)	Potassium	25–100 mmol
granular	–	Chloride	135 mmol
waxy	–	Calcium	Less than 3.8 mmol
red cell	–	Phosphate	30 mmol
white cell	–	Creatinine	9–15 mmol
epithelial	–	Creatinine clearance	90–125 ml/min
Leucocytes	Men 0–2/HPF; women 0–5/HPF	Amylase	25–75 U/ml
Erythrocytes	0–5/HPF (glomerular forms)	Albumen	Less than 0.15 g/24 h
Epithelial cells	Usually present in women	Glucose	0.3–1.7 mmol/24 h
Fat droplets	–		
Bacteria	As contaminants		

Erythropoietin

Polypeptide (normal blood level 10–20 mU/ml). Barely measurable in dialysis patients. Production probably in peritubular adventitial cells (90%); 10% extrarenal (lung).

Definition of renal anaemia:

Normocytic, normochromic anaemia with normal maturation and morphology of erythrocytes, but reduction of the erythrocyte survival time by 50%.
Reticulocyte count normal to low. Platelet count normal to low.
White cell count normal. Normal bone marrow morphology with normal iron content.
The cause of the anaemia is multifactorial, but erythropoietin is significantly involved, since erythropoietin therapy corrects the anaemia.

Use of erythropoietin:

i.v. or s.c. (practically identical action), intraperitoneal possible, but expensive.
Individual dosage very variable (mean value: 75 U/kg (25–500) per week), divided into three doses, building up initially. Maintenance dose with haematocrit about 30%.

Positive aspects of erythropoietin therapy, primarily subjective:

Intensified feeling of wellbeing, increased effort tolerance, improved appetite with weight gain (observe for hyperkalaemia), less depression, improved sexual function, less dyspnoea and better sleep.

Negative aspects as a result of improved haemoglobin:

Increased heparin consumption in dialysis, more frequent shunt thromboses, repeated use of dialysers restricted, hyperkalaemia/hyperphosphataemia.

Disadvantages:

Arterial hypertension (20–30% of treated patients), hypertensive crises (infrequent), arthralgia, bone pain, local urticaria, pruritus.

Summary of renal syndromes

Syndrome	Symptoms indicative of diagnosis	Further clinical findings	Urinary findings
Acute renal failure (cf. p. 165)	Oliguria to anuria, creatinine rising daily, weight ↑	Worsening of general condition, hypertension, oedema, uraemic symptoms	Haematuria, pyuria, proteinuria
Chronic renal failure (cf. p. 167)	Azotaemia >3 months, signs of uraemia, small kidneys (typically)	Polydipsia, polyuria, nocturia, hypertension, oedema, uraemic symptoms	Haematuria, proteinuria, broad casts, leucocyturia, isosthenuria
Acute nephritis	Haematuria, azotaemia, oliguria, oedema, pain	Hypertension	Haematuria, red cell casts, proteinuria, pyuria
Nephrotic syndrome	Proteinuria above 3.5 g/day, serum albumin <30 g/l. hyperlipidaemia, oedema	Nocturia	Lipiduria, oval fat globules, hyaline casts, haematuria
Tubular syndromes	Electrolyte and acid–base disturbances, large kidneys	Nocturia, polyuria	Tubular proteinuria, urine pH >7, glycosuria, aminoaciduria, uricosuria, phosphaturia
Calculi (cf. p. 168)	History of stones, colic, haematuria	Passage of stones, recurrent urinary infections	Haematuria, pyuria
Obstruction	Oliguria to anuria, retention of urine, azotaemia. Note: one or two kidneys	Dysuria, nocturia, enlarged prostate, dilated renal pelvis	Haematuria, pyuria
Urinary tract infection, pyelonephritis, urosepsis (cf. p. 170)	Bacteriuria, bacteraemia, pyuria, renal pain, pain in bladder	Dysuria, frequency, fever	Haematuria, leucocyturia, white cell casts

Differential diagnosis of acute renal failure

1. Prerenal	(Cause prior to the kidney) Hypoperfusion in (still) intact kidney Blood loss, gastrointestinal losses, renal losses (diuretics, osmotic diuresis in diabetes), sequestration (burns, decompensated cirrhosis of liver), antihypertensive therapy (reduction of filtration pressure), heart failure (arrhythmia or heart muscle failure), vascular pooling (anaphylaxis)
2. Renal	(Causes in the kidney) Tubular necrosis (all prerenal causes which are not corrected immediately), drug induced (cephalosporins, aminoglycosides, amphotericin B), contrast media, heavy metals and organic solvents, poisoning (paraquat), tetanus, haemolysis and rhabdomyolysis. Acute interstitial nephritis (penicillin and derivatives, cephalosporins, rifampicin, cotrimoxazole, tetracyclins, diuretics rarely, salicylates, NSAIDs and others), with infections Acute glomerulonephritis Acute renal failure in collagenoses Malignant nephrosclerosis Bilateral diffuse pyelonephritis Hypercalcaemia Hepatorenal syndrome in literal sense (but mostly prerenal) Pregnancy (abortion, toxaemia, premature separation of placenta, and placenta praevia, haemolytic-uraemic syndrome after pregnancy) Multiple myeloma Vascular obstruction
3. Postrenal	(Causes in disturbed drainage) Prostatic hypertrophy, carcinoma of prostate or bladder, retroperitoneal and pelvic floor lesions, urethral stricture/stenosis, unilalateral renal lesions with nonfunctioning or absent contralateral kidney: ureteric calculus, papillary necrosis

Urine findings in acute renal failure

	Urine volume	Urine osmolality	Urine sodium	Ratios		
				Urine/plasma creatinine	Urine/plasma urea	Urea/creatinine in plasma
Normal values	750–1500 ml/d	350 mosmol/l	15–40 mmol/l	~80	20	10
Prerenal	Oliguria	>500	<20	>40	>8	>10
Renal	Oliguria	<400	>40	<20	<2	~10
Postrenal	Oliguria/anuria	<400	>40		<8	~10

Subjective symptoms dependent on renal failure

Urine quantity	Symptoms
130–50 ml/min	None
50–20 ml/min	Headache (hypertension) Reduction of effort tolerance and rapid fatigue (anaemia)
20–10 ml/min	Nausea, vomiting, depression, pruritus
10–0 ml/min	**Dyspnoea** (pulmonary oedema and acidosis) **Haemorrhage** (nasopharynx, gastrointestinal tract, skin) **Neurological symptoms** (neuropathy, disturbance of consciousness to coma)

Management of renal failure

Independent of the cause:

Assessment of the potentially lethal complications of acute renal failure, i.e. hypervolaemia, disturbance of consciousness, hyperkalaemia, metabolic acidosis, pericarditis.

On this basis decision as to acute dialysis.

Initial measures	1. Rapid exclusion of pre- and postrenal causes (ultrasound) 2. Therapy: frusemide i.v., mannitol i.v. 3. Further search for aetiology
Clinical	Daily weighing, fluid balance, assessment of state of hydration, assessment of state of consciousness, investigation for pericarditis and pulmonary oedema, examination of ocular fundus, care of forearm veins, assessment of neuropathy and osteodystrophy[a], psychological and family assessment as well as assessment of place of work, possibly coronary artery assessment
Laboratory	Plasma: Electrolytes, renal parameters, osmolality, albumin, blood gases, amylase[a], lipid status[a] Urine: Urine status, urinary bacteriology, osmolality, 24-hour urine for: creatinine clearance, electrolyte/protein/uric acid excretion Haematology: White and red cells, platelets, coagulation state, bleeding time X-ray: Abdominal ultrasound, chest X-ray Others: ECG, hepatitis and HIV serology[a], CT scan, isotope renogram
Nutrition	Salt and fluid restriction (general rule: daily excretion + 500 ml, except with polyuria), protein: untreated renal failure (0.7–1.0 g/kg/day) <haemodialysis <CAPD
Principles of therapy	Adjust dose of drugs to current renal function (cf. pp. 294–326), correction of hyperkalaemia, treatment of hypertension, correction of acidosis, loop diuretics, phosphate binders, ulcer prophylaxis, control of anaemia[a], treatment of osteodystrophy[a], hepatitis vaccination[a]
Renal support measures	Absolute indications: cf. above Insert shunt[a], peritoneal catheter[a], tissue typing for possible transplantation[a]

[a] Additional investigations in chronic, terminal renal failure.

Uraemia

Main causes:
Chronic glomerulonephritis
Chronic interstitial nephritis (analgesics)
Polycystic kidneys
Diabetic nephropathy
Chronic pyelonephritis
Hypertensive nephropathy

1. Cardiovascular
Circulatory instability,
arterial hypertension,
heart failure,
cardiomyopathy,
pericarditis,
accelerated arteriosclerosis,
uraemic pulmonary oedema

2. Gastrointestinal
Anorexia, nausea, vomiting,
gastroenteritis,
ulcers and bleeding,
uraemic fetor,
hepatitis

3. Electrolyte and water balance
Metabolic acidosis,
variability of sodium, potassium,
phosphate, calcium,
magnesium concentrations,
volume instability

4. Locomotor system
Renal osteodystrophy,
secondary hyperparathyroidism,
growth disturbance,
myoclonus,
motor weakness,
muscular irritability

5. Metabolic
Carbohydrate intolerance,
protein deficiency,
hyperlipidaemia,
hyperuricaemia

6. Endocrine
Infertility,
sexual dysfunction,
amenorrhoea,
thyroid dysfunction,
hypothermia

7. Neurological
Central
Sleep disturbance,
headache,
memory disturbance,
lethargy,
flapping tremor,
hypertensive encephalopathy,
subdural haematoma,
epileptiform convulsions,
dysequilibrium syndrome,
dialysis dementia,
uraemic coma
Peripheral
Neuropathy (peripheral and autonomic),
restless legs

8. Psychological
Depression,
anxiety,
denial,
psychotic reactions

9. Haematological
Normochromic normocytic anaemia,
$\uparrow$ ferritin, $\downarrow$ erythropoietin,
haemolysis,
haemorrhagic diathesis,
splenomegaly, hypersplenism,
$\uparrow$ tendency to infection,
$\downarrow$ complement factors,
$\uparrow$ fibrinogen

10. Dermatological
Pallor,
hyperpigmentation,
pruritus,
ecchymoses

11. Ophthalmic
Retinopathy,
keratopathy,
'red eye' syndrome

Nephrolithiasis

Diagnosis by means of ultrasound or IVU during acute attack (of little value after colic).

Primary treatment with spasmolytics and NSAIDs.

Early relief of obstruction because of recurrent colic and threatening infection with persistent obstruction.

Possibilities: Spontaneous passage after conservative treatment with volume loading and spasmolytics
Removal with ureteric snare at cystoscopy
Percutaneous lumbar lithopexy
Extracorporeal shock wave lithotripsy (ESWL)
Open operation

Chemical analysis of the calculus recommended in every case (with view to recurrence).

Frequency: 30% of the population will have a calculus once during their lifetime.
With recurrence appropriate laboratory investigations according to stone analysis.

Prophylaxis: High fluid intake; possibly long-term treatment with thiazide diuretics for hypercalciuria and recurrent stone formation.

Frequency of urinary stone composition:
Calcium oxalate 75–85%
Uric acid 5–10%
Non-metabolic (infective) 10%
Cystine stone: rarity

Proteinuria

| **Renal parenchymatous** |
| Glomerulonephritis[a], interstitial nephritis[a], tubular disorders, polycystic kidneys, glomerulosclerosis (diabetic, hypertensive) |

| **Renovascular** |
| Renal vein thrombosis[a] |

| **Extrarenal** |
| Orthostatic, pronounced lumbar lordosis, infective |

| **Systemic illnesses** |
| Systemic lupus erythematosus[a], multiple myeloma, Waldenström's macroglobulinaemia, amyloidosis, benign monoclonal gammopathy |

[a] With haematuria.

Haematuria

| **Renal parenchymatous** |
| Glomerulonephritis[b], pyelonephritis[b], tuberculosis, renal cell carcinoma, carcinoma of renal pelvis, polycystic kidneys, trauma (including heavy physical exertion) |

| **Renovascular** |
| Renal vein thrombosis[b], renal infarct, renal cortical necrosis |

| **Urinary outflow tract and prostate** |
| Urogenital tuberculosis, cystitis (bilharzia), urethritis, carcinoma of bladder and prostate, trauma (including instrumentations), calculi |

| **Systemic illnesses** |
| Systemic lupus erythematosus[b], vasculitis, thrombo- and coagulopathies, polycythaemia |

| **Others** |
| Anticoagulant bleeding, benign familial haematuria |

[b] With proteinuria.

Red urine
(Modified after Sandoz (1988))

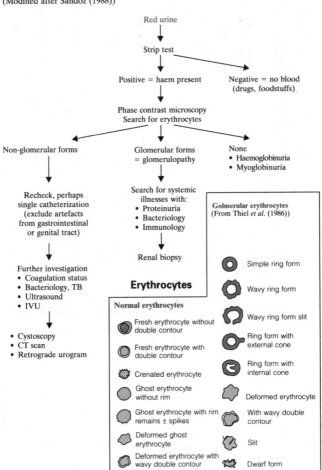

Red urine

↓

Strip test

Positive = haem present → Negative = no blood (drugs, foodstuffs)

↓

Phase contrast microscopy
Search for erythrocytes

Non-glomerular forms — Glomerular forms = glomerulopathy — None
- Haemoglobinuria
- Myoglobinuria

Recheck, perhaps single catheterization (exclude artefacts from gastrointestinal or genital tract)

↓

Further investigation
- Coagulation status
- Bacteriology, TB
- Ultrasound
- IVU

↓

- Cystoscopy
- CT scan
- Retrograde urogram

Search for systemic illnesses with:
- Proteinuria
- Bacteriology
- Immunology

↓

Renal biopsy

Golmerular erythrocytes
(From Thiel *et al.* (1986))

- Simple ring form
- Wavy ring form
- Wavy ring form slit
- Ring form with external cone
- Ring form with internal cone
- Deformed erythrocyte
- With wavy double contour
- Slit
- Dwarf form

Erythrocytes

Normal erythrocytes

- Fresh erythrocyte without double contour
- Fresh erythrocyte with double contour
- Crenated erythrocyte
- Ghost erythrocyte without rim
- Ghost erythrocyte with rim remains ± spikes
- Deformed ghost erythrocyte
- Deformed erythrocyte with wavy double contour

Urinary tract infection

Complaint (dysuria)	Leucocyturia	Bacteria (fungi)	Procedure
+	+	+	**Male:** Bacteriology and treatment, then investigation (ultrasound, IVU, urethrography, cystoscopy) **Female:** For first event: bacteriology and treatment Interpretation of culture: < 10^5 organisms/ml, mixed growth: contamination > 10^5 organisms/ml, pure growth: infective focus in urinary tract For recurrence: possibly comparison of simultaneous mid-stream urine (MSU) and bladder puncture for differentiation: genuine UTI v. genital infection
+	+	–	**Male:** Search for tuberculosis **Female:** Investigation UTI rather unlikely (vaginal discharge, colpitis!)
+	–	+	*** Male:** Balanitis, urethral problem **Female:** Probable genital infection, UTI rather unlikely
+	–	–	No UTI (look for other cause)
–	+	+	**Male:** Repeat urine examination If positive: repeat investigation as above **Female:** Compare MSU and bladder puncture With genuine UTI treat as such (renal parenchymatous illness, look for analgesic nephropathy) Chronic pyelonephritis, polycystic kidneys Otherwise gynaecological investigations
–	–	+	**Male:** Repeat urine examination, if positive No UTI (contamination) **Female:** Trial of treatment according to bacteriology (asymptomatic bacteriuria of older women)
–	+	–	**Male:** Repeat urine examination, if positive, exclude TB Idiopathic leucocyturia of the younger man Chronic prostatitis **Female:** Look for genital cause

Diuretics

Carbonic anhydrase inhibitors / Thiazides / Loop diuretics / Potassium-sparing diuretics / Cortex / Medulla — Site of action of diuretics within the nephron.

Preparation	Site of action	Ion excretion in urine					Plasma parameters			
		Na+/H2O	K+	Cl-	Ca2+	Mg2+	pH change	Uric acid	Blood glucose	
All diuretics		↑						↑	↑	Lead to dehydration, prerenal failure. Disturb Na^+, K^+, Cl^-, Mg^{2+}, Ca^{2+} balance. Interfere with acid–base balance. Can lead to hyperuricaemia and hyperglycaemia
Mannitol	Proximal tubule	↑	(↑)				−			Volume overloading (danger of pulmonary oedema)
Acetazolamide		↑	↑	(↑)	↑	↑	↓			Carbonic anhydrase inhibitor, ↑ HCO_3^- excretion (leads to metabolic acidosis). Watch for hepatic insufficiency
Frusemide Ethacrynic acid	Ascending limb of loop of Henle	↑↑↑	↑↑	↑	↑	↑	↑	↑		Loop diuretics, hypokalaemia, metabolic alkalosis, ototoxic. Watch out for hepatic insufficiency
Thiazide	Beginning of distal tubule	↑↑	↑	↑	−	↑	↑	↑	↑	Hypokalaemia, metabolic (hypochloraemic) alkalosis, potentiation of frusemide activity. Watch out for hepatic insufficiency
Metolazone		↑↑	↑	(↑)	−	−	↑	↑	(↑)	
Spironolactone	End of distal tubule	↑	↓	(↑)	−	−	↑			Potassium sparer, aldosterone antagonist, gynaecomastia, permissible in hepatic insufficiency
Amiloride		↑	↓	(↑)	−	↑	↓			Potassium sparer

Dialysis

Drug therapy for dialysis patients (haemodialysis and peritoneal dialysis)

Use of substances which are mainly (50–100%) eliminated by the liver, and control of dose by blood level determinations.
Dose of substances mainly (50–100%) eliminated through the kidneys: normal initial dose.
> Haemodialysis: half the daily dose immediately after dialysis.
> Peritoneal dialysis: half the usual daily dose.

Haemodialysis-associated problems

Acute: Exclusively iatrogenic.
Cardiovascular disturbances: volume depletion following inaccurate estimation of the ideal weight.
Too rapid volume reduction in extracellular space expansion. Bleeding due to anticoagulants. Incorrect or displaced position of the dialysis catheter. Drug-induced lowering of blood pressure during dialysis. Haemodynamically relevant rhythm disturbances with volume reduction or rapid changes of potassium.

Chronic: Aluminium-induced neuropathy and microcytic hypochromic anaemia, β_2-microglobulin-induced amyloidosis. Silicone deposition in practically all organs due to roller pump when using silicone-containing equipment.

Emergency measures with severe complications:
Discontinue dialysis and examination of blood and dialysate.

Peritoneal dialysis-associated problems

Acute: Peritonitis (turbid dialysate first and often only sign).

Chronic: Reduction of dialysing ability due to recurrent infective, chemical or allergic peritonitis.

Emergency measures:
Estimation of dialysate cell count at above 1000 (normal <100/ml).
Bacteriological examination including fungi. Contact the attending centre.

Treatment suggestions for peritonitis: rapid irrigation with 3 times 2 l (1.26% glucose). Inoculate 4th bag with cephalosporin (e.g. cephazolin 1 g) and aminoglycoside (e.g. tobramycin 80 mg). Continue the dialysis. Subsequent bags inoculated with cephazolin 200 mg and tobramycin 16 mg until bacteriological resistance is found (mostly staphylococci). Continue with cephalosporin or aminoglycoside in the same dose according to resistance until cell count <100/ml; after this only inoculate night bag. Treatment duration 10–14 days. With fungal infections removal of the catheter is usually required: temporary change to haemodialysis or trial of amphotericin B or ketoconazole, but never with flucytosine alone because of rapid development of resistance.

Inadequate outflow of the dialysate with good inflow and rapid weight gain:

Valve mechanism at the catheter tip

Measures: try a position change (standing or prone); enema (often satisfactory dialysis outflow after bowel emptying); removal of a possible fibrin clot with urokinase, 10 000 units in 5 ml and 1000 units heparin to fill the catheter overnight. If unsuccessful: plain abdominal X-ray, check of catheter position (normal: tip should lie at pelvic inlet). If there is displacement, attempt replacement with guide by an experienced operator. If unsuccessful: surgical change of catheter (temporary haemodialysis).

Perforation: persistent peritonitis with usually a mixture of organisms, without severe symptoms.

Ileus with adhesions, bowel volvulus (clinical picture of acute abdomen).

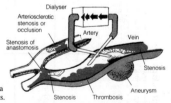

Causes of a Cimino shunt dysfunction. (After Schinz)

Organ donation

A code of practice concerning cadaveric organs for transplantation, including the diagnosis of brain death, has been drawn up by a working party on behalf of the Health Departments of Great Britain and Northern Ireland (Health Departments of Great Britain and Northern Ireland (1983)). This publication, from which the recommendations below have been taken, should be consulted.

Conditions under which the diagnosis of brain death should be considered:
1. The patient is deeply comatose.
   (a) There should be no suspicion that this state is due to depressant drugs.
   (b) Primary hypothermia as a cause of coma should have been excluded.
   (c) Metabolic and endocrine disturbances which can be responsible or can contribute to coma should have been excluded.
2. The patient is being maintained on a ventilator because spontaneous respiration had previously become inadequate or had ceased altogether.
   (a) Relaxants (neuromuscular blocking agents) and other drugs should have been excluded as a cause of respiratory inadequacy or failure.
3. There should be no doubt that the patient's condition is due to irremediable structural brain damage. The diagnosis of a disorder which can lead to brain death should have been fully established.

Diagnostic tests for the confirmation of brain death
All brainstem reflexes are absent:

(i) The pupils are fixed in diameter and do not respond to sharp changes in the intensity of incident light.
(ii) There is no corneal reflex.
(iii) The vestibulo-ocular reflexes are absent.
(iv) No motor responses within the cranial nerve distribution can be elicited by adequate stimulation of any somatic area.
(v) There is no gag reflex or reflex response to bronchial stimulation by a suction catheter passed down the trachea.
(vi) No respiratory movements occur when the patient is disconnected from the mechanical ventilator for long enough to ensure that the arterial carbon dioxide tension rises above the threshold for stimulation of respiration.

The diagnosis of brain death is to be made on the above criteria by two independent doctors, one a consultant, preferably the one in charge of the case, and the other a consultant or senior registrar clinically independent of the first. Diagnosis should not normally be considered until at least 6 hours after the onset of coma, or, if cardiac arrest was the cause of coma, until 24 hours after the circulation has been restored. The tests should be repeated after an interval adequate for reassurance of all directly concerned.

Once the diagnosis of brain death has been made, certain further criteria must be established to determine whether the patient is suitable as an organ donor.

Criteria   General
- Complete history (including HIV risk)
- State of health before acute cerebral event
- Laboratory: blood group, blood count, prothrombin time, plasma creatinine, liver function tests, blood sugar
- Blood gas analysis, serology (HIV, hepatitis, CMV, tissue typing)
Special
- Heart: ECG, echocardiogram, size and weight, no resuscitation
- Liver: prothrombin time, routine liver function tests, size and weight
- Kidneys: proteinuria (strip test)
- Pancreas: no special features
- Lungs: chest X-ray, normal blood gases, no resuscitation

Exclusion criteria for organ removal
Absolute:
- Wasting diseases (malignancy, except primary brain tumour – arguable)
- Insulin-dependent diabetes mellitus
- Positive HIV test or hepatitis B antigen
Relative:
- Arterial hypertension
- Bacterial infection
- Age

Renal transplantation

Renal transplantation is the treatment of choice for terminal renal failure. It requires the collaboration of all medical disciplines.

The measure of success of renal transplantation is the percentage of living patients (optimum: 95%) and still functioning organs (optimum: 80–90%) after 1 year.

Immunosuppression

Postoperative immunosuppression with combinations of cyclosporin, azathioprine, steroids and antilymphocyte products with the aim of a basic immunosuppression low in steroids.
Treatment of rejection primarily with methylprednisolone (0.5–1 g/day for 3 days by short-term infusion).

Acute problems in renal transplantation

Most are general medical problems which are to be recognized and treated as such, with consideration of the interaction with immunosuppressants. Consultation with the attending transplant centre.

Acute deterioration of transplant function

Treat as rejection until proof to the contrary. Consider the differential diagnosis of acute renal failure including cyclosporin nephrotoxicity.

Acute abdominal pain (especially in the early stage after transplantation)

Rejection, thrombosis of the renal artery or vein, primary or secondary in the course of rejection, obstruction, urinary leak, rupture of kidney, acute abdomen of general surgical nature.

Haematuria

From native urinary tract: cyst bleeding in polycystic kidneys, papillary necrosis (analgesic or diabetic nephropathy), calculi in chronic pyelonephritis, infection of the native urinary tract.

From the transplant: vascular catastrophe (rupture, infarct, arterial and venous thrombosis); stones (rarely), infection.

Pyrexia

Investigation plan

Establish: height, duration, type of fever (continuous, remittent, intermittent, periodic, undulant)
Clues to confirmation and localization of infection:

- **History**
  Cough, headache, abdominal pain, diarrhoea, dysuria, backache, joint pains, muscular pains, operations, i.m. injections, drugs, sexual behaviour, travel, animal contacts, profession, old TB.
- **Findings**
  Rash, inflamed mucous membranes, lungs (pneumonia?), heart (valve defect?), locomotor system, lymph nodes, focal neurological signs, meningism, peritonitis.
- **Laboratory**
  C-reactive protein, ESR, differential white cell count, liver function tests, chest X-ray. Bacteriological cultures and/or serology, according to case history details or physical findings (urine, sputum, blood, CSF).

Types of fever

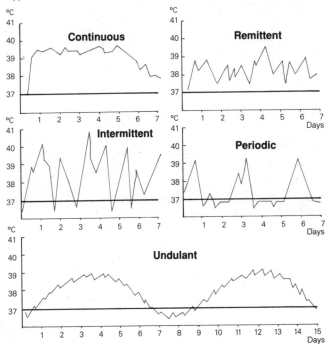

175

Pyrexia of undetermined origin

Definition: Fever $\geq 38°C$ lasting ≥ 3 weeks, for which no cause is found with the above-mentioned investigations after ≥ 1 week.

Causes

1. Infections (35%)
As a rule, infections with few local signs of inflammation.
Abscesses: intra-abdominal (liver, subphrenic, pancreas, spleen, also after abdominal surgery, diverticulitis, Crohn's disease, intrauterine pessary, curettage, dental abscess, brain abscess, muscle abscess after i.m. injection).
Biliary infections: cholecystitis, cholangitis, pancreatitis.
Osteomyelitis.
Urinary tract infections: rarely, as usually rapidly diagnosed, except in perinephric abscess or ureteric obstruction.
Subacute bacterial endocarditis.
Tuberculosis: note also miliary tuberculosis in the elderly patient.
Others: gonococcal sepsis, chronic meningococcal sepsis, Q fever, chlamydial infections, leptospirosis, brucellosis (history of travel and animal contact important).
Viral infections: HIV, cytomegalovirus, infectious mononucleosis, hepatitis.
Parasitic infections: toxoplasmosis, malaria, according to travel history.

2. Tumours (20%)
Hodgkin's and non-Hodgkin's lymphoma, leukaemias, solid tumours (renal cell carcinoma, hepatoma, cerebral tumour, atrial myxoma).

3. Collagen/vascular illnesses (15%)
Giant cell arteritis, Still's disease, polyarteritis nodosa, systemic lupus erythematosus.

4. Miscellaneous (15%)
Drug fever, sarcoidosis, granulomatous hepatitis, Whipple's disease, factitious fever, thyroiditis.

5. No diagnosis (15%)

Synopsis of nine studies from 1958–1980 (Good reviews include: Esposito *et al.* (1979) and Larson *et al.* (1982))

Bacteriological stains – direct preparations

Gram stain
- Dry specimen in air
- Fix (draw through flame 3 times)
- Crystal violet 1 min
- Rinse and stain with Lugol's iodine solution: 2 min
- Decolorize with acetone/alcohol until no colour is discharged
- Counterstain with safranin or diluted carbol-fuchsin solution: $\frac{1}{2}$–1 min
- Rinse with tap water

Result
Gram-positive bacteria: dark blue
Gram-negative bacteria: red

Ziehl–Neelsen stain
- Heat with concentrated carbol-fuchsin solution until steaming
- Rinse with water. Decolorize with HCl (3% alcohol)
- Counterstain with methylene blue: 1–5 min
- Rinse with tap water

Result
Mycobacteria: red

The commonest pathogens in Gram stain preparations

| Material* | Gram-positive | | Gram-negative | |
	Cocci	Rods	Cocci	Rods
CSF	Strep. pneumoniae	Listeria	N. meningitidis	Haemophilus influenzae
Sputum	Strep. pneumoniae		Moraxella catarrhalis	Haemophilus influenzae Klebsiella pneumoniae
Pleural effusion	Strep. pneumoniae Staph. aureus Anaerobic streptococci			Haemophilus influenzae Enterobacteriacae
Ascites	Strep. pneumoniae			E. coli
Liver abscess	Streptococci			E. coli Klebsiella pneumoniae Bacteroides
Intra-abdominal abscess	Anaerobic streptococci Enterococci			Enterobacteriacae Bacteroides

* Note: Any organisms demonstrable in specimens which are physiologically sterile (e.g. CSF) are pathological. In sputum, however, demonstration of organisms by Gram stain is only relevant when numerous organisms **and** leucocytes are found. If TB is suspected, a Ziehl–Neelsen stain is essential.

Interpretation of aspirates

I. Cerebrospinal fluid (p. 267)

	Normal	Viral meningitis	Bacterial meningitis	Tuberculous meningitis
Appearance	Water-clear	Clear	Turbid	Clear-turbid
Pressure (cm H$_2$O)	5–12	Normal or raised	>20	Normal or raised
Cells (per litre)	1–4 × 10^6	<10^9 (lymphocytes raised)	>1.2 × 10^9 Polymorphs raised	<1 × 10^9 (monocytes and lymphocytes raised)
Glucose (% of serum concentration)	50–80%	50–80%	<40%	<40%
Protein (g/l)	0.1–0.45	Normal or raised	Mostly >1.0	Mostly 0.5–5.0
Lactate (mmol/l)	<1.6	<1.6	>1.6	>1.6
Direct stain	Negative	Negative	80% positive	35% positive

Note: The findings mentioned are typical, but their absence does not exclude the corresponding aetiology. For example, while a cell count >1.2 × 10^9 l points to a bacterial meningitis, a count of less than this value does not by any means exclude it.

II. Pleural effusion

Findings in favour of an infective effusion:
- Protein   >30 g/l
- Rel. protein   (% of serum value) >50%
- Rel. LDH   (% of serum value) >60%
- pH   <7.0
- Leucocytes   >1 × 10^9/l (>50% polymorphonuclear)
- Gram stain   see p. 177

III. Ascites

Findings in favour of a bacterial peritonitis:
- Protein >25 g/l (>30 g/l never cardiac or cirrhotic)
- Lactate >3.7 mmol/l, or, more reliably[a]:
  Lactate (ascites) − lactate (blood) <2.2 mmol/l: sterile
                                         >2.2 mmol/l: infected
- Leucocytes:
  <300 × 10^9/l, infection excluded, but sterile ascites possible up to 2 × 10^9
  <25% granulocytes: infection excluded, but >25% granulocytes in ca. 50% of cases with sterile ascites
  Gram stain: see p. 177

IV. Joint aspirate (p. 260)

[a] Permits the evaluation of ascitic lactate even with raised serum lactate.

Common viral infections

Syndrome/illness	Commonest pathogen	Mode of transmission
Common cold Pharyngitis Laryngitis Croup	Rhinoviruses RS virus (respiratory syncytial) Influenza virus Parainfluenza virus Adenovirus	Droplet Hands Fomites
Hepatitis	Hepatitis A (HAV) Hepatitis B (HBV) Hepatitis C (HCV) Cytomegalovirus (CMV) Epstein–Barr virus (EBV) Herpes simplex (HSV) Varicella-zoster (VZV)	Faecal Blood, sexual Blood, sexual Blood, sputum, sexual Sputum, blood Lesion Lesion
CNS infection	Herpes simplex (HSV) Varicella-zoster (VZV) Measles virus Mumps virus Tick-borne encephalitis HIV	Mostly reactivation Droplet/lesion Droplet Droplet Ticks (zoonosis) Blood, sexual
Lymphadenopathy	Epstein–Barr virus (EBV) Cytomegalovirus (CMV) Rubella virus HIV	Sputum, blood Blood, sputum, sexual Droplet Blood, sexual

Methods of laboratory diagnosis in viral illnesses
(Bundesamt für Gesundheitswesen (1985))

Clinical picture	Virus isolation	Direct virus detection	Serology
Vesicle-forming eruption	Yes, vesicle fluid or smear from lesion, crusts not useful Time: 1–10 days	Yes, in herpes and smallpox. Not in coxsackie Time: 2–24 h	No. Except: varicella-zoster: Rising titre or demonstration of IgM
Diarrhoeal illnesses	No	Yes, essentially only rotavirus. Time: 4–72 h	No
Central nervous system	Yes, only mumps and enteroviruses. Pharyngeal material, stool, possibly CSF Time: 3–15 days	Yes, only herpes and possibly measles Biopsy material	Yes: mumps, measles, polio Rising titre No: all other viruses
Tick-borne encephalitis	No	No	Yes: IgM demonstration or rising titre
Respiratory tract	Yes, nasal, pharyngeal, bronchial secretions Time: 3–15 days	Yes, rhinopharyngeal aspiration Time: 4–24 h	Yes: rising titre
Eye conditions	Yes, only herpes (and possibly chlamydia). Smear Time 3–20 days	No (*Chlamydia* yes)	No
Hepatitis	No	No	Yes: Hep. A: IgM demonstration; Hep. B: HBs-Ag, Anti-HBc, Anti-HBc-IgM Supplement: anti-HBs, Anti-HBe Hep C: total Ig
Prenatal infections	Yes. Pharyngeal material, urine Time: up to 6 weeks	No	Yes for rubella and CMV: IgM and IgG in mother and child simultaneously

Collection and dispatch of material for investigation

Material	Collection	Dispatch for virus isolation	Dispatch for direct demonstration
Nasal smear	With swab under turbinate	0°C, in VTM[a]	–
Nasopharyngeal secretion	Aspiration	0°C, no additive	As for isolation
Throat swab	With swab from tonsils and pharynx	0°C, in VTM[a]	–
Pharyngeal washings	Gargle with pharyngeal rinsing fluid[a]	0°C, fluid without additive	–
Bronchial secretion	Use as little fluid as possible	0°C, fluid without additive	As for isolation
Eyes (conjunctiva)	With swab from upper and lower lid	0°C, in VTM[a], for *Chlamydia* in special transport medium	(*Chlamydia*: smear on microscope slide)
Vesicle fluid	Isolation: with swab or needle. Direct demonstration: puncture with needle (not disposable needle with silicone coating!) or glass pipette	0°C, in VTM[a]	Without additive, direct in needle or glass pipette
Mucosal erosions	With swab, after removal of necrotic material, from edge and floor of lesion	0°C, in VTM[a]	–
Urine	Terminal stream	0°C, use of VTM[a] only after discussion with laboratory	Without additive
Stool	–	Without additive	Without additive
CSF	Puncture	0°C, in VTM[a]	–
Tissue (biopsy, autopsy)	–	Only after discussion with laboratory	–
Blood: virus isolation	Puncture	–70°C, anticoagulant, special transport!	–
Blood: serology	Puncture without additive	Room temperature	–

[a] VTM (virus transport medium) or rinsing fluid should be requested from the laboratory that performs the examination.

Antiviral agents

Drug	Spectrum, indication	Daily dose*	Most important side effects
Acyclovir†	HSVI and II, also VZV: HSV primary infection (mucocutaneous) Suppression in recurrent HSV infection VZV disseminated or ophthalmic zoster HSV encephalitis HSV in immunoin-competence	5 times 200 mg (5 days) oral 2 times 400 mg oral OR 4 times 200 mg oral 5 times 800 mg (7 days) oral OR 30 mg/kg (10 days) i.v. in 3 doses	Nephrotoxicity Neurotoxicity Adjust according to renal function
Ganciclovir‡	CMV (HSV, VZV, EBV) Retinitis Colitis Pneumonia Maintenance therapy for retinitis	10 mg/kg (14–21 days) i.v. in 2 doses 6 mg/kg i.v. on 5 days/week OR 5 mg/kg i.v. daily	Neutropenia Thrombocytopenia Neurotoxixity Adjust according to renal function
Zidovudine§	HIV IV A HIV IV B HIV IV C1 HIV II + CD4 < 200/µl or 2 of the following criteria: CD4-Ly 200–500/µl CD4-Ly 200–500/µl + 30% fall β_2-microglobulin >5 mg/l Positive HIV-p24 antigen	500–600 mg in 2–5 divided doses OR 6–12 mg/kg (2 weeks) i.v. in 6 doses	Anaemia Neutropenia Nausea **Note:** cumulative toxicity with high doses of sulphona-namides, trimethoprim, pyrimethamine, ganciclovir In general, avoid combined therapy

Abbreviations:
HSV, herpes simplex virus; VZV, varicella-zoster virus; CMV, cytomegalovirus; EBV, Epstein–Barr virus; HIV, human immunodeficiency virus; CD4-Ly, T helper cells.

* For adults; refer to detailed prescibing information for children's doses.
† Alternative treatments for HSV or VZV include famciclovir, recommended for herpes zoster and genital herpes, and valaciclovir for herpes zoster only. Idoxuridine may be used for topical treatment of herpes simplex.
‡ Foscarnet is also active against cytomegalovirus, but indicated only for retinitis in AIDS patients for whom ganciclovir is inappropriate.
§ Didanosine is indicated for treatment of HIV in adults intolerant of zidovudine; zalcitabine has similar indications.

Tribavirin is used to treat bronchiolitis caused by respiratory syncytial virus in infants.

The immunocompromised patient

Malignant tumours and their therapy lead to an increased risk of infection. This risk to the patient is related to the nature of the underlying disease and the type of immunological defect.

Immunological defect	Illness/therapy	Commonest pathogens
Neutropenia (< 1000/µl)	Leukaemias (blast cell crisis) Advanced lymphomas, myelomas Solid tumour chemotherapy causing aplasia Bone marrow transplantation	*Staph. aureus* *Staph. epidermis* Gram-negative bacteria *Candida albicans* *Aspergillus*
Disturbed granulocyte function	Chronic granulomatous illness Job syndrome (recurrent cold staphylococcal abscesses) Bone marrow transplantation (graft-versus-host disease) Antithymocyte globulin Adriamycin and others	*Staph. aureus* *Staph. epidermis* Gram-negative bacteria *Candida albicans* *Aspergillus*
Disturbed barriers	Cytotoxic drugs Catheter Surgery Burns and others	*Staph. aureus* *Staph. epidermis* *Pseudomonas aeruginosa* *Candida albicans*
Disturbed cell-mediated immunity	Hodgkin's and non-Hodgkin's lymphoma AIDS Status after transplantation (cyclosporin, steroids, azathioprine, etc.)	Cytomegalovirus Herpes simplex Herpes zoster *Pneumocystis carinii* *Toxoplasma gondii* *Listeria* *Nocardia* *Cryptococcus neoformans* *M. tuberculosis* Atypical mycobacteria
Hypogamma-globulinaemia, dysgamma-globulinaemia	Chronic lymphatic leukaemia Multiple myeloma Bone marrow transplantation	*Strep. pneumoniae* *Haemophilus influenzae* *N. meningitidis*
Splenectomy	Hodgkin's lymphoma and others	*Strep. pneumoniae* *Haemophilus influenzae*

Note: In the febrile immunocompromised patient the investigation and empirical therapy must be directed against the commonest pathogens, i.e. a patient with disturbed cell-mediated immunity requires different investigation and therapy from a neutropenic patient.

Literature: Hughes *et al.* (1990) (Neutropenia)
Colonna *et al.* (1988) (Liver transplantation)
Oh *et al.* (1988) (Renal transplantation)
Zimmerli *et al.* (1991) (Bone marrow transplantation)

AIDS: definition and classification

Human immunodeficiency virus (HIV) infection and acquired immune deficiency syndrome (AIDS)

Definition

HIV demonstration in tissue or body fluid
HIV antibody demonstration (cf. illustration)
AIDS: acquired immune deficiency syndrome without other cause
(neoplasia, immunosuppressive therapy) and demonstration of an opportunistic infection or tumour
(see CDC classification)

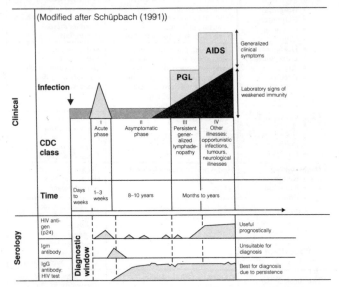

Classification

1. CDC classification

Group I   **Acute infection:** mononucleosis-like picture, meningoencephalitis, seroconversion

Group II   **Asymptomatic infection:**
    A Laboratory tests normal
    B Laboratory tests abnormal (lymphopenia, thrombocytopenia, reduced CD4 lymphocytes)

Group III   **Persistent generalized lymphadenopathy:**
    Lymph nodes above 1 cm in at least 2 places apart from inguinal region lasting more than 3
    months without other explanation

Group IV
A   **Constitutional clinical picture:**
- Weight loss > 10% and/or
- Unexplained pyrexia over 1 month (continuous or intermittent) and/or
- Diarrhoea over 1 month

B Neurological clinical picture:
- Dementia
- Myelopathy without other cause
- Peripheral neuropathy

C Secondary illness: opportunistic infections
C1 • *Pneumocystis carinii* pneumonia
- Toxoplasmosis of CNS
- Cryptosporidiosis with diarrhoea >1 month
- Isosporiasis with diarrhoea >1 month
- Extraintestinal strongyloides infection
- Candidiasis (oesophagus, bronchi, lungs)
- Cryptococcosis, extrapulmonary
- Histoplasmosis, extrapulmonary
- Extrapulmonary tuberculosis
- Atypical mycobacterial infections (disseminated)
- Recurrent *Salmonella* bacteraemia (except *S. typhi*)
- Cytomegalovirus infections (not liver, spleen or lymph nodes)
- Chronic mucocutaneous or disseminated herpes simplex infection
- Progressive multifocal leucoencephalopathy
C2 • Oral leucoplakia
- Herpes zoster
- Nocardiosis
- Pulmonary tuberculosis
- *Candida* stomatitis

D Secondary illnesses: neoplasia
- Kaposi's sarcoma
- Non-Hodgkin's lymphoma
- Primary CNS lymphoma

E Other HIV-associated illnesses, e.g.
- Chronic lymphoid pneumonia
- Recurrent bacterial pneumonia

2. Walter Reed classification

The Walter Reed classification, introduced in 1985, divides the HIV infection into clinical–immunological functional disturbances (Redfield *et al.*, 1986).
The stages WR3–WR6 indicate the progression towards AIDS.

Stage	HIV antibodies and/or virus demonstration	Chronic lymphadenopathy	CD4 lymphocytes	Skin test	Stomatitis	Opportunistic infections
WR0	−	−	>400	Normal	−	−
WR1	+	−	>400	Normal	−	−
WR2	+	+	>400	Normal	−	−
WR3	+	±	<400	Normal	−	−
WR4	+	±	<400	P	−	−
WR5	+	±	<400	A and/or P	±	−
WR6	+	±	<400	P/A	±	+

P, partial anergy in Mérieux Multitest.
A, complete anergy in Mérieux Multitest.
The parameters that are important for the classification are shown in red.

Investigation of AIDS

Laboratory parameters for immune state

CD4 lymphocytes, CD8 lymphocytes, lymphocyte transformation test, immunoglobulins, p24 antigen, β_2-microglobulin, leucocytes, haemoglobin, platelets, Mérieux Multitest

Investigations of infections according to clinical problems

1. **Respiratory syndrome**
   - If CD4 lymphocytes >200/µl: sputum bacteriology → probably bacterial pneumonia, including *Strep. pneumoniae, H. influenzae, Staph. aureus, Legionella, M. tuberculosis*
   - If CD4 lymphocytes <200/µl: provoked sputum or bronchial lavage for bacteriology (including *M. tuberculosis*); also: *Pneumocystis carinii*, cytomegalovirus, *Candida, Aspergillus*, cryptococci, histoplasma, cytology (inclusion bodies), if indicated transbronchial biopsy (Kaposi's sarcoma)

2. **CNS syndrome**
   - If meningitic syndrome: lumbar puncture for general bacteriology, cryptococcus neoformans, virology (CMV, HSV, HZV), p24 antigen, CSF/serum antibodies (CMV, HSV, HZV, HIV), protein, glucose, lactate, cells
   - If encephalitic syndrome: CT without/with contrast. If CT lesion with nodular or ring enhancement: serology (toxoplasma, HSV, HZV, CMV) → empirical toxoplasma therapy (p. 187)

3. **Retinitis**
   - Fundoscopy
   - CMV serology, CMV demonstration in urine, sputum, heparinized blood (leucocytes)

4. **Oesophagitis, gastroenteritis, colitis**
   - In case of dysphagia and *Candida* stomatitis: empirical therapy against *Candida* oesophagitis. If no repsonse: endoscopy with biopsy (histology, cytology, CMV, HSV demonstration, *Candida*)
   - In case of diarrhoea: stool bacteriology, including Ziehl–Neelsen stain, stool parasites (cryptosporidia, *Isopora belli*, amoebae, *Giardia lamblia, Blastocystis hominis*, etc.), stool virology (adenoviruses)

5. **Hepatitis**
   - Serology: HAV, HBV, HCV, CMV, EBV, HSV, HZV
   - Heparinized blood for mycobacteria and CMV
   - Possibly liver biopsy for histology, mycobacterial culture, CMV, HSV demonstration

6. **Generalized symptoms**
   - Blood cultures
   - CMV demonstration in urine, sputum and heparinized blood
   - Mycobacterial demonstration (heparinized blood, stool, lymph node biopsy)
   - Serology (CMV, HSV, HZV, *Toxoplasma gondii, Leishmania, Strongyloides*)

Therapy of the most important pathogens in HIV infection

Site of infection	Pathogen	Initial therapy	Dose	Duration	Suppressive therapy
Respiratory tract	*M. tuberculosis*	Triple therapy, e.g. Rifater[a] followed by rifampicin + isoniazid	4–5 tab./day oral 10mg/kg/day 300mg/day	2 months } 4–7 months	If necessary, isoniazid
	Pneumocystis carinii	Trimethoprim + sulphame-thoxazole or dapsone + trimethoprim or pentamidine	20mg/kg/day 100mg/kg/day 100mg/day 20mg/day oral 4mg/kg/day i.v.	} oral/i.v. 3 weeks } 3 weeks	Pentamidine inhalation (300mg every 3 weeks) or trimethoprim + sulphame-thoxazole (1 forte tab. b.d. 3 times per week)
	Cytomegalo-virus	Ganciclovir	7.5–15mg/day i.v.	2–3 weeks	If necessary, ganciclovir (5mg/kg/day)
	Legionella sp.	Erythromycin	3g/day oral/i.v.	3 weeks	None
CNS Brain abscess	*Toxoplasma gondii*[b]	Pyrimethamine + sulphadiazine + calcium folinate + sodium bicarbonate or pyrimethamine + clindamycin	100mg/day oral 1 week, followed by 50–75mg/day oral 4(–6)g/day oral 5–15mg/day oral urine>pH7 as above >2400mg/day oral or i.v.	} 2–4 months	Pyrimethamine (25mg/day) + sulphadiazine (3g/day) Lifelong
Meningitis	*Cryptococcus neoformans*	Amphotericin B	0.5mg/kg/day i.v.	ca. 6–8 weeks	Fluconazole (100–200mg/day oral)
Retinitis	Cytomegalo-virus[c]	Ganciclovir or foscarnet	10mg/kg/day i.v. 180mg/kg/day i.v.	2–3 weeks	Ganciclovir (5mg/kg/day or higher) 90–120mg/kg/day i.v.
Encephalitis	Herpes	Acyclovir	3× 10mg/kg i.v.	10 days	

[a] Combined antituber as to US treatment
[b] Dannemann *et al.* (1992)
[c] ACTG (1992)

Site of infection	Pathogen	Initial therapy	Dose	Duration	Suppressive therapy
Oesophago-gastro-intestinal	*Candida* spp. Herper simplex	Fluconazole Acyclovir	400 mg/day 400 mg q.i.d. oral or 15 mg/kg/day i.v.	Single dose 10 days	None ?
Oesophagitis	Cytomegalo-virus	Ganciclovir	10 mg/kg/day i.v.	14 days	?
Colitis	*Isospora belli*	Trimethoprim + sulphame-thoxazole	10 mg/kg/day 50 mg/kg/day	14 days or longer	?
Skin/mucous membranes	Herpes simplex	Acyclovir	200–400 mg 5 times per day oral	7–10 days	Individually
	Herpes zoster	Acyclovir	800 mg 5 times per day oral	7–10 days	None
	Candida spp.	Fiuconazole or amphotericin B lozenges	150 mg/day 4–5/day	Single dose 2–3 weeks	None
Systemic	HIV	Zidovudine	500–(1000) mg/day	Lifelong	
	Cytomegalo-virus	Ganciclovir	10 mg/kg/day i.v.	2–3 weeks	Ganciclovir at least 5 mg/kg/day i.v.
	M. avium complex[a]	Clofazymine + rifampicin + ciprofloxacin + amikacin or ethambutol	100 mg/kg/day oral 600 mg/day oral 1500 mg/day oral 10 mg/kg/day i.v. 15 mg/kg/day oral	Stop Amikacin after 4–6 weeks	Lifelong

[a] Horsburgh (1991)

Empirical therapy of infections

I **Checklist before therapy**
   The following questions should be answered before any antibiotic therapy is prescribed:
   - Is antibiotic indicated on clinical grounds?
   - Have microbiological samples been taken?
   - Is immediate chemotherapy essential, or can the microbiological results be awaited?
   - Best antibiotic for empirical therapy? (Spectrum, pharmacokinetics, toxicity, price)
   - Is synergistic combination necessary?
   - Additional problems (immunosuppression)?
   - Drug allergies?
   - Method of administration?
   - Dose?
   - Duration?

II **Indication for empirical therapy**
   Antibiotic therapy should, as a rule, be directed against the causative organism(s). In certain bacterial infections the prognosis is, however, dependent on the start of adequate therapy. These therapies are summarized below. For infections where the start of therapy can be delayed until the culture results are available, consult the relevant textbooks. Empirical therapy is especially appropriate in the following infections:
   Sepsis with unknown primary site; endocarditis; pneumonia; intra-abdominal infection; urinary tract infection; CNS infections; fever with neutropenia.

III **Empirical therapy according to clinical diagnosis**
   Note: only one of the several alternatives is given for the empirical therapy.

Sepsis with unknown primary site

History: Short hospital stay? Intravenous drug abuse? Alcohol abuse? Additional symptoms? Travel, animals? Epidemiological situation? Underlying diseases?

Findings: Catheter? Puncture sites? Abnormal organ findings? Septic emboli?

Commonest organisms (O) and therapy (T), if no additional symptoms and no abnormal organ findings:

a) No pointers: O: mostly *Staphylococcus aureus*
                 T: Flucloxacillin and aminoglycoside

b) Drug abuse   O: *Staphylococcus aureus* or Gram-negative aerobes
                 T: Cephazolin and aminoglycoside

c) Alcohol abuse O: *Streptococcus pneumoniae*, *Escherichia coli*, *Klebsiella pneumoniae*
                 T: Ceftriaxone or co-amoxiclav and aminoglycoside

d) Intravascular O: Coagulase-negative staphylococci, *Staphylococcus aureus*
   catheter   T: Cephamandole

Endocarditis

Before therapy:
- With acute endocarditis:
  3 blood cultures over approx. 30 min
- With subacute endocarditis:
  3–6 blood cultures over approx. 24 h
- After previous antibiotic therapy:
  5–10 blood cultures over several days, if clinical condition stable

Commonest organisms (O) and therapy (T):

a) Acute endocarditis
   O: *Staphylococcus aureus*, group A or B staphylococci (less often),
      Gram-negative rods (less often)
   T: Flucloxacillin (2 g 6 times daily i.v.)+ aminoglycoside

b) Acute endocarditis with prosthetic heart valve
   O: *Staphylococcus aureus*, coagulase-negative staphylococci, other
      organisms
   T: Vancomycin (0.5 g q.i.d. as short infusion) + netilmycin

c) Subacute endocarditis
   O: *Streptococcus viridans*, enterococci, *Haemophilus* spp.
   T: Penicillin G (20 megaunits/day) + gentamicin or ceftriaxone (2 g/
      day)

Literature
Scheld and Sande (1990)

Pneumonia

Before therapy:
- Empirical therapy necessary (neutropenia, sepsis)?
- Exclude other causes (pulmonary embolus, cardiac
  decompensation)
- Bacterial pathogen (purulent sputum)?
- Non-bacterial pathogen (unproductive cough)?
- Underlying illnesses (alcoholism, condition after TB)?
- Necessary cultures taken (blood cultures, sputum)?

Commonest organisms (O) and therapy (T):
(a) No underlying illness, good general condition
    O: *Streptococcus pneumoniae*
        Mycoplasma pneumoniae (in younger patients)
    T: Penicillin G i.v. or
        amoxicillin orally or
        erythromycin (in younger patients)

(b) Respiratory insufficiency
    O: additionally Gram-negative organisms
    T: Penicillin G, i.v.+ aminoglycoside
        or ceftriaxone

(c) Additional symptoms (diarrhoea, CNS symptoms, hyponatraemia)
    O: *Legionella* species
    T: In addition to ceftriaxone,
        erythromycin (3–4 g/day)

(d) With underlying illness
    • Alcohol abuse
        O: *Klebsiella pneumoniae*
        T: Cephalosporin (2nd or 3rd generation)
    • Chronic obstructive airways disease
        O: *Haemophilus influenzae*
            Streptococcus pneumoniae
        T: Co-amoxiclav
    • With history of influenza
        O: *Haemophilus influenzae*
            Staphylococcus aureus
        T: Co-amoxiclav or
            ceftriaxone
    • HIV infection with purulent sputum
        O: *Haemophilus influenzae*
            Streptococcus pneumoniae
        T: Co-amoxiclav or
            ceftriaxone
    • HIV infection without purulent sputum
      (when CD4 lymphocytes $<200–400/mm^3$)
        O: *Pneumocystis carinii*
            ($\rightarrow$ bronchoalveolar lavage!)
        T: Cotrimoxazole (20/100 mg/kg/day)
    • Cystic fibrosis
        O: *Staphylococcus aureus*
            Pseudomonas aeruginosa
        T: Quinolone (e.g. ciprofloxacin, ofloxacin)

Note: In hospital-acquired pneumonia the therapy must be individually chosen. In the ventilated patient surveillance cultures are useful as a basis for decision-making.

Literature
Sanford (1991)

Intra-abdominal infection

Before therapy: Clarification: cholecystitis (stone?), pancreatitis, perforated ulcer, diverticulitis, appendicitis, ulcerative colitis, Crohn's disease, infectious enterocolitis

Commonest organisms (O) and therapy (T):
a) Proximal to jejunum

> O: Streptococci, enterococci, Gram-negative rods
> T: • Surgery, when indicated
> • Co-amoxiclav + aminoglycoside

b) Distal

> O: *Escherichia coli*, Gram-negative anaerobes, etc.
> T: • Surgery, when indicated
> • Piperacillin + tobramycin + perhaps metronidazole
> or
> • Cefoxitin + tobramycin
> or
> • Imipenem (perhaps + aminoglycoside)
> (Still unclear whether aminoglycoside necessary)

Urinary sepsis

Before therapy: Symptoms of urinary tract infection (dysuria, frequency, loin pain, pyuria)?
Symptoms of sepsis (high pyrexia, rigors, hypotension, tachycardia)?

Commonest organisms (O) and therapy (T):

> O: *Escherichia coli, Enterococcus, Klebsiella pneumoniae, Proteus mirabilis, Pseudomonas aeruginosa* (esp. after instrumentation or with calculi)
> T: • Younger patients with normal renal function: amoxicillin + tobramycin
> • Older patients and/or disturbed renal function: ciprofloxacin, ofloxacin or other newer quinolone

Note: This choice of antibiotics is valid for urinary sepsis, not for simple urinary tract infection. With rapid response, therapy can be changed from intravenous to oral after 3–5 days.

Literature
Stamm *et al.* (1989)
Zimmerli (1990)

Infections of the central nervous system

Before therapy: decide if meningitic or encephalitic syndrome

- Meningitic syndrome: meningism, pyrexia, photophobia, headache
- Encephalitic syndrome: clouding of consciousness, delirium, confusion, convulsions, focal neurological signs, pyrexia

→ **If meningitis:** lumbar puncture (interpretation, see p. 178), blood cultures, differential white cell count, lactate, venous blood gas analyses, search for primary focus (sinusitis, otitis, mastoiditis, etc.)

→ **If brain abscess or encephalitis:**
 CT scan without/with contrast (lumbar puncture contraindicated)
- If brain abscess: search for primary focus (sinusitis, otitis, after skull trauma, endocarditis, bronchiectasis, AIDS)
- If encephalitis: serology (mumps, measles, poliomyelitis, coxsackie, echoviruses, rabies, tick-borne encephalitis, HSV, CMV, HIV)

Commonest organisms (O) and therapy (T):

(a) **Meningitis**

O:
- Newborn: Streptococci, group B, *E. coli*, *Listeria monocytogenes*
- Child: *H. influenzae*, *Strep. pneumoniae*, *Neisseria meningitidis*
- Adult: *Strep. pneumoniae*, *Neisseria meningitidis*

T:
• Infant:	amoxicillin, 100 mg/kg/day + ceftriaxone, 100 mg/kg/day
• Young child:	ceftriaxone, 100 mg/kg/day
• Adult without underlying illness:	penicillin G, 24 megaunits/day
• Underlying ENT illness:	ceftriaxone, 2 g b.d.
• After organ transplantation:	amoxicillin, 2 g 6 times/day + gentamicin 5–7.5 mg/kg/day
• Neurosurgical shunt:	rifampicin 450–600 mg b.d. + ceftriaxone 2 g b.d.

Note: If a conclusive result on Gram preparation or if culture positive, treatment should be targeted appropriately.

Literature
Schaad (1986)
Talan *et al.* (1988)

(b) **Brain abscess**

O: *Streptococcus* sp. (anaerobic, aerobic),
H. influenzae, Strep. pneumoniae, Bacteroides sp.,
Staph. aureus, Nocardia, Toxoplasma gondii

T: • Unknown or ENT focus:
  ceftriaxone   2 g b.d. i.v.
  +
  metronidazole   0.5 g t.d.s. i.v.
• After skull or brain injury or neurosurgical operation:
  flucloxacillin   2 g 6 times/day i.v.
  or
  rifampicin   450–600 mg b.d. i.v.
  +
  ceftriaxone   2 g b.d. i.v.
• HIV infection
  Empirical toxoplasma therapy

Literature
Chun *et al.* (1986)

(c) **Encephalitis**

O: treatable: Herpes simplex, varicella-zoster, cytomegalovirus,
Mycoplasma, Brucella, Borrelia burgdorferi,
Treponema pallidum, M. tuberculosis, Cryptococcus,
Toxoplasma gondii, Plasmodium falciparum

T: • Herpes simplex and varicella-zoster
  acyclovir, 30 mg/kg/day i.v. in 3 doses
• Cytomegalovirus
  ganciclovir 10 mg/kg/day in 2 doses

For remaining therapies see textbook.

Literature
Whitley (1990)

Pyrexia with neutropenia

Before therapy:
- Document pyrexia
- Actual number of neutrophil granulocytes?

Definition:
Pyrexia: single measurement above 38°C
Persistent pyrexia: temperature ≥ 38°C for ≥ 1 h
Neutropenia: < 1000 neutrophil granulocytes/µl
Note: The danger of infection increases greatly if < 500/µl, and very greatly if < 100/µl. Rapid fall in neutrophil count and long duration of the neutropenia are risk factors.

Clinical examination:
Gums, pharynx, perianal region, cannula puncture sites, fingernails, chest auscultation, abdominal palpation.

Laboratory:
Two aerobic/anaerobic blood cultures, Gram stain and culture of skin lesions, culture of nasal smear, oropharynx, urine, stool, possibly sputum.

Commonest organisms (O) and therapy (T):

O: *Staph. aureus*, coagulase-negative staphylococci, Gram-negative bacilli (*Ps. aeruginosa*, *E. coli*, *Klebsiella*), *Candida albicans*, *Aspergillus*.

T: Anti-pseudomonas betalactam antibiotic (e.g. ceftazidime **or** piperacillin) + aminoglycoside (e.g. amikacin), possibly + vancomycin if methicillin-resistant *Staph. aureus* in control culture or if indication of cannula infection.

Procedure after initial empirical therapy:
Reassessment after 72 h:
If good response: continue empirical therapy.
If deterioration: change of empirical therapy on day 4:
+ Vancomycin, if not used previously,
+ Amphotericin B if *Candida* or *Aspergillus* in control cultures.

For further procedures (antiviral therapy, duration of therapy, etc.) see Hughes *et al.* (1990).

Antituberculous drugs

Drug	Dose per day	Most important side effects and interactions	Control tests, precautions	Mode of action
Isoniazid	5–10 mg/kg max. 300 mg	Hepatitis Peripheral neuropathy CNS symptoms GIT disturbances Interaction with phenytoin, barbiturates	SGOT, SGPT Prophylaxis of neuropathy with 50 mg vitamin B_6 in case of poor nutrition	Intra- and extracellularly bactericidal
Rifampicin	10 mg/kg max. 600 mg	Hepatitis, jaundice, nausea, anorexia, pruritus Interaction with coumarins, contraceptives (!), steroids, digitalis Red discoloration of all body fluids (contact lens staining!)	SGOT, SGPT, bilirubin	Intra- and extracellularly bactericidal
Pyrazinamide	25 mg/kg max. 2.5 g	Hepatitis, nausea, vomiting, hyperuricaemia, arthralgia	SGOT, SGPT, uric acid	Intra- and extracellularly bactericidal at pH $\leq$ 5.5
Ethambutol	25 mg/kg max. 2 g	Optical neuritis	Vision, visual field, colour vision	Bacteriostatic
Streptomycin	15–20 mg/kg max. 1 g	Ototoxicity Nephrotoxicity	Audiogram, vestibular function tests, creatinine	Extracellularly bactericidal

Note: The duration of therapy can be limited to a total of 6 months if the three intra- and extracellularly bactericidal drugs are used. Without rifampicin the treatment must be prolonged. Patients with open TB must be isolated for at least the first 2 weeks of treatment. With poor response to therapy (persistent cough), isolation must be prolonged.

Recommended dosage for standard unsupervised 6-month regimen

Isoniazid (for 6 months)	Adult 300 mg daily
	Child 10 mg/kg (max. 300 mg) daily
Rifampicin (for 6 months)	Adult under 50 kg, 450 mg daily; 50 kg and over, 600 mg daily
	Child 10 mg/kg daily
Pyrazinamide (for first 2 months only)	Adult under 50 kg, 1.5 g; 50 kg and over, 2 g daily
	Child 35 mg/kg

Syphilis

Test	Positive result in % Prim.	Sec.	Tert.	Specificity	Test indication	Persistence over years
Non-specific antibody tests (cardiolipin)						
VDRL — Flocculation test, Quantitative result	70	100	0	Low	Screening	Decreasing
RPR — Agglutination, Automated, screening survey	80	100	0		Screening	
Specific treponemal antibody tests						
TPHA — Haemagglutination	65	100	95	High	Screening	Remains positive
FTA Abs — Immunofluorescence	85	100	98		Confirmation	
TPI (Nelson) — Immobilization	50	100	97			

Interpretation of syphilis test results

TPHA	VDRL	FTA	Interpretation
Pos.	Pos.	Pos.	Syphilis requiring treatment
Pos.	Neg.	Pos.	Differential diagnosis: treated syphilis or syphilis I
Neg.	Neg.		No syphilis (but note incubation period)
Pos.	Neg.	Neg. }	Check after 14 days
Neg.	Neg.	Pos. }	
Neg.	Pos.	Neg.	Non-specific reaction

Spontaneous course of untreated syphilis

Infection → 9–90 days Incubation → 2–6 weeks Primary syphilis → 4–6 weeks → 2–6 weeks Secondary syphilis → 2 years Latent phase → 5–20 years Tertiary syphilis

Infectious

Syphilis I: 'Soft chancre'; bilateral inguinal lymphadenopathy

Syphilis II: 'Non-irritating', generalized, symmetrical eruption; many systemic symptoms and findings

Infectious recurrence in 25% in 1st year

Syphilis III: Gummata, Cardiovascular syphilis, Tabes dorsalis

VDRL, venereal disease research laboratory; RPR, rapid plasma reagin; TPHA, *Treponema pallidum* haemagglutination; FTA, fluorescent *Treponema* antibody; TPI, *Treponema pallidum* immobilization.

Immunization recommendations for children and adults

Note: Advice on vaccination and immunization varies from country to country.

In most countries there is an advisory schedule of immunizations for children (from birth to around school-leaving age).

Further immunizations are performed in adults when it is important to reinforce childhood immunizations or to make up for any omitted for which natural immunity has not been acquired (e.g. diphtheria, tetanus, rubella, measles). Other immunizations may be considered in special epidemiological circumstances or risks in children and adults. Some immunizations are required for travel in certain areas by international health regulations or are desirable for individual protection. The decision concerning the nature and extent of the immunizations requires the physician to weigh the indications and contraindications in each individual case. This also applies to passive and active immunization against hepatitis A.

There are no maximum intervals for killed vaccine immunizations. After a completed basic immunization there is no need for a repeated basic programme.

Childhood immunization schedule

Age (years)	Vaccine	Notes
0–1	Diphtheria, tetanus and pertussis *and* *Haemophilus influenzae* b *and* Poliomyelitis (oral)	First doses to be given at 2 months
1–2	Measles/mumps/rubella (MMR) (live) *Haemophilus influenzae* b	At 12–15 months At 13 months to 4 years if not previously given
Entry to nursery school or school (3–5 years)	Diphtheria and tetanus *and* Poliomyelitis (oral) Measles/mumps/rubella (MMR) (live)	Preferably allow interval of at least 3 years after basic course Unless history of measle/mumps/rubella immunization or contraindication or immunity
10–14 10–14 (females)	BCG Rubella (live)	For tuberculin-negative children allow at least 3 weeks between BCG and rubella immunization
On leaving school or before employment or higher education	Poliomyelitis (oral) *and* Diphtheria and tetanus	

Adult immunizations important for individual and public health

Vaccine	Notes
Poliomyelitis (oral) if previously unimmunized	No adult should remain unimmunized
Rubella (live)	Women of child-bearing age, if sero-negative (pregnancy should be excluded)
Tetanus if previously unimmunized	Reinforcing dose 10 years after primary course, then 10 years later
Hepatitis A and B *Influenza Pneumococcal*	For all individuals in high-risk groups

Other vaccines and anti-sera available in special epidemiological circumstances and required or recommended for travel to certain areas

Vaccine	Notes
Anthrax	Available to those subject to high exposure, e.g. infected hides and carcasses, imported bone-meal, fishmeal and feedstuffs
Botulism antitoxin	Post-exposure prophylaxis
Cholera	No longer required for travel to any country. Efficacy limited
Meningococcal polysaccharide	Indicated for travel in parts of Africa and the Indian subcontinent
Rabies	Use prophylactically for those at high risk of exposure
Smallpox	No longer required for travel. For laboratory workers subject to potential exposure
Typhoid	
Yellow fever	Certificate of vaccination required travel to much of Africa and South America

In the UK, information and advice on immunization required for international travel is issued by the Department of Health.
(The guidelines above reflect those of the UK Joint Committee on Vaccination and Immunization, modified from the British National Formulary.)

Sedimentation rate

Reaction	Tumour	Infection	Connective tissue disorder/others
↑↑↑ Raised (above 100 mm after 1 h)	Plasmacytoma Waldenström's macroglobulinaemia Hodgkin's disease	Rheumatic fever Sepsis Peritonitis	Polymalgia rheumatica Vasculitis Polyarthritis Nephrotic syndrome
↑↑ Raised (above 50 mm after 1 h)	Metastasizing tumours	Bacterial infections	Tissue necroses Myocardial infarct Chronic liver diseases
↑ Raised (up to 50 mm after 1 h)	Leukaemia	Tuberculosis	Postoperative, anaemia, hyperlipidaemia, pregnancy (after 8th week), menstruation, oral contraceptives, incorrect measurement technique
↓ Lowered	Polycythemia vera		Polycythemia, heart failure, cryoglobulinaemia, dehydration, anabolic agents, plasma expanders, incorrect measurement technique

ESR
Normal values:
Men ♂
after 1 h 3–8 mm
after 2 h 5–18 mm
Women ♀
after 1 h 6–11 mm
after 2 h 6–20 mm

Plasma:
(fluid blood component):
Serum + fibrinogen + coagulation factors
Serum:
Albumin + globulin
(McMorran and Paraskevas, 1981)

Protein electro-phoresis

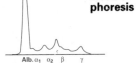

Alb. α_1 α_2 β γ

Total protein 60–84 g/l	Albumin	Globulins			
		α_1	α_2	β	γ
Concentration g/l	35–40	0.6–1.5	0.4–3.4	2.1–4.9	2.5–7.1
Proportion %	52–68	2.4–4.4	6.1–10.1	8.5–14.5	10–21
Proteins	Carrier protein for bilirubin, hormones, fatty acids, drugs Maintainance of colloidal osmotic presssure	α_1/α_2-lipoprotein α_1-antitrypsin α_2-macroglobulin Haptoglobulin Caeruloplasmin Thyroxine-binding globulin		β-lipoproteins Transferrin	Immunoglobulins
Significance of low values	↓ Synthesis ↑ Losses (renal, enteral) Tumour, inflammation	Chronic liver disorders, deficiency dysproteinaemia		Chronic hepatic disorders	Antibody deficiency, tumour of lymphatic system, corticosteroids, immunosuppressive agents, nephrotic syndrome, exudative enteropathy
Significance of high values	Dehydration, hypoglobulinaemia	Acute inflammation, nephrotic syndrome		Paraproteinaemia, hyperlipidaemia, nephrotic syndrome	Rheumatic disorders, collagenoses, chronic infections, chronic liver disorders, paraproteinaemia
Acute inflammation	Albumin reduced, alphaglobulins increased				
Chronic inflammation	Albumin reduced, alpha- and gammaglobulins increased				

Peripheral blood and bone marrow cells

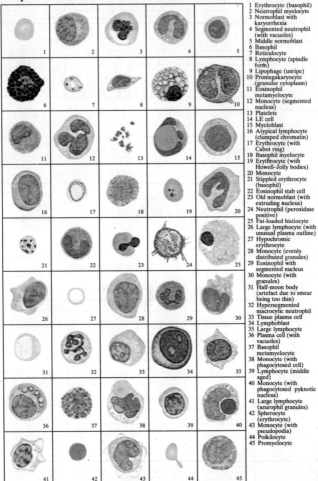

1 Erythrocyte (basophil)
2 Neutrophil myelocyte
3 Normoblast with karyorrhexia
4 Segmented neutrophil (with vacuoles)
5 Middle normoblast
6 Basophil
7 Reticulocyte
8 Lymphocyte (spindle form)
9 Lipophage (unripe)
10 Promegakaryocyte (granular cytoplasm)
11 Eosinophil metamyelocyte
12 Monocyte (segmented nucleus)
13 Platelets
14 LE cell
15 Myeloblast
16 Atypical lymphocyte (clumped chromatin)
17 Erythrocyte (with Cabot ring)
18 Basophil myelocyte
19 Erythrocyte (with Howell-Jolly bodies)
20 Monocyte
21 Stippled erythrocyte (basophil)
22 Eosinophil stab cell
23 Old normoblast (with extruding nucleus)
24 Neutrophil (peroxidase positive)
25 Fat-loaded histiocyte
26 Large lymphocyte (with unusual plasma outline)
27 Hypochromic erythrocyte
28 Monocyte (evenly distributed granules)
29 Eosinophil with segmented nucleus
30 Monocyte (with granules)
31 Half-moon body (artefact due to smear being too thin)
32 Hypersegmented macrocytic neutrophil
33 Tissue plasma cell
34 Lymphoblast
35 Large lymphocyte
36 Plasma cell (with vacuoles)
37 Basophil metamyelocyte
38 Monocyte (with phagocytosed cell)
39 Lymphocyte (middle aged)
40 Monocyte (with phagocytosed pyknotic nucleus)
41 Large lymphocyte (azurophil granules)
42 Spherocyte (erythrocyte)
43 Monocyte (with pseudopodia)
44 Poikilocyte
45 Promyelocyte

(Reprinted with permission of Firma Ortho Diagnostic Systems GmbH, D-6903 Neckargemünd)

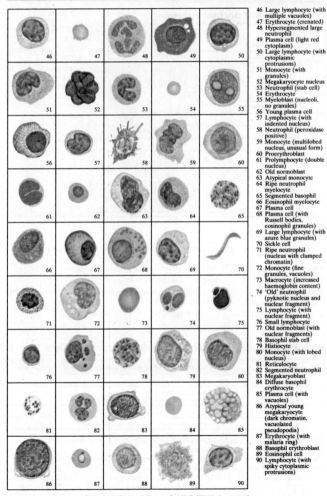

46 Large lymphocyte (with multiple vacuoles)
47 Erythrocyte (crenated)
48 Hypersegmented large neutrophil
49 Plasma cell (light red cytoplasm)
50 Large lymphocyte (with cytoplasmic protrusions)
51 Monocyte (with granules)
52 Megakaryocyte nucleus
53 Neutrophil (stab cell)
54 Erythrocyte
55 Myeloblast (nucleoli, no granules)
56 Young plasma cell
57 Lymphocyte (with indented nucleus)
58 Neutrophil (peroxidase positive)
59 Monocyte (multilobed nucleus, unusual form)
60 Proerythroblast
61 Prolymphocyte (double nucleus)
62 Old normoblast
63 Atypical monocyte
64 Ripe neutrophil myelocyte
65 Segmented basophil
66 Eosinophil myelocyte
67 Plasma cell
68 Plasma cell (with Russell bodies, eosinophil granules)
69 Large lymphocyte (with azure blue granules)
70 Sickle cell
71 Ripe neutrophil (nucleus with clumped chromatin)
72 Monocyte (fine granules, vacuoles)
73 Macrocyte (increased haemoglobin content)
74 'Old' neutrophil (pyknotic nucleus and nuclear fragment)
75 Lymphocyte (with nuclear fragment)
76 Small lymphocyte
77 Old normoblast (with nuclear fragments)
78 Basophil stab cell
79 Histiocyte
80 Monocyte (with lobed nucleus)
81 Reticulocyte
82 Segmented neutrophil
83 Megakaryoblast
84 Diffuse basophil erythrocyte
85 Plasma cell (with vacuoles)
86 Atypical young megakaryocyte (dark chromatin, vacuolated pseudopodia)
87 Erythrocyte (with malaria ring)
88 Basophil erythroblast
89 Eosinophil cell
90 Lymphocyte (with spiky cytoplasmic protrusions)

Haematological normal values

Hb g/dl Hct % Erythrocytes (RBC) ($\times 10^6$)	♂ 14–18 41–51 4.5–6.0	♀ 12–16 37–47 4.0–5.5	**Blood count** MCV, mean corpuscular volume;
MCV fl $\quad \dfrac{\text{Hct} \times 10}{\text{RBC}}$	87 ± 7		MCH, mean corpuscular haemoglobin;
MCH pg $\quad \dfrac{\text{Hb} \times 10}{\text{RBC}} (= \text{Hb}_e)$	29 ± 2		MCHC, mean corpuscular haemoglobin concentration
MCHC g/dl $\quad \dfrac{\text{Hb} \times 100}{\text{Hct}}$	34 ± 2		
Reticulocytes $\quad$ 7–15 ‰	35 000–75 000/µl		
Platelets	150 000–400 000/µl		
Leucocytes	4 000–10 000/µl		

Differential white cell count		Percentage	Absolute
Neutrophils	Segmented	40–70	2 000–7 000
	stab cells	5–15	200–800
Eosinophils		2–10	100–600
Basophils		0–1	0–100
Lymphocytes		20–40	1 500–5 000
Monocytes		2–10	100–800

Iron metabolism

Transported from duodenum/jejunum to erythropoietic sites by **transferrin** (transport protein).
Superfluous iron is stored by binding to **iron storage protein** (ferritin).

Daily iron loss $\qquad\qquad$ = 1 mg/day; 2 ml blood ~ 1 mg Fe

Minimal daily iron $\qquad\;\;$ = 12 mg/day (normal absorption 10–20%, absorption during
requirement for adults $\qquad$ pregnancy ca. 40%)

Loss during menstruation $\;$ ~ 15–45 mg; in pregnancy ~ 300–400 mg

(1 unit stored red cells = 200 mg iron)

Important laboratory parameters for iron metabolism

Ferritin		(Normal **15–200 ng/ml**) correlated with total body iron
	↓	Iron deficiency anaemia
Normal	↑	Anaemia of chronic illness (tumour, infection, renal, chronic polyarthritis)
	↑	Liver disorders, pernicious anaemia, leukaemia
	↑↑↑	Haemochromatosis, liver necrosis, iron infusion

Transferrin: behaves in reciprocal fashion to ferritin (raised in iron deficiency)
Oral iron replacement is treatment of choice
Only ferrous iron (Fe^{2+}). Sulphate salts are well absorbed (absorption about 20% of the administered amount, preferably taken fasting): because of side effects 100 mg once, later 100 mg twice daily orally (after ca. 10 days reticulocytes ↑, Hb rise daily ca. 0.1–0.2 g%). After correction of blood count continue 50–100 mg daily for a further 2 months to replenish iron stores. Parenteral iron therapy very rarely.

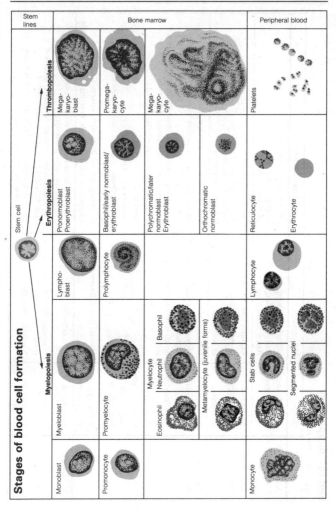

Stages of blood cell formation

Red cell morphology

(After Wintrobe et al. (1981))

	Description	Morphology	Clinical significance
Alteration of coloration	Anisochromia Polychromasia	Differing staining Basophil shading Basophil stippling	Possible in all anaemias Young erythrocytes Lead poisoning
Alterations in size	Anisocytosis Macrocytes Microcytes	Erythrocytes of different sizes Ø over 8.5 µm Ø below 7 µm	Pernicious anaemia Accelerated erythropoiesis Macrocytic anaemia Microcytic anaemia
Alterations in shape	Poikilocytosis Target cells Acanthocytes Elliptocytes Crenated cells Sickle cells Spherocytes Schistocytes Stomatocytes	Different shapes Hypochromia with central pigmentation Small spikes on the red cell surface Helmet forms, fragmentation	Sign of disordered erthropoiesis Microcytic anaemia, post-splenectomy, cirrhosis of liver Abetalipoproteinaemia, uraemia, liver disorders with haemolysis, pyruvate kinase deficiency Elliptocytosis, megaloblastic anaemia Artefact due to drying Sickle cell anaemia Spherocytosis, acquired autoimmune haemolytic anaemia Microangiopathic haemolytic anaemia Alcoholic hepatic cirrhosis, hereditary stomatocytosis
Inclusions	Siderocytes Heinz bodies Howell–Jolly bodies	Iron granules Haemoglobin denaturation products Nuclear remnants	Sideroblastic anaemia, pernicious anaemia, post-splenectomy, lead poisoning Post-splenectomy, phenacetin abuse, glucose-6-phosphate dehydrogenase deficiency Post-splenectomy, myelofibrosis, erythroleukaemia, megaloblastic anaemia

Investigation of anaemia

Reticulocytes	Smear	Bone marrow	Other tests	Diagnosis
Normal	Hypochromic	No iron	$\downarrow$ Fe; $\downarrow$ ferritin	Iron deficiency
		Ring sideroblasts	$\uparrow$ HBA$_2$, $\uparrow$ HBF $\downarrow$ HBA$_2$	β-thalassaemia Sideroblastic anaemia
	Macrocytic	Megaloblastic	$\downarrow$ B$_{12}$	B$_{12}$ deficiency
			$\downarrow$ B$_{12}$; achlorhydria	Pernicious anaemia
			$\downarrow$ Fe; $\uparrow$ ferritin	Chronic inflammation
			$\uparrow$ Creatinine	Uraemia
			Disturbed liver function	Liver disease
			$\downarrow$ T$_4$	Hypothyroidism
		Aplastic		Panmyelopathy
	Normoblasts	Infiltration		Disseminated malignancy
		Fibrosis	$\uparrow$ Leucine aminopeptidase	Myelofibrosis
Increased	Spherocytes	Erythroid hyperplasia	+ve Coombs' test	Autoimmune haemolytic anaemia
			$\uparrow$ Osmotic fragility	Hereditary spherocytosis
	–		Internal/urogenital bleeding	Anaemia of bleeding
	Heinz bodies		Altered Hb electrophoresis	Heinz body anaemia
	Heinz bodies		G-6-PDH	Enzyme deficiency
	Polychromasia		+ve Sucrose test	Paroxysmal nocturnal haemoglobinuria
	Sickle cells		+ve Sickling test	Sickle cell anaemia
	Target cells		Altered Hb electrophoresis	HbC, D and others
	Schistocytes			Traumatic haemolysis
	Acanthocytes		Disturbed liver function	Abetalipopro- teinaemia, liver disease

(Modified after Franklin Bunn (1983))

Diagnostic criteria of polycythaemia vera
(After the guidelines of the Polycythemia Vera Study Group)

A1. Red cell mass $\uparrow$ ($\male$ >36 ml/kg) ($\female$ >32 ml/kg)	**B1.** Thrombocytosis (>400 000/µl)
A2. O$_2$ saturation >92%	**B2.** Leucocytosis (>12 000/µl)
A3. Splenomegaly	**B3.** LAP* $\uparrow$ or vitamin B$_{12}$ $\uparrow$
Diagnosis confirmed when **A1 + A2 + A3** or **A1 + A2 + 2B criteria** are fulfilled	

Coombs' test

Direct Coombs' test

Diagnostic test (when positive, perform indirect Coombs' test). Indication of incomplete antibodies bound to patient's red cells.

Red cell with bound antibodies (washed) + Coombs' serum = Agglutination (bivalent antibodies against human globulin)

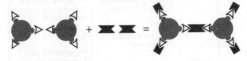

Indirect Coombs' test

Indication of antibodies circulating in patient

Serum with incomplete antibodies to be tested + Red cells with known antigen = Binding of antibodies to test red cells

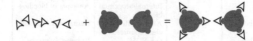

Occurs in:

Acquired haemolytic anaemias, after transfusion reactions, in leukaemia, lymphoma, systemic lupus erythematosus, primary chronic polyarthritis, CMV infection, infectious mononucleosis, viral pneumonia, therapy with penicillin, methyldopa; haemolytic disease of the newborn (infant: direct Coombs' test positive; mother: indirect Coombs' test positive).

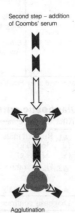

Second step – addition of Coombs' serum

Agglutination

Differential diagnosis of enlarged lymph nodes

Infection
Streptococcal, staphylococcal and *Salmonella* infection, tuberculosis, brucellosis, syphilis, mononucleosis, cytomegalovirus infection, hepatitis, rubella, malaria, toxoplasmosis, histoplasmosis, coccidioidomycosis

Systemic illnesses
Rheumatoid arthritis, SLE, dermatomyositis, sarcoidosis

Neoplasia
Lymphomas, chronic lymphatic leukaemia, myeloproliferative syndrome, acute leukaemia, histiocytosis; metastases from breast, bronchus, ENT and urogenital tumours

Endocrine
Hyperthyroidism, Addison's disease

Others
Serum sickness, hydantoin reaction, lymph node hyperplasia, histiocytosis, dermatopathic lymphadenitis, Gaucher's disease, Niemann–Pick disease

---

Differential diagnosis of splenomegaly

Infection
Endocarditis, TB, brucellosis, mononucleosis, cytomegalovirus infection, syphilis, malaria, histoplasmosis, schistosomiasis, kala-azar

Systemic illnesses
Rheumatoid arthritis, Felty's syndrome, SLE

Neoplasia
Lymphomas, CLL, myeloproliferative syndrome, acute leukaemia, histiocytosis

Haematological
Spherocytosis, autoimmune haemolytic anaemia, haemoglobinopathies, angioimmunoblastic lymphadenopathy with dysproteinaemia (AILD)

Congestion
Hepatic cirrhosis, portal vein/splenic vein thrombosis, extramedullary erythropoiesis, vinyl chloride

Metabolic
Amyloidosis, Gaucher's disease, Niemann–Pick disease

Others
Abscess, cysts, haemangiomas, aneurysms

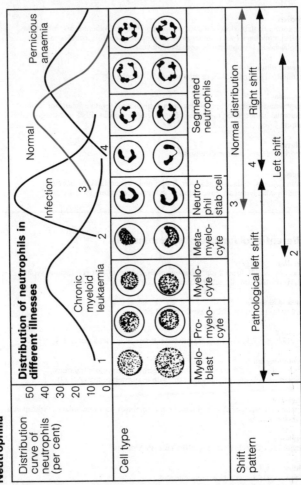

Neutrophilia

Distribution curve of neutrophils (per cent): 50, 40, 30, 20, 10, 0

Distribution of neutrophils in different illnesses

Pernicious anaemia

Normal

Infection

Chronic myeloid leukaemia

1, 2, 3, 4

Cell type: Myelo-blast | Pro-myelo-cyte | Myelo-cyte | Meta-myelo-cyte | Neutro-phil stab cell | Segmented neutrophils

Shift pattern: Pathological left shift | Left shift | Normal distribution | Right shift

1, 2, 3, 4

(Modified after Haden (1935))

Leukaemia

Leukaemia type	Acute		Chronic	
	Lymphoblastic leukaemia (ALL)	Myeloid leukaemia (AML)	Lymphocytic leukaemia (CLL)	Myeloid leukaemia (CML)
Age	Children 85% Adults 15%	Adults 82% Children 10%	Over 50 years	25–45 years
Incidence per 100 000	2–3	2–3	Below 50 years 5 Over 60 years 20	Over 60 years 3
Blood count Leucocytes	Lymphoblasts Leukaemic hiatus	Myeloblasts Leukaemic hiatus	↑↑ Lymphocytes	↑↑ All maturation stages
Platelets	↓↓	↓↓	n↓	n↑
Erythrocytes	Anaemia	Anaemia	Anaemia	Anaemia
Others		Auer rods	Gumprecht's nuclear shadow	↓↓ Leucocyte alkaline phosphatase Philadelphia chromosome
Therapy	**Emergency** admission to treatment centre Urgent cytoreductive therapy		Treat according to stage (see below)	1. Leucocytes should be <20 000 (e.g. chlorambucil) 2. Introduction to a treatment cantre

FAB classification of acute leukaemias (French–American–British Cooperative Group (1976))

Acute lymphoblastic leukaemia
L-1 Acute lymphoblastic leukaemia in children, homogeneous cell population
L-2 Acute lymphoblastic leukaemia in adults, heterogeneous cell population
L-3 Leukaemia resembling Burkitt's lymphoma, large cells, homogeneous cell population

Acute myeloblastic leukaemia
M-1 Little granulocytic differentiation, no maturation
M-2 Granulocytic differentiation with promyelocytes
M-3 Granulocytic differentiation with hypergranular promyelocytes (often disseminated intravascular coagulation (DIC))
M-4 Myelomonocytic differentiation
M-5 Monocytic cells of differing degrees of differentiation
M-6 Predominantly erythroblasts with severe dyserythropoiesis
M-7 Acute megakaryocytic leukaemia (acute myelofibrosis)

Myelodysplastic syndrome

Definition: Maturation defect of myelopoiesis with, usually, normo- to hypercellular marrow and ineffective haemopoiesis (thrombopenia and/or leucopenia)

Classification	Abbreviation	Peripheral blood count	Marrow
Refractory anaemia	RA	Anaemia, reticulocytopenia, dyserythropoiesis, dysgranulopoiesis, blasts <1%	Normo- or hypercellularity, predominant dyserythropoiesis, blasts <5%
Refractory anaemia with ringed sideroblasts	RAS	As RA	As RA and: >15% sideroblasts in marrow
Refractory anaemia with excess of blasts	RAEB	At least bilinear cytopenia, blasts <5%	Hypercellularity. Blasts 5–20%
Refractory anaemia with excess of blasts in transformation	RAEB-t	RAEB criteria and >5% blasts	Either 20–30% blasts or Auer rods
Chronic myelomonocytic leukaemia	CMML	Monocytes >1000/µl Blasts <5%	As in RA or RAEB: blasts up to 20%. Increase in monocyte precursors

Therapy: supportive (erythrocyte and/or platelet transfusions).

Hodgkin's lymphoma

Clinical staging (Ann Arbor classification)

I: Involvement of a single lymph node region or of a single extralymphatic organ or site

II: Two or more lymph node regions, or lymph node regions and one extralymphatic organ on the **same** side of the diaphragm

III: Lymph node regions on both sides of the diaphragm, involvement of one extralymphatic organ or splenic involvement possible

IV: Diffuse extralymphatic organ involvement

E: Extranodal involvement

S: Splenic involvement

A: No general symptoms

B: General symptoms:
     Fever above 38°C (Pel-Ebstein), night sweats, loss of weight (more than 10% of body weight in 6 months)

Histological classification

Lymphocyte predominant, giant cell deficient, nodular sclerosing, mixed cellularity, lymphocyte depleted, giant cell rich.

Staging of CLL after Rai (1975)

Stage	Definition
0	Lymphocytosis >15000/mm³ Bone marrow infiltration >40%
I	Lymphocytosis and adenopathy
II	Lymphocytosis and hepatomegaly and/or splenomegaly (with or without adenopathy)
III	Lymphocytosis and anaemia (Hb <110g/l) (with or without adenopathy and/or organomegaly)
IV	Lymphocytosis and thrombocytopenia (<100000/mm³) (with or without anaemia, adenopathy, organomegaly)

Therapy: from stage III and/or with **symptomatic** lymphomas

Kiel classification of non-Hodgkin's lymphoma

Low malignancy grade

Lymphocytic
- B cell
- T cell
- Hairy cell leukaemia
- Mycosis fungoides/Sézary syndrome
- T zone lymphoma

Lymphoplasmocytic/cytoid (LP-immunocytoma)
Plasmocytic
Centrocytic
Centroblastic/centrocytic
Unclassified (low malignancy)

High malignancy grade

Centroblastic
Lymphoblastic
- B lymphoblastic, Burkitt type and others
- T lymphoblastic, convoluted cell type and others
- Unclassified

Immunoblastic
- with plasmoblastic/plasmocytic differentiation (B-immunoblastic)
- without plasmoblastic/plasmocytic differentiation (B- or T-immunoblastic)

Unclassified (high malignancy)

Clinical staging of plasmacytoma

(After Durie and Salmon)

Stage	Criteria	Tumour cell mass/m² body surface
I	All of the following: 1. Hb >100 g/l 2. Serum Ca normal (≤10.5 mmol/l) 3. Radiologically normal bony skeleton; or only a single solitary plasmacytoma localized in bone 4. Low concentration of paraprotein a) IgG <50 g/l b) IgA <30 g/l c) Light chains in urine <4 g/24 h	$<0.6 \times 10^{12}$
II	Not fitting into either stage I or stage III	$0.6–1.2 \times 10^{12}$
III	One or more of the following: 1. Hb <85 g/l 2. Serum Ca >8.5 mmol/l 3. Advanced osteolytic bone changes 4. High concentration of paraprotein a) IgG >70 g/l b) IgA >50 g/l c) Light chains in urine >12 g/24 h	$>1.2 \times 10^{12}$
Subclassification:	A Relatively normal renal function: serum creatinine <180 µmol/l B Impaired renal function: serum creatinine ≥180 µmol/l	

Therapy: from stage II and/or for local problems (e.g. danger of fracture)

Types of allergic reactions (After Coombs and Gell)

Type	Time	Agent	Illnesses
I Immediate anaphylaxis	Minutes	IgE	Anaphylaxis (shock), bronchial asthma, allergic rhinitis, urticaria, angioneurotic oedema
II Cytotoxic	4–8h	IgG (IgM)	Transfusion reaction, autoimmune haemolytic anaemia, Goodpasture's syndrome
III Immune complex	4–8h	IgG (IgA, IgM)	Serum sickness, allergic alveolitis, vasculitis, systemic lupus erythematosus, glomerulonephritis
IV Late type, cell mediated	24–72h	T cells	Tuberculin reaction, contact eczema, transplant rejection, chronic hepatitis

Assessment of immune system illnesses

(After Lawton and Cooper (1983))

	T cell system	B cell system
History	Fatigue, deterioration of general condition, fever, infections, loss of weight	
	Reaction against nettles, atypical infections, chronic diarrhoea	Reaction against vaccinations
Laboratory (simple)	ESR, red and white cell counts, chest X-ray, immunoelectrophoresis, complement C3, C4, CH50	
	Skin test (multitest: diphtheria, tetanus, streptococcal, tuberculin, *Candida*, *Trichophyton*, *Proteus*, glycerine)	Antibodies against rubella, influenza, tetanus, diphtheria
Laboratory (specialized)	T lymphocyte count, surface markers, lymph node biopsy	B lymphocyte count, membrane markers (for γ-globulins, C3, Epstein–Barr virus) Immunofluorescence investigation of bone marrow, lymph node biopsy

Anaphylaxis

Classification of anaphylactic/anaphylactoid reactions by degree of severity
(After Ring and Messmer (1977))

Grade	Skin	Abdomen	Respiratory tract	Heart circulation
I		–	–	–
II	Itching Flush Urticaria Angioneurotic oedema	Nausea Cramps	Rhinorrhoea Hoarseness Dyspnoea	Tachycardia ($\Delta > 20$/min) Hypotension ($\Delta > 20$ mmHg systolic) Arrhythmia
III	(not obligatory)	Vomiting Defecation	Laryngeal oedema Bronchospasm Cyanosis	Shock
IV			Respiratory arrest	Cardiac arrest

Emergency measures in anaphylactic/anaphylactoid reaction of different degrees of severity

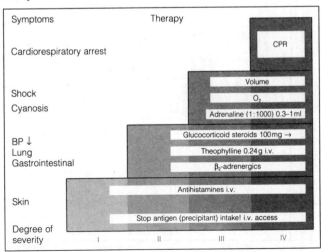

Haemorrhagic diatheses

		Vasculopathy	Thrombopathy	Coagulopathy
Illnesses	Hereditary	Osler–Rendu–Weber syndrome Ehlers–Danlos syndrome Cavernous haemangioma	Glanzmann's disease Giant thrombopathies Thrombocytopenia	Haemophilia A/B (I) Von Willebrand's disease (I) Coagulation factor deficiency (E + I) Afibrinogenaemia
	Acquired	Drug toxicity With infections (e.g. meningococcal) Metabolic (Cushing's disease, vitamin C deficiency, corticosteroid treatment) Autoimmune (Henoch–Schönlein's purpura)	Idiopathic thrombocytopenic purpura (ITP) (Werlhof's disease) Drugs (Acetylsalicylic acid, dipyridamole phenylbutazone sulphinpyrazone heparin) Uraemia	Anticoagulant bleeding (E + I) Fibrinolytic therapy (I) Liver diseases Vitamin K deficiency (E + I) Disseminated intravascular coagulopathy (DIC)
Symptoms	Petechiae	++	+++	–
	Haematomata	++	+++	++
	Epistaxis	+++	+++	++
	Gastrointestinal bleeding	+++	+++	++
	Menorrhagia	(+)	+++	(+)
	Haematuria	–/+	+	+++
	Visceral haematomata	–	–	+++
	Haemarthroses	–		+
	Cerebral haemorrhage	–/+	+++	+++
	Post-traumatic bleeding		+++	+++
	Postoperative bleeding			+++
	Positive tourniquet test	n/path.	path.	n
Laboratory				Extrinsic (E) — Intrinsic (I)
	Platelets	n	n/↓	n — n
	Quick's test	n	n	path. — n
	PTT	n	n	n — path.
	Bleeding time	n/↑↑	↑↑	n/↑ — n ↑
	Clotting time	n	n	n — ↑

I, disturbance of intravascular coagulation; E; disturbance of extravascular coagulation.

Coagulation cascade

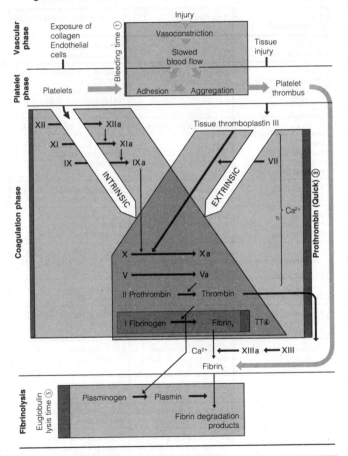

Coagulation tests: ① Bleeding time, ② PTT, ③ Prothrombin time (Quick), ④ Thrombin time (TT), ⑤ Euglobulin lysis time

Coagulation tests

Test (normal values)	Test function	Causes of abnormal test result
Platelets 150 000–400 000		Thrombocytosis Thrombocytopenia
Quick's test (Thromboplastin time, prothrombin time) 70–100%	Global test of extrinsic system, control of coumarin therapy	Deficiency or inhibition of I, II, V, VII, X. Vitamin K deficiency. Anticoagulation with coumarins, liver diseases
PTT Partial thromboplastin time Standard: 68–82s Activated: 11–15s (method dependent)	Global test of intrinsic system	Deficiency or inhibition of I, II, V, VIII, IX, X, XI, XII. Vitamin K deficiency, anticoagulation with coumarins
Thrombin time 13–17s	Control of heparin therapy	Afibrinogenaemia, thrombin inhibitors, heparin therapy
Bleeding time Ivy: 1–9min Duke: 1–4min	Global test of platelet function	Thrombocytopenia, von Willebrand's disease, thrombasthenia, aspirin
Clotting time Lee-White: 8–18min	Global test of extrinsic and common coagulation systems	Factor deficiency (less than 3%): I, II, V, VIII, IX, X, XI, XII
Coagulation factors 50–200% of normal		Hereditary deficiency, liver diseases, DIC
Fibrinogen 150–450mg% 1.5–4.5g/l		Afibrinogenaemia, DIC, infections
Fibrinogen degradation products (FDP) Over 8mg/ml	Semiquantitative latex demonstration of FDP (X, Y, D, E)	DIC, fibrinolytic therapy, liver diseases
Ethanol test	Demonstration of fibrin monomer	DIC, fibrinolytic therapy
Euglobulin lysis time Over 2 hours	Global test of fibrinolytic activity	DIC, fibrinolytic therapy, liver diseases
Reptilase time 18–22s	Heparin independent: demonstration of DIC in heparinized patient	Prolonged with fibrin–fibrinogen degradation products: DIC

DIC, disseminated intravascular coagulation.

Coagulation factors (cf. p. 217)

Factor	Synonyms	Site of action in coagulation system	Illnesses
I	Fibrinogen	Common	Afibrinogenaemia
II	Prothrombin	Common	Vitamin K deficiency, liver disease
III	Tissue thromboplastin	Extrinsic	
IV	Calcium ions	Universal	
V	Labile factor, proaccelerin	Common	Hereditary deficiency
VII	Proconvertin	Extrinsic	Vitamin K deficiency, liver disease, hereditary
VIII	Antihaemophilic factor	Intrinsic	Haemophilia A
IX	Christmas factor (antihaemophilic factor B)	Intrinsic	Haemophilia B (Christmas disease), vitamin K deficiency, liver diseases
X	Stuart Prower factor	Common	Vitamin K deficiency, liver disease, hereditary
XI	Plasma thromboplastin antecedent (PTA)	Intrinsic	Hereditary
XII	Hagemann factor	Intrinsic	Hereditary
XIII	Fibrin stabilizing factor	Common	Hereditary

Drugs affecting coagulation and their antidotes in the coagulation system

Drug	Antidote
Heparin Main action: antithrombin. Inactivates: IIa, IX, X; inhibits the conversion of prothrombin to thrombin. Develops its activity in the presence of heparin cofactor (antithrombin III). Short half life	Protamine
Coumarins Main action: vitamin K antagonist. Inactivates: II, VII, IX, X. Long half life	Vitamin K_1 Is used in liver for synthesis of factors II, VII, IX, X
Fibrinolytics **Streptokinase, Urokinase, t-PA, APSAC** Main action: promote the conversion of plasminogen to plasmin	Antifibrinolytics Tranexamic axid (AMCA) Main action: inhibits the activation of plasminogen

Thromboembolism

Clinical risk factors for venous thromboembolism	Congenital, in part also acquired disturbances of the haemostatic and fibrinolytic systems which can cause increased tendency to thrombosis
Age (>40 years)	Antithrombin III deficiency (type I defect) or abnormal AT III molecule (type II defect)
Surgery (dependent on nature and duration of operation, esp. hip surgery!)	Protein C deficiency
Trauma, burns	Protein S deficiency Dysfibrinogenaemia Factor XII deficiency Plasminogen deficiency/abnormal plasminogen
Immobilization (confinement to bed; e.g. also immobilization of limb in plaster, or long car/air journeys)	
Malignancy	Diminished fibrinolytic capacity due to a) reduced liberation of tissue plasminogen activator (t-PA) from the vessel wall or b) increased plasma activity of the plasminogen activator inhibitors (PAI)
Previous venous thrombosis	
Varicose veins	
Obesity	
Pareses and paralyses of legs	Appearance of a lupus anticoagulant[a]
Oral contraceptives (oestrogen content)	[a] The designation anticoagulant is misleading and refers to the *in vitro* inhibitory activity of this immunoglobulin on clotting. Patients more commonly develop a tendency to thrombosis than to bleeding.
Pregnancy, puerperium	

(After Kienast and van de Loo (1991))

Thrombolytics

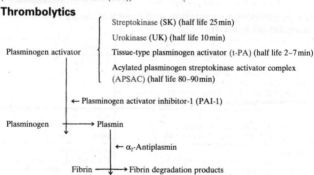

Plasminogen activator
- Streptokinase (SK) (half life 25 min)
- Urokinase (UK) (half life 10 min)
- Tissue-type plasminogen activator (t-PA) (half life 2–7 min)
- Acylated plasminogen streptokinase activator complex (APSAC) (half life 80–90 min)

← Plasminogen activator inhibitor-1 (PAI-1)

Plasminogen ──→ Plasmin

← α_2-Antiplasmin

Fibrin ──→ Fibrin degradation products

Scheme of the fibrinolytic systems

Standardization of thromboplastins; INR/Quick's test

Calculation of the International Normalized Ratio for therapy control under stable anticoagulation with vitamin K antagonists
(After Kienast and van de Loo (1991))

$$INI = R^{ISI}$$

INR International Normalized Ratio
R Quotient from thromboplastin time (prothrombin time) of the patient's plasma divided by thromboplastin time of a normal plasma pool (usually commercial calibration or standard human plasma)
ISI International Sensitivity Index
This index is determined by the manufacturer for the respective thromboplastin batch by calibration against an international reference thromboplastin

If a thromboplastin with a sensitivity factor of 1.1 (e.g. Thromborel S) is used, the INR range of 2.0–3.0 is equivalent to a Quick's test value of 24–48%

Thromboplastins

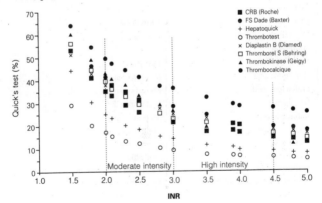

Oral anticoagulants – interfering factors

Enhancement of activity (Quick's test falls, danger of bleeding)	**Reduction** of activity (Quick's test rises, inadequate protection against thrombosis)
Drugs:	**Drugs:**
Allopurinol	Activated charcoal
Amiodarone	Acetylcholine
Anabolic steroids	ACTH
Antibiotics (oral)	Adrenaline
Aperients, especially those containing paraffin	Antithyroid drugs
	Atropine
Aspirin[a]	**Barbiturates**[a]
Azapropazone[a]	Biguanides
Bezafibrate	**Carbamazepine**
Carbamazepine	Cholestyramine
Chloral hydrate[b]	**Contraceptives** (oral)
Chloramphenicol	(Digitalis)
Chlorpropamide	(Diuretics)
Cimetidine	Ganglion blockers
Clofibrate	**Glutethimide**
Dextran preparations	Griseofulvin
Disulfiram	Haloperidol[b]
Ergot alkaloids	**Laxatives**
Ethacrynic acid	Meprobamate
Flufenamic acid[a]	Mercaptopurine
Glucagon	Metformin
Indomethacin[a]	Metronidazole
Local anaesthetics	Multivitamin preparations
Mefenamic acid[a]	Neuroleptics[b]
Methyldopa	**Penicillins**
Metronidazole	**Phenytoin** (with prolonged treatment)
Monoamine oxidase inhibitors	Propylthiouracil
Nalidixic acid	Purine derivatives
	Rifampicin
	Steroids[a]
	Strophanthin (ouabain)

Enhancement of activity (Quick's test falls, danger of bleeding)	Reduction of activity (Quick's test rises, inadequate protection against thrombosis)
Naproxen	
Neomycin	
Nicotinic acid derivatives	
Nortriptyline	Vitamin K (preparations)
Oxyphenbutazone[a]	
Phenothiazine preparations	**Foodstuffs containing large amounts of vitamin K***
Phenylbutazone[a]	(>0.1 mg vitamin K/100 g):
Phenytoin (at start of therapy)	Spinach (3–4.6)
Piroxicam	Cabbage, sauerkraut
Probenecid	Tomatoes (0.4–0.8)
Propafenone	(Pig's) liver (0.4–0.8) offal
Quinine, quinidine	Soya beans, also bean sprouts (0.2)
Ranitidine	Bean (0.3), peas (ca. 0.3)
Salicylates[a]	Pork and other meats (ca. 0.2)
Sulphinpyrazone	Sunflower seed oil (ca. 0.5)
Sulphonamides	
Sulphonylureas	* also dependent on fat consumption; avoid excessively fatty foods
Thyroid hormones (thyroxine, triiodothyronine)	
Tolbutamide	
Tricyclic antidepressants	
Others:	**Others:**
Alcoholism	Obesity
Hepatic illness of other types	Hypothyroidism, myxoedema
Gall bladder disease	
Fever	
Heart failure with hepatic congestion	
Hyperthyroidism	
Old age	
Malabsorption	
Radiotherapy	

Alternative drugs:

[a] **Analgesics:** paracetamol, centrally acting analgesics;
  Antirheumatic agents: diclofenac, sulindac, ketoprofen, tolmetin.

[b] **Hypnotics:** diazepam, flurazepam, nitrazepam.

Blood replacement

	Fresh blood	Plasma-depleted blood	Concentrated red cells	Platelet concentrate	FFP
Definition	Whole blood	Whole blood (minus 100 ml plasma)	Concentrated red cells (minus 200 ml plasma)	Platelet concentrate pooled from 4–6 donors	Fresh frozen plasma
Indication	Not used in practice: single preparations preferred	Major haemorrhage	RBC replacement (little circulatory load) Hct rise/ concentrate: 2–3%	Bleeding with thrombocytopenia	Bleeding with deficiency of clotting factors, anticoagulants or DIC
Hct	40 ± 7%	47 ± 3%	70 ± 10%		
Volume	500 ml	400 ml	300 ml	250 ± 50 ml	250 ± 50 ml

Procedure in case of transfusion reaction
- Repeated typing of donor and recipient blood
- Detection of free Hb, haemoglobinuria, haptoglobin fall
- Hyperbilirubinaemia, search for intravascular coagulation

Complications of blood transfusion
- Cooling, air embolism, hypervolaemia
- Citrate intoxication, hyperkalaemia, acidosis
- Contamination with bacteria, viruses, parasites

Exclusion criteria for own blood donation

1. Hb below 120 g/l

2. Poor general condition, signs of hypovolaemia

3. Acute infection

4. Less than 48 h before surgery

5. 24 h after contrast medium administration

6. Further invasive measures on day of own blood donation

7. Tendency to convulsion: epilepsy

8. Haematological illnesses: e.g. leukaemia, autoimmune haemolytic anaemia

9. Manifest cardiac failure

10. Myocardial infarct within last 3 months (time interval dependent on general condition and cardiac catheterization findings)

11. Aortic stenosis (moderate to severe)

12. Unstable angina pectoris

13. Severe arrhythmias: bradycardia

(Johannesson *et al.* 1990)

Basic tumour therapy

Preconditions for all tumour therapy

- **Confirmation of diagnosis**
  Histology? Stage? Prognosis?

- **Assessment of progress**
  Measurable parameters (X-ray, ultrasound, markers)? Side effects?

- **Treatment strategy**
  Curative? Aggressive to total remission; 2 consolidation treatments; but: change of therapy if failure of response!
  Palliative? Low side effects, aimed at symptoms
  Modality? Local (surgery, radiotherapy)? Systemic?

- **No contraindication**

Clinical trial of cytostatic agents

Phase I	Determination of maximum tolerable dose
Phase II	Determination of toxicity **and** effectiveness of a drug for **one** tumour type
Phase III	Comparison with established therapy

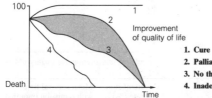

1. Cure
2. Palliative therapy
3. No therapy
4. Inadequate therapy

Definitions of response of solid tumours to therapy

Definition	Measurable disease	Non-measurable disease	Bony metastases
Complete response **(CR)**	Disappearance of all known manifestations of disease for at least 4 weeks	Disappearance of all known manifestations of disease for at least 4 weeks	Complete disappearance of all lesions on X-ray or bone scintigram for at least 4 weeks
Partial response **(PR)**	Reduction of measurable tumour mass by at least 50% for at least 4 weeks. No new lesions or progression of a solitary lesion	Estimated reduction of tumour mass by at least 50% in 4 weeks	Partial size reduction of lytic lesions, recalcification of lytic lesions, density reduction of sclerotic lesion for at least 4 weeks
No change **(NC)**	PR and PD criteria not fulfilled	PR and PD criteria not fulfilled	An assessment is only possible after 8 weeks
Progressive disease **(PD)**	Enlargement by at least 25% or appearance of new lesions	Estimated enlargement by at least 25% or appearance of new lesions	Enlargement of existing lesions, appearance of new lesions

(After Miller, Hoogstraten, Staquet and Winkler (1981))

Prognoses

Curable tumours (10–20% of all neoplasms)

Tumour	Complete remissions (%)	% Survival after ⩾ 5 years
Chorioncarcinoma (women)	80–90	80–90
Testicular carcinoma	90–90	75–90
Acute lymphatic leukaemia (< 20 years)	90–90	50–90
Hodgkin's disease III–IV	80–90	50–80
Burkitt's lymphoma III–IV	80–90	50–70
Non-Hodgkin's lymphoma II–IV	70–90	30–40
Acute myeloid leukaemia	70–90	10–20
Small cell carcinoma of bronchus	60–90	⩽ 10

Palliative therapy with prolongation of life (ca. 40% of all neoplasms)

Tumour	Response rate (%)	Mean survival time with remission (years)
Chronic leukaemias (CML, CLL)	90–100	3–5
Carcinoma of prostate	70–80	2–3
Multiple myeloma	60–70	2–3
Carcinoma of breast	60–70	2
Carcinoma of ovary, FIGO III–IV	60–70	1–2
Carcinoma of endometrium	50	1–2
Sarcoma of supporting tissue	40	1(–2)
Squamous carcinoma of ENT region	50	1–2

Palliative chemotherapy without increased survival, but improvement in quality of life (ca. 30% of all tumours)

Tumour	Remission rate (%)	Mean survival time with remission (months)
Adenocarcinoma of stomach	40(–50)	10–12
Urothelial carcinoma	40(–50)	8–10
Non-small cell carcinoma of bronchus	30(–40)	8–12
Carcinoma of adrenal cortex	30–40	8–12
Other carcinomas of gastrointestinal tract	20(–30)	6–8
Malignant melanoma	20–40	6–8
Squamous carcinoma in gynaecological region	(10–)20	5–6

Tumours hardly responsive to chemotherapy

Tumour (inoperable, metastasizing)	Partial remission rate
Carcinoma of kidney	10–25%
Primary CNS tumours (except medulloblastoma)	10–20%
Carcinoma of liver	10–20%
Slow-growing sarcomata (e.g. chondrosarcoma)	10%
Anaplastic carcinoma of thyroid	10–20%

(After Handschuh and Diehl (1986))

Early warning symptoms of tumours

- Loss of weight (>10%)
- Frequent attacks of fever
- Alteration of bowel or bladder habit; frequent digestive disturbances
- Persistent hoarseness, intractable (bloody) cough
- Persistent dysphagia
- Changes in warts or naevi
- Bleeding or discharge from body orifices (extramenstrual bleeding)
- Development of lumps or hardening (breast, testicular swelling, etc.)
- Non-healing wounds; persistent swellings

Tumour markers

Employment	Aftercare
Diagnostic:	• Within follow-up programme (e.g. quarterly)
• In symptomatic patients	• Postoperative after curative resection
• Supervision of risk groups	• Prior to extensive therapeutic measures
• Not in asymptomatic partients	• Before change of therapy
	• In case of unclear changes in clinical picture
	• With renewed staging

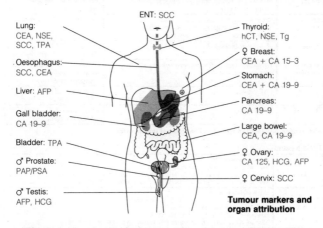

ENT: SCC

Lung:
CEA, NSE,
SCC, TPA

Oesophagus:
SCC, CEA

Liver: AFP

Gall bladder:
CA 19–9

Bladder: TPA

♂ Prostate:
PAP/PSA

♂ Testis:
AFP, HCG

Thyroid:
hCT, NSE, Tg

♀ Breast:
CEA + CA 15–3

Stomach:
CEA + CA 19–9

Pancreas:
CA 19–9

Large bowel:
CEA, CA 19–9

♀ Ovary:
CA 125, HCG, AFP

♀ Cervix: SCC

**Tumour markers and
organ attribution**

SCC, squamous cell carcinoma antigen; CEA, carcinoembryonic antigen; NSE, neuron-specific enolase; TPA, tissue polypeptide antigen; hCT, human calcitonin; Tg, thyroglobulin; AFP, alpha-fetoprotein; HCG, human chorionic gonadotrophin; PAP, prostatic acid phosphatase; PSA, prostate-specific antigen; ENT, tumours in ENT region

(After Lamerz (1986))

Tumour staging

Tumour	Tissue identification (non-operative)/laboratory (Tumour markers see p. 227)	X-ray/ultrasound (MRI indications cf. pp. 45–7)
Lung	Sputum cytology, bronchoscopy with biopsy, trans-thoracic biopsy, mediastinoscopy, pleural biopsy, tapping of pleural effusion, lung function tests, blood gas analysis, cf. p. 128	CT thorax CT skull Bone scintigram Sonogram
Breast	Biopsy/hormone receptors, lymph node biopsy	Mammography, chest X-ray, sonogram, bone scintigram
Prostate	Transrectal biopsy, cystoscopy, prostate-specific acid phosphatase	IVU, X-ray pelvis, bone scintigram, transrectal sonography
Oesophagus	Endoscopy + biopsy, mediastinoscopy	CT thorax, barium swallow
Stomach	Endoscopy + biopsy (laparotomy), stool occult blood	Ultrasound, chest X-ray, CT abdomen
Colon	Endoscopy + biopsy (laparotomy), stool occult blood	Ultrasound, CT abdomen
Pancreas	Needle biopsy	Barium enema ultrasound, CT abdomen, ERCP (i.v. cholangiogram)
Liver	Laparoscopy + biopsy, hepatitis serology	Ultrasound, CT abdomen
Lymph nodes	Lymph node biopsy, biopsy with contrast medium, liver biopsy, laparotomy, possibly splenectomy, lymphocyte typing	CT thorax, CT abdomen, lymphography, skeletal scintigraphy
Ovary, uterus	Laparoscopy + biopsy, cervical smear, cytology of washings, curettage, proctoscopy, possibly oophoropexy, hormone receptors	Ultrasound, CT abdomen (IVU)
Testes	(Testicular biopsy)	CT pelvis, CT thorax, CT skull, lymphography
Kidney, bladder	Urine cytology, cystoscopy, proctoscopy, erythropoietin	Ultrasound, IVU, chest X-ray, CT abdomen, cavogram, arteriography
CNS	CSF cytology	CT skull, cerebral arteriography
Thyroid	Needle biopsy	Chest X-ray, radioiodine uptake, ultrasound

Aim: Staging: histological diagnosis and recording of tumour extent

TNM System

T	Primary tumour size
Tis	Non-invasive carcinoma (carcinoma *in situ*)
T1, T2, T3, T4	Increasing size and extent of the primary tumour (all sizes in 2 dimensions)
TX	Minimal requirements for assessment of primary tumour not fulfilled

N	Regional lymph nodes
N0	No evidence of regional lymph node involvement
N1, N2, N3	Regional lymph node involvement
N4	Involvement of juxtaregional lymph nodes
NX	Minimal requirements for assessment of regional lymph nodes not fulfilled

M	Metastases
M0	No distant metastases
M1	Distant metastases
MX	Minimal requirements for assessment of distant metastases not fulfilled

G	Histopathological grading	
G1–3	Increasingly undifferentiated tumour	
GX	Grading not ascertainable	(Modified after UICC (1982))

Occult primary tumour with metastases

Histology	Search for tumour in:
Squamous cell	ENT area, lung, oesophagus, bladder, rectum
Adenocarcinoma	Breast, gastrointestinal tract, lung, pancreas, uterus, prostate, kidney, thyroid
Undifferentiated	Lymphoma, breast, skin, thyroid, germ cells
Others	Adrenal, APUD system, small intestine

Anatomy	Search for tumour in:
Cervical lymph nodes	ENT area, thyroid, lung, stomach
Axillary lymph glands	Breast, lung, gastrointestinal tract
Periumbilical mass	Gastrointestinal tract, ovary, uterus
Inguinal mass	Rectum, prostate, testis

Metastases and possible primary tumour

Metastasis	Thyroid	Lung	Breast	Stomach	Colon	Pancreas	Biliary system	Kidney	Bladder	Prostate	Testis	Ovary	Uterus/cervix	Melanoma	Lymphoma	Undetermined aetiology
Brain		+++	++		+									++		++
Lung	+		+++	+	+	+	+	++	+	+	++		+	++	+	++
Malignant pleural effusion		++	+++			+									++	+
Liver			++	++	++	+	+++	+				+	++	++	+	+
Bone	++	++	+++		+				++	+++			+	+		+

Scales for assessment of the physical condition of tumour patients

ECOG – Eastern Cooperative Oncology Group; AJC – American Joint Commission for Cancer Staging and End Results Reporting

Description of condition	Karnofsky scale (%)	Zubrod scale (ECOG)	Description of condition (ECOG, AJC)
No complaints, no evidence of the illness	100	0	Normal activity
Can perform normal activities, minor symptoms of illness	90	1	Symptoms of illness, patient is ambulant, and can master the activities of everyday life
Some symptoms on exertion	80		
Self-caring: Can perform neither normal activities nor active work	70	2	Symptoms; less than 50% of time in bed; self-caring
Requires occasional assistance, but can still look after own personal bodily functions	60		
Needs considerable assistance and frequent medical attention	50	3	In bed more than 50% of time; requires assistance
Handicapped, requires specialized nursing and support	40		
Severely disabled, admission to hospital indicated, not in immediate danger of death	30	4	Bedridden, requires admission to hospital
Very ill, requires admission to hospital, requires active and supportive therapy	20		
Moribund	10		
Dead	0		

Mode of action of cytostatic drugs

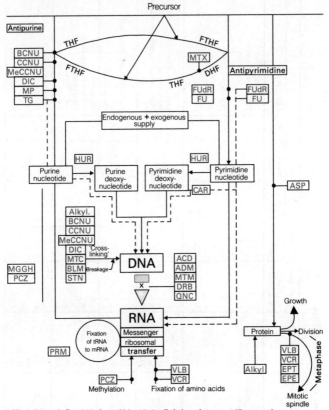

ACD, actinomycin D; ADM, doxorubicin; Alkyl., alkylating substances; ASP, asparaginase;
BCNU, carmustine; BLM, bleomycin; CAR, cytarabine; CCNU, lomustine; DHF, dihydrofolic acid;
DIC, dacarbazine; DRB, daunorubicin; EPE, etoposide; EPT, teniposide; FU, fluorouracil;
FUdR, 5-fluorodesoxyuridine; HUR, hydroxyurea; MeCCNU, methyl-CCNU; MGGH, methyl-GAG;
MP, mercaptopurine; MTC, mitomycin C; MTM, plicamycin; PCZ, procarbazine; PRM, puromycin;
QNC, quinacrin; STN, streptonigrin; TG, thioguanine; THF, tetrahydrofolic acid; VCR, vincristine;
VLB, vinblastine

(After Pfreundschuh and Diehl (1986))

Side effects of cytostatic drugs

Class	Generic name	Abbreviations	Elimination L Liver K Kidney	Toxicity Leuco-cytes	Platelets	Nausea/vomiting	Hair loss	Other organs
Alkylating agents	Busulphan	BSF/BUS	L	++	++	+		Pulmonary fibrosis
	BCNU (carmustine)	BCNU	L	+++	+++	++	+	Pulmonary fibrosis
	CCNU (lomustine)	CCNU	L	+++	+++	++		
	Chlorambucil	CLB		++	++	+		
	Cisplatin	CDDP	L/K	(+)	(+)	+++		Nephro-/ototoxic
	Carboplatin	CBCDA		+++	+++	++	++	
	Cyclophosphamide	CMP/CTX	L	+++	+++	++	++	Cystitis
	Melphalan	MEL	L	+++	+++	+		
	Thiotepa	TTP	L	+++	+++	+	+	
Antimeta-bolites	Cytarabine	ARA-C	L	+	+	++	++	Diarrhoea, stomatitis
	Fluorouracil	FU	L	++	+	++	++	Hepatotoxic
	Mercaptopurine	MP	L	++	+	+	+	Mouth ulcers, neuro-/hepatatoxic
	Methotrexate	MTX	K	+++	++	++	++	
	Thioguanine	TG	L	++	+	+	+	
Alkaloids	Vinblastine	VLB	L	++	++	(+)	(+)	Neurotoxic, paralytic ileus
	Vincristine	VCR	L	(+)	(+)	(+)	++	
	Vindesine	VDS		+		++		
	Etoposide	VP 16	L/K	+	+	++		Neurotoxic
Antibiotics	Actinomycin	AC	L/K	++	++	+++	++	Stomatitis
	Bleomycin	BLM	K	(+)	(+)	(+)	+++	Pulmonary fibrosis
	Doxorubicin	ADM	L	+++	+++	+++	+++	Cardiotoxic
	Mitozandrone	MIT	L	++	++	++	+	Cardiotoxic
	Mitomycin	MM	L	++	++	++	(+)	Nephro-/neurotoxic
Others	Asparaginase	ASP	L			+		Pancreatitis, allergy
	Dacarbazine	DIC	L	++	++	+++	++	Pseudo-influenza
	Estramustine	EMP		++	++	++		
	Hydroxyurea	HUR		+++	++	+++		
	Procarbazine	PCZ	L	++	++	++		Neurotoxic

Dose reduction of cytostatic drugs

	Bone marrow function — Leucocytes and/or platelets		Renal function — Creatinine			Liver function — Bilirubin / GOT		
	2 500–4000 / 75 000–100 000	<2500 / <75 000	120–180 µmol/l / 1.3–2 mg/dl	180–300 / 2–3.3	>300 / >3.3	25–50 µmol/l / 1.5–3 mg/dl / 2–5 × Norm	50–85 / 3–5 / >5 × Norm	>85 / >5
Alkylating agents								
BCNU/CCNU	50	0				75	50	0
Chlorambucil	50	0						0
Cisplatin	100	0	100	0	0	100	50	0
Cyclophosphamide	50	0	100	100	0	100	75	0
Melphalan	50	0			0			
Procarbazine	50	0	75	50	0			
Antimetabolites								
Cytarabine	50	0			75–50			
Fluorouracil	50	0			75–50			
Mercaptopurine	50	0	100	100	50	100	100	0
Methotrexate	50	0	50	0	0	100	75	0
Alkaloids								
Vinblastine	50	0	100	75	75	50	25	0
Vincristine	100	100	100	100	75	150	25	0
Etoposide	50	0	100	75	0	75	50	0
Antibiotics								
Actinomycin	50	0						
Doxorubicin	50	0	100	100	75	50	25	0
Mitomycin	50	0	50	0	75	50	0	0

Antiemetics

For degree of vomiting to be expected see p. 232

Basic programme	Antiemetics			
		Mild		
Sedative the evening before (diazepam, 5–10 mg, supp.)	Before administration of cytostatic Metoclopramide, 10–20 mg p.o. /supp.; perhaps methotrimeprazine 10 mg p.o.			
			Moderate	
	Before administration of cytostatic Prochlorperazine 10(–20) mg p.o./supp.; repeat if necessary every 4 h (until 24 h after therapy); if necessary metoclopramide, 10–20 mg			
				Severe
If therapy includes cortisone: first dose the evening before, last dose the following day	30 min before administration of cytostatic Dexamethasone, 8 mg slowly over 15 min i.v. In addition Odansetron 3 doses 8 mg p.o./i.v.; 15 min before, 4 and 8 h after chemotherapy; (alternatively 1 dose granisetron 3 mg)			

Endocrine system – summary

Hypothalamus

Hormone	GHRH	TRH	CRH	Gn-RH
Inhibited by	Somatostatin	Thyroxine	Cortisol	Oestradiol
Hypofunction	Retarded growth	Tertiary hypothyroidism	Tertiary adrenal insufficiency	Kallmann's syndrome, hypothalamic amenorrhoea, idiopathic delayed puberty
Stimulation test	Insulin test, physical stress, arginine test	None known	Insulin test (metopirone test)	Clomiphene test

Anterior pituitary

Hormone	STH (GH)	TSH	ACTH	LH, FSH
Stimulated by	GHRH	TRH	CRH	Gn-RH
Inhibited by	Somatostatin	Thyroxine	Cortisol	Oestradiol, testosterone, inhibin
Stimulation test	GHRH test	TRH test	CRH test	Gn-RH test
Hypofunction	In children: retarded growth	Secondary hypothyroidism	Secondary adrenal insufficiency	Secondary hypogonadism: subfertility, oligo-/amenorrhoea, impotence, delayed puberty
Excessive function	STH-secreting anterior pituitary adenoma; in children: gigantism; in adults: acromegaly	TSH-secreting anterior pituitary adenoma: secondary hyperthyroidism	ACTH-secreting anterior pituitary adenoma: Cushing's disease	Gonadotrophin-secreting anterior pituitary adenoma: oligo-/amenorrhoea, impotence

Effector gland

Effector gland	Liver	Thyroid	Adrenals	Ovaries, testes
Hormone	Somatomedin C	Thyroxine Triiodothyronine	Cortisol Adrenal androgens	Oestradiol, testosterone
Stimulated by	STH (GH)	TSH	ACTH	LH: Steroid secretion FSH: Follicle ripening, spermatogenesis
Excessive function	–	Primary hyperthyroidism	Cortisol-secreting adrenal adenoma	Testotoxicosis (rare) Polycystic ovary syndrome
Hypofunction	Laron dwarfism	Primary hypothyroidism	Primary adrenal cortical insufficiency: Addison's disease	Primary hypogonadism, menopause, Turner's syndrome (♀:X0), Klinefelter's syndrome (♂:XXY)
Principal action	Bone growth	Energy metabolism	Immune modulation Stress response	Oestrogens: feminization Androgens: virilization Gonadotrophins: fertility
End-organ resistance (rare)	Dwarfism	Partial effects only anterior pituitary or complete (rare)	Very rare	Testicular feminization (Reifenstein's syndrome: 5α-reductase deficiency)

Abbreviations:

GHRH	Growth hormone releasing hormone;	STH (GH)	Growth hormone (somatotrophin);
TRH	Thyrotrophin releasing hormone;	TSH	Thyrotrophic hormone (thyrotrophin);
CRH	Corticotrophin releasing hormone;	ACTH	Adrenocorticotrophic hormone (corticotrophin);
Gn-RH	Gonadotrophin releasing hormone	LH	Luteinizing hormone (luteotrophin);
		FSH	Follicle stimulating hormone

Gland	Anterior pituitary	Posterior pituitary	Parathyroid	Thyroid C-cells
Hormone	Prolactin	AVP (ADH)	Parathormone (PTH)	Calcitonin
Stimulated by	TRH	Osmolarity ↑ Hypovolaemia	Calcium ↓	Calcium ↑ Gastrin
Inhibited by	Dopamine	Osmolarity ↓	Calcium ↑	Calcium ↓
Effect	Lactation	Renal water retention	Calcium liberation from bone	Calcium retention by bone
Stimulation test	TRH test if urine osmolarity < 350 mosmol/kg	Water deprivation test	–	Pentagastrin test
Hypofunction	Disturbed lactation	Diabetes insipidus	Hypocalcaemia, tetany	–
Hyperfunction	Prolactinoma: ♀: Sterility Oligomenorrhoea Galactorrhoea ♂: Impotence Hypogonadism	SIADH: usually paraneoplastic Syndrome of inappropriate ADH secretion (oedema, hyponatraemia)	Hypercalcaemia (nephrolithiasis, pancreatitis, psychiatric disturbances)	C-cell carcinoma of thyroid, e.g. with multiple endocrine neoplasia (diarrhoea)

Abbreviations:

AVP Arginine vasopressin; TRH Thyrotrophin releasing hormone; ADH Antidiuretic hormone

Gland	Kidney (juxtaglomerular apparatus)	Adrenal cortex	Adrenal cortex	Adrenal medulla Sympath. ganglia
Hormone	Renin liberates angiotensin by proteolysis	Aldosterone	DHEAS, DHEA, 17α-OH-progesterone, testosterone	Adrenaline (esp. in adr. medulla), dopamine, noradrenaline
Stimulated by	Renal perfusion ↓ Hyponatraemia	Angiotensin (ACTH)	ACTH	Neuronal control
Inhibited by	Hypernatraemia Hypokalaemia	–	–	Neuronal control
Effect	Arteriolar constriction Aldosterone ↑	Renal potassium loss, sodium retention	Slight androgenic action	Cardiovascular
Stimulation test	Frusemide test Captopril test	(ACTH test)	ACTH test	All stimulation tests are obsolete
Hyperfunction	Secondary hyperaldosteronism	Primary hyperaldosteronism (Conn's syndrome)	Adrenogenital syndrome (complete or incomplete)	Phaeochromocytoma, paraganglioma
Hypofunction	Very rare	Often in primary adrenal cortical insufficiency (Addison's disease)	–	Shy–Drager syndrome (very rare)

Abbreviations:

ACTH Adrenocorticotrophic hormone (corticotrophin)   DHEA Dehydroepiandrosterone
DHEAS Dehydroepiandrosterone sulphate

Endocrine normal values[a]

Plasma concentration Gland and measurement	Unit	Normal value		Comments, normal values in SI units and conversion factors (CF)	
Thyroid					
Total thyroxine	µg/dl	4.5–12.0		nmol/l 60–160	(CF: × 12.9)
Total triiodothyronine	ng/ml	0.45–2.0		pmol/l 0.6–3.0	(CF: × 1.54)
TBG	µg/ml	12.0–30.0		↑ in pregnancy, with oral contraceptives, etc.	
T4/TBG ratio	µg/dl	0.2–0.5		nmol/l 200–500	
Free thyroxine	ng/dl	0.8–2.4		pmol/l 10–31	(CF: × 12.9)
Free triiodothyronine	pg/dl	230–660		pmol/l 3.5–10.2	(CF: × 0.0154)
TSH (basal)	U/l	0.3–4.0			
Thyroglobulin antibodies (**TAb**)	U/ml	< 500			
Microsomal antibodies (**MAb**)	U/ml	< 500			
TRAb (TSH receptor Ab)	U/l	< 5.0			
Thyroglobulin	ng/ml	< 50		After thyroid ablation < 5	
Parathyroid					
Parathormone peptide 44–68	pg/ml	< 300		Interpretation in relation to	
Intact PTH	pg/ml	< 50		plasma calcium concentration	
Osteocalcin	ng/ml	3.0–16.0		Age dependent! nmol/l 0.6–3.0	
25-hydroxy vitamin D₃	ng/ml	15–120		nmol/l 40–300	(CF: × 2.5)
1,25-dihydroxy vitamin D₃	pg/ml	25–45		pmol/l 60–110	(CF: × 2.4)
Adrenal					
Cortisol	µg/dl	5.0–25.0		nmol/l 140–700	(CF: × 27.6)
ACTH	pg/ml	< 100		pmol/l < 25	(CF: × 0.23)
Cortisone-binding globulin (CBG) (transcortin)	µg/ml	30–50		↑ in pregnancy	
Dehydroepiandrosterone	ng/ml	< 10		nmol/l < 35	(CF: × 3.47)
DHEA sulphate'	ng/ml	< 5000		µmol/l < 13	(CF: × 0.0026)
17-α-hydroxyprogesterone	ng/dl	< 150		nmol/l < 4.5	(CF: × 0.03)
11-desoxycortisol	ng/ml	< 10		nmol/l < 30	(CF: × 2.9)
Aldosterone	ng/ml	< 120		pmol/l < 330	(CF: × 2.77)
Plasma renin activity	ng/ml/h	0.2–2.0		Resting value (recumbent), increased by standing, diuretics, low-salt diet	
Noradrenaline	ng/l	< 500		pmol/l < 3000	(CF: × 5.91)
Adrenaline	ng/l	< 120		pmol/l < 700	(CF: × 5.46)
Dopamine	ng/l	< 120		pmol/l < 800	(CF: × 6.53)
				↑↑ by stress and standing	

Gonads		Men	Women	Men Women	
Testosterone	ng/ml	> 3.0	< 3.0	nmol/l > 10 < 3	(CF: × 3.47)
Sex hormone binding globulin (SHBG)	µg/ml	6–16	12–23	Increased in pregnancy	
Oestradiol (E2)	pg/ml	< 60	> 40	pmol/l < 200 > 150 } In 2nd phase of cycle	
Oestrone (E1)	pg/ml	< 80	> 40	pmol/l < 300 > 150 } increased to approx.	
Total oestrogens	pg/ml	< 120	> 80	nmol/l < 8 > 5 double value	
Progesterone	ng/ml		6–20	nmol/l 20–100 In 2nd phase of cycle,	
LH	U/l	< 15	< 15	Around ovulation briefly strongly ↑	
FSH	U/l	< 10	< 10		
Prolactin	ng/ml	< 20	< 25	↑↑ through stress (e.g. phlebotomy)!	

Metabolism					
Growth hormone (STH)	ng/ml	< 5.0		↑ through stress and physical exercise	
Insulin	U/l	10.0–30.0		Fasting value	
C-peptide	ng/ml	1.5–5.0		pmol/l 0.6–1.3 Fasting value	
Glucagon	pg/ml	< 100		Fasting value	
Gastrin	pg/ml	< 100		Zollinger–Ellison syndrome > 300 pg/ml	

Urine determinations (urine assays are superior to plasma determinations for screening!)					
Cortisol excretion	µg/24 h	< 75.0		Important if suspicion of Cushing's syndrome	
Aldosterone excretion	µg/24 h	< 14.0		Important if suspicion of Conn's syndrome	
C-peptide	nmol/24 h	< 14.0		Important if suspicion of insulinoma	
Vallinylmandelic acid (VMA)	mg/24 h	< 7.0		Liable to interference, better:	
Noradrenaline	µg/24 h	< 40.0		Unequivocally abnormal > 100.0 µg/24 h	
Adrenaline	µg/24 h	< 16.0		Unequivocally abnormal > 50.0 µg/24 h	
Dopamine	µg/24 h	< 430.0		Unequivocally abnormal > 500.0 µg/24 h	

[a] Beware local laboratory differences.

Endocrine tests

Indication, method, assay requirement and normal ranges

TRH test

I: Suspicion of borderline hyperthyreoidism
   Suspicion of borderline hypothyreoidism
M: <u>1 amp. TRH (200 µg) i.v.</u>
A: 0 min   TSH   >0.2   < 4.0   U/l
    30 min   TSH   >2.0   <25.0   U/l

Gn-RH test

I: Suspicion and DD of
   hypogonadotrophic hypogonadism
M: <u>1 amp. Gn-RH (100 µg) i.v.</u>
A: 0 min   LH   ....   FSH
    30 min   (*2) LH   ....   FSH

CRH test

I: DD of Cushing's syndrome and
   secondary adrenal insufficiency
M: <u>1 amp. CRH (100 µg) i.v.</u>
A: 0 min   ACTH   Cortisol
    15 min   ACTH   ....   Cortisol
    30 min   >25   ACTH   >15   Cortisol
    45 min   ....   ACTH   ....   Cortisol
    60 min   pg/ml   ACTH   µg/dl   Cortisol

GHRH test

.I: DD of growth retardation
M: <u>GHRH (1 µg/kg) i.v.</u>
A: 0 min   ......   STH
    15 min   ......   STH
    30 min   >5 ng/ml   STH
    45 min   ......   STH
    60 min   ......   STH

Dexamethasone suppression test

I: 1. Suspicion of Cushing's syndrome
   2. Suspicion of androgen-secreting
      adrenal tumour
M: <u>2 mg dexamethasone p.o. at 2300 hrs</u>
   (3 mg if > 70 kg)
A: The following morning (0800–0900 hrs)
   for 1. <5 µg/dl cortisol
   for 2. ↓↓ DHEA, testosterone

Synacthen test

I: 1. Suspicion of adrenal insufficiency
   2. Suspicion of adrenogenital syndrome
      (poss. heterozygote)
M: <u>250 mg Synacthen</u>
   <u>i.v.</u>
A: Cortisol   17α-
   (for 1. and 2.)   hydroxyprogesterone
   0 min   (for 2.)
   60 min > 20 µg/dl   < 260 ng/dl
   120 min ....

Insulin hypoglycaemia test

I: 1. Suspicion of secondary adrenal insufficiency
   2. Suspicion of growth hormone deficiency
   3. Suspicion of pseudo-Cushing's syndrome
M: <u>0.15 IU insulin/kg i.v.</u>

min	BS	ACTH	Cortisol	/	STH (for 2.)
0				/	
15				/	
30	<2.0	>100	>20	/	>5
45		....	....	/	....
60		....	....	/	....
90		....	....	/	....
120	mmol/l	pg/ml	µg/dl	/	ng/ml

Combined anterior pituitary test
(without insulin hypoglycaemia)

I: Test of all anterior pituitary functions
M: <u>Simultaneous i.v. 1 amp. each of Gn-RH, TRH and CRH</u>

min	LH	TSH	PRL	ACTH	Cort.	poss. STH
0						
15				....		
30	(*2)	>2.0	↑↑	>25	>15	>5
45	–		–	....	....	....
60	–	U/l	–	pg/ml	µg/dl	ng/ml

Combined anterior pituitary test
(with insulin hypoglycaemia)

I: Test of all anterior pituitary functions and in part of
   hypothalamic regulation
M: <u>Simultaneous i.v. 1 amp. each of Gn-RH and TRH</u>
   <u>and 0.15 IU insulin/kg</u>

min	LH	THS	PRL	BS	ACTH	Cort.	STH
0							
15							
30	(*2)	>2.0	↑↑	<2.0	>100	>20	>5
45	–				....	....	....
60	–						
90	–			mmol/l	....	....	....
120	–	U/l			....	....	....

Abbreviations:

I	Indication, question to be answered
M	Method
A	Time of phlebotomy Required assay
XYZ	Result to be considered normal
(*2)	Normal response is a doubling
.....	Optional assay (increases sensitivity in individual cases)

DD, differential diagnosis

Blood samples:

5 ml heparinized blood/hormone assay
5 ml EDTA blood on ice/ACTH assay

Thyrotoxicosis and hypothyroidism

	Thyrotoxicosis	Hypothyroidism
Aetiology and differential diagnosis	Autoimmune thyroid disease (e.g. Graves' disease), toxic nodular goitre (multinodular or single toxic adenoma), thyroxine intoxication. Rarely: TSH-secreting anterior pituitary adenoma, carcinoma of thyroid	Autoimmune thyroid disease, thyroidectomy, radioiodine therapy, iodine deficiency, anterior pituitary insufficiency
Symptoms (older patients often monosymptomatic)		
General	Metabolism ↑ Weight ↓, appetite ↑, heat intolerance, sweating	Metabolism ↓ Weight ↑, appetite ↓, cold intolerance, hypothermia
Skin	Warm, moist	Cool, dry, bloated faces, swollen tongue, pretibial myxoedema
Hair	Fine, hair loss	Coarse, rough
Eyes	Possibly ophthalmopathy with lid lag, lid retraction and exophthalmos	Swollen lids (Ophthalmopathy also possible!)
Neurology and psychiatry	Fine tremor Reflexes ↑, hyperactivity, insomnia, restlessness, anxiety, psychosis	Carpal tunnel syndrome Reflexes ↓, delayed relaxation phase, activity ↓, marked somnolence, apathy, lethargy
Circulation	Palpitation, supraventricular tachycardia, atrial fibrillation, RR ↑ (RR amplitude ↑)	Bradycardia, heart failure, pericardial effusion RR ↓
Respiration	Possibly tachypnoea	Respiratory insufficiency
Gastrointestinal	Diarrhoea	Constipation
Breasts	♂: Gynaecomastia	♀: Galactorrhoea
Gonads	♀: Oligomenorrhoea	♀: Menorrhagia, subfertility
Laboratory	↑: T_4, T_3, FT_4 ↓: TSH (except in secondary form) TRH test: negative	↓: T_4, T_3, FT_4 ↑: TSH (except in secondary form) TRH test: excessive response
For DD	History, measurement of TAb, MAb, TRAb, thyroid scintigram, thyroid ultrasound	History, measurement of TAb, MAb, TRAb
Therapy	Antithyroid drugs Radioiodine therapy Thyroid surgery	Thyroxine (T_4) replacement

Abbreviations:

TAb	Thyroglobulin antibodies	TSH	Thyroid-stimulating hormone
TRAb	TSH receptor antibodies	T_3	Triiodothyronine
TRH	Thyrotrophin-releasing hormone	FT_4	Free thyroxine (not bound to
T_4	Thyroxine		thyroxine-binding globulin)
MAb	Microsomal antibodies	DD	Differential diagnosis

Adrenal cortex

Underactivity	Overactivity		Failure of function
Addison's disease	Hypercortisolism	Hyperaldosteronism	Adrenogenital syndrome
Aetiology and differential diagnosis			
Autoimmune disorder >80% Tuberculosis <10% Adrenalectomy, metastases <10% DD: Adrenal atrophy after glucocorticoid therapy	**Primary (ACTH ↓)** Adrenal adenoma <20% Adrenal carcinoma <10% **Secondary (ACTH ↑)** <10% Ectopic ACTH secretion ACTH-secreting pituitary adenoma (Cushing's syndrome) >65%	**Primary (Renin ↓)** Adrenal adenoma 80% (Conn's syndrome) Adrenal hyperplasia 15% Adrenal carcinoma 5% **Secondary (Renin ↑)** On diuretics, with renal artery stenosis, cirrhosis of liver, heart failure, etc.	21-hydroxylase deficiency >90% 11β-hydroxylase deficiency Rare 3β-hydroxysteroid dehydrogenase deficiency Rare 17α-hydroxylase deficiency Rare
Symptoms			
Fatigue, weakness, weight ↓, anorexia, vomiting, hypotension, salt craving	Truncal obesity, moon face, nuchal hump, hypertension, osteoporosis, ecchymoses, psychosis	Hypertension (especially diastolic), muscular weakness, polyuria, oedema	♀: Virilization, hirsutism, oligomenorrhoea, adrenal insufficiency ♂: Precocious puberty, adrenal insufficiency
Investigations			
↑: ACTH, renin, potassium, ↓: Cortisol, pH, sodium, blood sugar	↑: Cortisol, Hb, blood sugar, pH ↓: Potassium	↑: Aldosterone, pH ↓: Potassium	↑: 17α-hydroxy-progesterone, ACTH, renin ↓: Cortisol

Cushing's syndrome

Step 1:	**Clinical suspicion**
Procedure:	Search for typical somatic symptoms
History:	Exclusion of an iatrogenic Cushing's syndrome

Step 2:	**Confirmation of the diagnosis of Cushing's syndrome**
Tests:	1. Urinary cortisol ↑ (>100µg/24h)
	2. Morning plasma cortisol ↑ (>5µg/dl) after taking 2 mg dexamethasone orally the previous evening

Step 3:   **Differential diagnosis of Cushing's syndrome**

A ACTH-secreting pituitary adenoma (Cushing's disease)

Tests:
1. Plasma ACTH (collect sample on ice) normal – ↑
2. ACTH and cortisol response obtained in CRH test
3. Suppression of urinary cortisol into normal range after administration of 2 mg dexamethasone 6-hourly over 48 h (Liddle test)
4. MRI scan demonstration of pituitary adenoma (positive in only 50–70%)
5. ACTH gradient >1.4 between inferior petrosal sinus and peripheral vein (reserve diagnostic test)

B Cortisol-secreting adrenal adenoma or carcinoma

Tests:
1. Plasma ACTH (collection on ice) normal – ↓
2. No ACTH or cortisol response in CRH test
3. Negative Liddle test
4. Demonstration of an adrenal tumour by ultrasound or CT. Carcinomas are usually large (>>4cm), adenomas are small (<4cm). Note: the demonstration of an adrenal tumour does not exclude a pituitary tumour!

C Cushing's syndrome with paraneoplastic ACTH secretion

Tests:
1. Plasma ACTH (collection on ice) ↑ – ↑↑
2. No ACTH or cortisol response in CRH test
3. Negative Liddle test
4. Demonstration of a carcinoid, bronchial carcinoma, phaeochromocytoma or medullary thyroid carcinoma, e.g. with ultrasound, CT, etc.
5. ACTH gradient <1.4 between inferior petrosal sinus and peripheral vein (reserve diagnostic test)

Stage 4:	**Therapy**
for A:	Transsphenoidal ablation of the pituitary adenoma
for B:	Unilateral adrenalectomy, for metastasizing carcinoma o,p'-DDD therapy
for C:	Operative removal of the tumour, possibly chemotherapy, possibly palliative bilateral adrenalectomy

Replacement therapy

Deficient hormone	Replacement therapy	Preparation	Aim of treatment, control parameters
ACTH	Hydrocortisone 25–30 mg/day		Provides complete substitution
STH (GH)	Recombinant human GH		Only in children by specialists
TSH	L-thyroxine 50–150 µg/day		Dose according to clinical picture
LH, FSH	♀: hMG, then hCG, until pregnancy		hCG, hMG therapy by specialists Only if fertility required, otherwise ♂: testosterone, ♀: oestrogens and progestogens
	♂: hCG plus hMG, ca. 3–6 months		
ADH (AVP)	Desmopressin 5–20 µg once or twice daily intranasally		Dose adjusted according to fluid intake and urine volume
Prolactin	–		No substitution
Thyroxine	l-thyroxine 50–150 µg/day		TSH should be within normal range
Parathormone	Dihydrotachysterol 0.5–1.5 mg/day or 1.25-hydroxy-D_3 0.5–1.0 µg/day		Plasma calcium should be at lower end of normal range
Calcitonin	–		No substitution
Cortisol	Hydrocortisone 25–30 mg/day		No control by ACTH or cortisol
Aldosterone	Fludrocortisone 0.1–0.3 mg/day		Control by BP and renin activity
Adrenal androgens	–		No substitution
Catecholamines	–		No substitution
Testosterone	Testosterone proprionate (oily) 250 mg i.m. every 3–6 weeks		No control by LH, FSH or testosterone necessary
Oestrogens	Conjugated oestrogens 0.6–1.25 mg/day		Always replace oestrogens in combination with progestogens (otherwise ↑ risk of carcinoma)
Progestogens	e.g. Medroxyprogesterone acetate 5 mg/day (days 15–24)		

Abbreviations: hCG human chorionic gonadotrophin; hMG human menopausal gonadotrophin

Endocrine crises

Thyrotoxic crisis	1. Fluid and electrolyte correction 2. Nutrition (glucose) 3. Temperature lowering (physical), antipyretics (no salicylates) 4. O_2 5. Betablockers: propranolol 1–5 mg i.v. or 20–80 mg 6-hourly p.o. 6. Hydrocortisone, 300 mg i.v. initially, then 100 mg i.v. 8-hourly 7. Antithyroid drugs: 60–120 mg carbimazole or 600–1200 mg propylthiouracil p.o., if necessary by nasogastric tube
Myxoedema coma	1. Correction of hypoventilation, if necessary intubation and ventilation 2. Treatment of hypothermia with blankets (beware peripheral vasodilatation, avoid active warming) 3. T_3, 100 µg i.v./12h, then 25 µg/12h 4. Hydrocortisone 100 mg i.v. 6-hourly 5. Careful fluid and electrolyte correction (hyponatraemia, beware fluid overload) 6. Dobutamine if heart failure 7. If necessary, antibiotic cover
Addisonian crisis	1. Hydrocortisone 100 mg i.v. as bolus, then 100 mg 8-hourly i.v. 2. Rehydration with 0.9% NaCl and glucose i.v.; ca. 20% of extracellular volume on first day Beware heart failure
Hypercalcaemic crisis	1. Infusion of 200–300 ml 0.9% NaCl per hour 2. Frusemide 80–200 mg/12h after diuresis 3. Electrolyte replacement 4. Salcatonin 5–10 units/kg daily to 400 units every 8 h according to clinical and biochemical response s.c. or i.m.; by slow i.v. infusion 5–10 units over at least 6 h (avoid phosphate or EDTA administration) 5. If due to hyperparathyroidism: surgery 6. If resistant to therapy, consider haemodialysis
Hypocalcaemic crisis	1. Calcium gluconate 20 ml 10% solution i.v., if necessary followed by 50 ml in 500 ml 0.9% NaCl as infusion 2. Later oral calcium therapy and/or vitamin D
Hypertensive crisis	1. Nifedipine, glyceryl trinitrate or sodium nitroprusside i.v. (dose according to effect) if cause unclear 2. Phentolamine 0.25–1 mg/min i.v. continuously if phaeochromocytoma confirmed 3. Usual therapy for cardiac arrhythmias

Corticosteroids

Generic name	Biological half life	Relative potency		Equivalent doses in mg[a]				
		Anti-inflammatory Glucocorticoid activity	Sodium retention Mineralocorticoid activity					
Cortisone	Short 8–12h	0.8	0.8	25	50	100	200	500
Cortisol (Hydrocortisone)		1	1	20	40	80	160	400
Fludrocortisone		10	125	5	10	20	40	100
Prednisone/ Prednisolone	Medium 12–36	4	0.8	5	10	20	40	100
Methyl- prednisolone		5	0.5	4	8	16	32	80
Triamcinolone		5	0	4	8	16	32	80
Dexamethasone	Long 36–72h	20	0	1	2	4	8	20
Betamethasone		25	0	0.75	1.5	3	6	15

Sources: Haynes and Murad (1985) Kaiser (1977)
[a] With reference to the indicated biological half life, i.e. 1 mg dexamethasone/48h is approximately equivalent to 4 × 25 mg hydrocortisone/48h or 2 × 5 mg prednisolone/48h.

Classification of renal osteodystrophy

Type	Morphology	Cause
I II III	Osteitis fibrosa Osteomalacia Osteitis fibrosa and osteomalacia	Secondary hyperparathyroidism Mineralization defect Secondary hyperparathyroidism and mineralization defect
a b c	Reduced bone turnover Normal or increased bone turnover Greatly increased bone turnover } Activity	
− +	Osteoporosis Osteosclerosis	

Types of multiple endocrine neoplasia (MEN)
(Identification of one of the disorders requires exclusion of the others)

Type	Affected organ	Illness
I	Parathyroid adenoma and pancreatic tumours and pituitary adenomas	Primary hyperparathyroidism Gastrinoma, insulinoma, vipoma, etc. Acromegaly, prolactinoma, Cushing's disease
IIa	Thyroid carcinoma and adrenal medullary tumours and parathyroid adenomas	(medullary) C-cell carcinoma (bilateral) Phaeochromocytomas Primary hyperparathyroidism
IIb	Thyroid carcinoma and adrenal medullary tumours and mucosal neuromas	(medullary) C-cell carcinoma (bilateral) Phaeochromocytomas (intestinal) Ganglion neuromatosis (Megacolon in Hirschsprung's disease)

Classification of diabetes mellitus

A Manifest diabetes Mellitus
- Type I: insulin-dependent diabetes (IDDM)
- Type II: non-insulin-dependent diabetes (NIDDM)
    - Type IIa: without obesity
    - Type IIb: with obesity
- MODY (NIDDY): Maturity onset diabetes of young patients

B Gestational diabetes

C Abnormal glucose tolerance

D Secondary diabetes
- In pancreatic disorders (pancreatitis, postoperative, etc.)
- With endocrinopathies (cortisol excess, acromegaly, etc.)
- Due to toxic influences (drugs, etc.)
- With genetic syndromes (insulin receptor abnormalities, etc.)

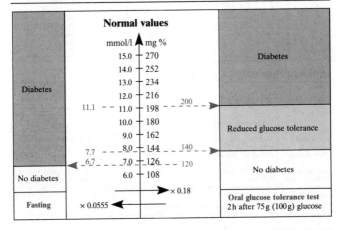

Gestational diabetes	
Glucose tolerance	Screening
fasting: > 90 mg/dl > 5.0 mmol/l and 1 h > 190 mg/dl > 10.6 mmol/l or 2 h > 160 mg/dl > 8.9 mmol/l	1h after 50g glucose independent of time of day or meals > 140 mg/dl > 7.8 mmol/l = diagnostic suspicion

Data after:
National Diabetes Data Group (1979)
American Diabetes Association (1985)
WHO Expert Committee on Diabetes Mellitus (1980)
Mehnert (1990)

Diabetic therapy

Type I	Insulin Adjustment of diet	**Diet** Well-balanced energy provision, slimming diet if overweight
Type II	1. Dietary treatment If necessary, weight reduction (possibly with absorption retarders for postprandial blood sugar peaks) 2. Diet + sulphonylureas 3. Diet + sulphonylureas + biguanide (especially for obese patients, biguanide monotherapy?) 4. Diet + combined therapy (sulphonylureas and insulin) or Diet and insulin monotherapy (especially for patient of normal weight)	1. Distribution of carbohydrate intake over several (5–7) meals throughout the day 2. Avoidance of rapidly absorbable carbohydrate (CHO) (sugar-free diet, etc.) 3. Calculation of carbohydrate consumption and exchange according to Bread Units (1 BU = 12 g CHO) if necessary with reference to the glycaemic index (blood sugar effectiveness of the CHO) **Gestational diabetes:** Insulin treatment if postprandial BS is not below 140 mg/dl (7.7 mmol/l) after dietary treatment for 2 weeks

Oral hypoglycaemics

Sulphonylureas
Main action: liberation of insulin from β cells

Product (selection)	Usual dose (adjusted according to response)	Half life (h)	Side effects
Gliquidone Glipizide Tolbutamide	45–60 mg in 2–3 doses/day Up to 40 mg daily in 2–3 doses 500 mg 1–2 times/day	ca. 1.4 ca. 3.5 ca. 4	Blood disorders. Skin changes (allergy, photodermatosis) Rarely gastrointestinal symptoms
Gliclazide Glibenclamide	Up to 320 mg daily in 2 doses 5–15 mg	ca. 10–12 ca. 8–16	Prolonged hypoglycaemia (especially glibenclamide)

Biguanide
Main action: enhancement of peripheral glucose utilization
Contraindications: impaired renal function, chronic renal disease, hypoxic conditions (operations,
heart failure, etc.), chronic liver disease, pregnancy

Product	Usual dose	Half life	Side effects
Metformin	500 mg 1–3 times daily	ca. 2 h	(possible lactic acidosis) Gastrointestinal symptoms

Absorption retardant
(α-glucosidase inhibitor)
Main action: retardation of carbohydrate absorption; possible addition to dietary treatment

Product	Usual dose	Half life	Side effects
Acarbose	50 mg 1–3 times daily	Practically no absorption	Gastrointestinal symptoms

Insulin therapy

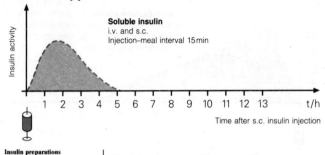

Soluble insulin
i.v. and s.c.
Injection–meal interval 15 min

Insulin preparations All 100 units/ml (H) Human insulin (P) Porcine insulin (B) Bovine insulin	Hypurin Neutral Velosulin Human Actrapid Human Velosulin Humulin S Pur-In Neutral	(B) (P) (H) (H) (H) (H)	CP Novo Nordisk, Wellcome Novo Nordisk Novo Nordisk, Wellcome Lilly CP

Intermediate- and long-acting insulins

Only s.c. Injection–meal interval: 30 min (absorption profile after s.c. administration dependent on injection amount, insulin type, etc.)

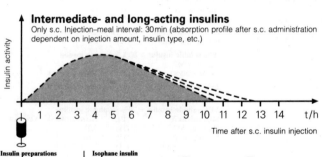

Insulin preparations All 100 units/ml (H) Human insulin (P) Porcine insulin (B) Bovine insulin	**Isophane insulin** Hypurin Isophane Insulatard Human Insulatard Human Protaphane Humulin Pur-In Isophane **Insulin Zinc Suspension** (mixed) Hypurin Lente Lentard MC Human Monotard Humulin Lente **Insulin Zinc Suspension** (amorphous) Semitard MC **Insulin Zinc Suspension** (crystalline) Human Ultratard Humulin Zn	 (B) (P) (H) (H) (H) (H) (B) (B,P) (H) (H) (P) (H) (H)	 CP Novo Nordisk, Wellcome Novo Nordisk, Wellcome Novo Nordisk Lilly CP CP Novo Nordisk Novo Nordisk Lilly Novo Nordisk Novo Nordisk Lilly

Biphasic insulins

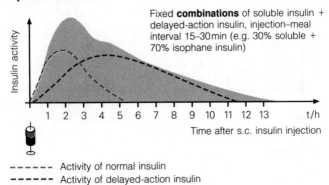

Fixed **combinations** of soluble insulin + delayed-action insulin, injection–meal interval 15–30 min (e.g. 30% soluble + 70% isophane insulin)

– – – – – Activity of normal insulin

– – – – – Activity of delayed-action insulin

▬▬▬ Total activity

Insulin preparations
All 100 units/ml
(H) Human insulin
(P) Porcine insulin
(B) Bovine insulin

10% soluble insulin + 90% isophane insulin

Humulin M1	(H)	Lilly
PenMix 10/90	(H)	Novo Nordisk

15% soluble insulin + 85% isophane insulin

Pur-In Mix 15/85	(H)	CP

20% soluble insulin + 80% isophane insulin

Humulin M2	(H)	Lilly
PenMix 20/80	(H)	Novo Nordisk

25% soluble insulin + 75% isophane insulin

Pur-In Mix 25/75	(H)	CP

30% soluble insulin + 70% isophane insulin

Mixtard 30/70	(P)	Novo Nordisk, Wellcome
Humulin M3	(H)	Lilly
PenMix 30/70	(H)	Novo Nordisk
Human Actraphane	(H)	Novo Nordisk
Human Mixtard	(H)	Novo Nordisk, Wellcome

40% soluble insulin + 60% isophane insulin

Humulin M4	(H)	Lilly
PenMix 40/60	(H)	Novo Nordisk

50% soluble insulin + 50% isophane insulin

Initard 50/50	(P)	Novo Nordisk, Wellcome
PenMix 50/50	(H)	Novo Nordisk
Pur-In Mix 50/50	(H)	CP
Human Initard 50/50	(H)	Novo Nordisk, Wellcome

Crystalline bovine in soluble porcine insulin

Rapitard MC	(B+P)	Novo Nordisk

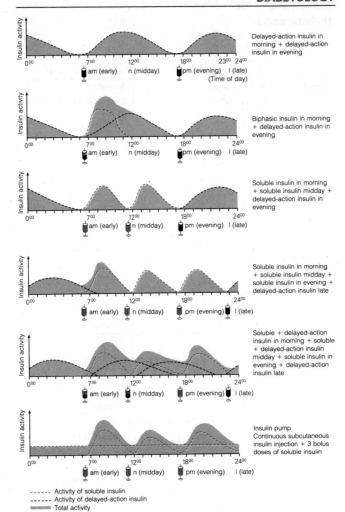

Delayed-action insulin in morning + delayed-action insulin in evening

Biphasic insulin in morning + delayed-action insulin in evening

Soluble insulin in morning + soluble insulin midday + delayed-action insulin in evening

Soluble insulin in morning + soluble insulin midday + soluble insulin in evening + delayed-action insulin late

Soluble + delayed-action insulin in morning + soluble + delayed-action insulin midday + soluble insulin in evening + delayed-action insulin late

Insulin pump
Continuous subcutaneous insulin injection + 3 bolus doses of soluble insulin

----- Activity of soluble insulin
----- Activity of delayed-action insulin
▨ Total activity

Diabetic coma

Incidence: ca. 3–5 cases/1000 diabetics/year
Association with type not always clear-cut

	Hyperglycaemic ketoacidotic coma	Hyperglycaemic hyperosmolar coma
Clinical	Mostly <60 years	Mostly >60 years
	Commonly type I diabetes known	Commonly type II diabetes known
	Rapid development	Protracted development
	Dehydration +	Dehydration + +
	Intestinal symptoms (diabetic pseudoperitonitis)	
	Kussmaul respiration	
	Fetor of acetone	
	Clouding of consciousness +	Clouding of consciousness + + Often few symptoms (picture of cerebrovascular accident)
	BP ↓ Heart rate ↑	BP ↓↓ Heart rate ↑
Precipitating factors	Infections (>40%)	Severe coexisting illness (cardiovascular, etc.)
	First manifestation of insulin-deficient diabetes (ca. 20%)	Diabetes not previously recognized (>20%)
	Treatment failure type I diabetes (including 'technical defects', pump failure, etc.)	Drugs (diuretics)
		Infections

Typical laboratory findings

17–45 mmol/l	BS	>33 mmol/l
<7.2	pH	>7.2
310–330	Osmolality	>330, often >400

Approximate calculation:

$$2 \times (Na + K) + BS\ (mmol) + urea\ (mmol/l)$$

+ +	Acetone in urine	(+)
<10 mmol/l	Bicarbonate	>10 mmol/l
Normal to ↓	Na	Normal to ↑
Normal to ↑	K	Normal to ↓

Hyperglycaemic ketoacidotic coma	Hyperglycaemic hyperosmolar coma

Treatment
1. Correction of fluid deficit
(Total deficit ca. 10–15% of body weight)

	Hyperglycaemic ketoacidotic coma	Hyperglycaemic hyperosmolar coma
Initial	1000 ml 0.9% NaCl/hour	1000 ml 0.9% NaCl/hour
		(Na > 155 mmol/l = NaCl 0.45%)
Subsequently	500 ml 0.9% NaCl/hour or according to CVP:	500 ml 0.9% NaCl/hour <0 = 1500 ml/hour 0–3 = 1000 ml/hour 4–8 = 500 ml/hour

2. Insulin dosage
(soluble insulin i.v.)

Initial	(Bolus 10 units) + continuous infusion 6–10 units/hour	No bolus + continuous infusion 3–6 units/hour
Course	Aim: Fall of blood glucose (initially hourly) 2.5–5 mmol/hour; More rapid reduction → danger of cerebral oedema!	

3. Correction of acidosis
Consider if signs of acidotic heart failure, i.e. hypotension with raised central venous pressure, are present

(only if pH < 7.0; stop when pH > 7.2)

1/3 of calculated base deficit = 0.1 base deficit × body weight (kg) as sodium bicarbonate 8.4%

4. Electrolyte replacement

Potassium	>5.5 mmol/l:	no replacement, monitor
	4.0–5.5 mmol/l:	10–20 mmol/h
	<4.0 mmol/l:	20–40 mmol/h
Sodium	>155 mmol/l:	1/2 electrolyte solution
Phosphate	<0.40 mmol/l:	4–10 mmol/h

Differential diagnosis
Other causes of disturbed consciousness (coma)

Hypoglycaemia: Rapid diagnosis by quick blood glucose determination → glucose i.v.

Lactic acidosis: Kussmaul respiration, but no acetone fetor
Anion gap: $Na^+ - (Cl^- + HCO_3^-) > 30$ mmol/l

Modified after: Krebs and Otto (1986)
Haslbeck (1989)

Check-up of the rheumatological patient

1. **Family history**

   Arthropathies (polyarthritis, ankylosing spondylitis), metabolic disorders (gout), allergies, skin diseases (psoriasis), osteoporosis.

2. **Past history**

   Previous joint inflammations and other disorders of the locomotor system (course), skin and mucous membrane conditions (psoriasis, aphthous ulcers, balanitis), ophthalmic conditions (conjunctivitis, iritis, iridocyclitis).

   Infections (TB, throat infections, urethritis, gonorrhoea, syphilis, tick bites (*Borrelia* infection)).

   Gastrointestinal tract: peptic ulcer, ulcerative colitis, Crohn's disease.

   Occupational history: dependence on activity, accidents.

   Psychosocial history (including pension).

3. **Present complaint**

   - **Pain**

     Localization:
     Joints: mono-, polyarticular, small or large joints, symmetrical or asymmetrical. Joint involvement in sequence.
     Pain in tendon insertions, musculature, adipose tissue.
     Backache (especially cervical and small of back), radiation.

     Temporal relation:
     Onset acute or gradual, pain progressive, diminishing or recurrent. Maximum intensity: nocturnal pain, morning pain, continuous pain. Morning stiffness.

     Relation to exertion:
     Spontaneous pain: pain on movement (at onset or on exercise), rest pain. Pain on coughing or sneezing. Pain in certain postures (lying, sitting, standing).
     Combination of the pain with other symptoms (paraesthesia, swelling, redness, heat).

   - **General symptoms**

     Therapy
     Previous physiotherapeutic, medicinal (especially corticosteroids and NSAIDs), orthopaedic and surgical treatments.

Rheumatological status

1. Axial skeleton

Inspection:
Posture, gait (limping), asymmetry of pelvis and shoulders (oblique pelvis: shortening of leg?), scoliosis (torsion of spine?), muscular atrophy, foot deformities, obesity. Height (especially with osteoporosis).

Palpation:
Pain on percussion or pressure, pain on agitation of individual vertebrae, Mennel manoeuvre (painful in sacroiliitis). Muscle spasm.

Functional examination:
Mobility test in three planes (finger–ground distance, Schober measurement (lumbar spine), thoracic spine rotation, sideways flexion and backward extension (blockages? laxity? harmonic flexion?)).
Thoracic circumference inspiration/expiration, examination of muscle function.

2. Joints

Inspection:
Redness, swelling, deformity, abnormal position, muscular atrophy.

Palpation:
Heat, swelling (differential dignosis: intra-articular effusion, synovial swelling, osteophytes, periarticular swelling, extra-articular swelling (ganglion, tenosynovitis, bursitis, exostosis)). Pressure pain of the joints and its localization. Periarticular pressure pain with insertion tendinitis/tendinosis. Crepitus.

Functional examination:
Measurement of active and passive excursion angle for flexion/extension, abduction/adduction, internal/external rotation, pronation/supination (neutral-null method).
Movement and end-phase pain. Crepitus. Instability. Combination movements. At the shoulder joints: C7–thumb distance; at the hand: fist closure and dynamometer values.

General medical examination

Skin (psoriasis, erythema, tophi, signs of vasculitis, peau d'orange). Mucous membranes (aphthous ulcers, ulcers, balanitis). Eyes: iritis, conjunctivitis, keratitis. Rheumatic nodules. Scleroderma.

Neurological status

Motor system (power and coordination), sensation (superficial and deep), reflexes, Lasègue's sign (sciatic stretch test).

Examination of the range of joint mobility (neutral-null method)

(After recommendations of the German and Swiss Orthopaedic Society)

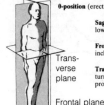

0-position (erect, feet parallel, arms extended at side of body, thumbs to front)

Sagittal plane: Flexion = bending, extension = straightening (plantar flexion = lowering of tip of foot, dorsal extension = elevation of tip of foot)

Frontal plane: Abduction = inclination away from midline, adduction = inclination towards midline

Transverse plane: Outward rotation = turning outwards, inward rotation = turning inwards (shoulder, hip), supination = palm towards front, sole inwards, pronation = palm towards back, lateral border of foot upwards/outwards.

Transverse plane

Frontal plane

Sagittal plane

Recording by the null-point transit method
1st Number: Movement towards body (flexion, adduction, inward rotation, anteversion)
2nd Number: 0-position (if not attained, 1st or 3rd number)
3rd Number: Movement away from body (extension, abduction, outward rotation, retroversion)

Normal values shoulder joint			
Anteversion/retroversion	150–170/0/40	Inward/outward rotation with forearm against body	40–60/0/95
Adduction/abduction	20–40/0/180	Inward/outward rotation with upper arm elevated sideways to 90 degrees	70/0/70

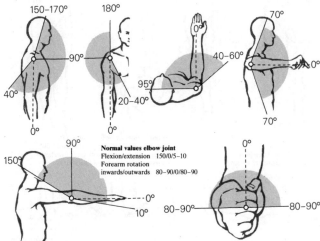

Normal values elbow joint
Flexion/extension 150/0/5–10
Forearm rotation inwards/outwards 80–90/0/80–90

Normal values wrist joint

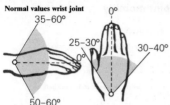

Palmar flexion/dorsiflexion   50–60/0/35–60
Radial abduction/ulnar abduction   25–30/0/30–40

Fingers
Metacarpophalangeal
joint of thumb
abduction/adduction
in palmar plane 70/0

Abduction/adduction
at right angle to
palmar plane 70/0

Terminal joint of thumb
Flexion/extension 80/0

Basal joint of thumb
Flexion/extension 50/0

Finger tip–palm
distance (in cm)

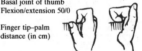

Normal values hip joint

Flexion/extension	130–140/0/10
Inward/outward rotation with hip flexed to 90 degrees	40–50/0/40–50
Inward/outward rotation with extended hip joint	30–40/0/40–50
Adduction/abduction	20–30/0/30–45

Normal values knee joint
Flexion/extension 120–150/0/5–10

Normal values ankle/foot joints
Plantar flexion/dorsiflexion 40–50/0/20–30
Pronation/supination (with fixed calcaneum) 15/0/35
Eversion/inversion (total) 30/0/60

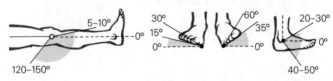

Classification of inflammatory illnesses

Chronic polyarthritis (cP)
• Felty's syndrome (seropositive cP with splenomegaly and leucopenia)
• Caplan's syndrome (pneumoconiosis and cP)
Juvenile chronic arthritis (types: systemic (Still's disease), mono- or polyarticular ± iridocyclitis, polyarticular)
Still's disease of adults
Palindromic rheumatism
Chronic atrophic polychondritis
Giant cell arteritis (temporal arteritis/polymyalgia rheumatica)
Behçet's syndrome
Eosinophilic fasciitis (Shulman's syndrome)
Eosinophilic myalgic syndrome (with L-tryptophan)
Sarcoidosis (Löfgren's syndrome: arthritis in acute sarcoidosis)
Amyloidosis; vasculitides
Collagenoses (in the strict sense)
Systemic lupus erythematosus (SLE)
• Drug-induced lupus
• Antiphospholipid syndrome (lupus anticoagulant – anticardiolipin antibody with arterial and venous
thromboses, abortion, thrombopenia)
Mixed connective tissue disease (MCTD), Sharp's syndrome
Systemic sclerosis (progressive systemic scleroderma (PSS))
• CREST syndrome (calcinosis, Raynaud's syndrome, oesophageal dysfunction, sclerodactyly, telangiectasia)
Dermato-/polymyositis
Polyarteritis nodosa
Wegener's granulomatosis, Churg–Strauss syndrome
Sjögren's syndrome

Reactive arthritides and seronegative spondylarthritides in
Ankylosing spondylitis (Pierre–Marie–Strümpell–Bechterew disease)
Psoriatic arthropathy
Enterogenous arthritides (with ulcerative colitis, Crohn's disease, Whipple's disease (probably through
Corynebacterium-induced jejunitis)) post-bypass syndrome
Reiter's syndrome (urethro-oculo-synovial syndrome)
Reactive arthritides: after enteral (*Yersinia, Shigella, Salmonella, Campylobacter, Clostridium difficile*), urogenital
(*Chlamydia*), pharyngeal (streptococci, rheumatic fever) infections
SAPHO syndrome (synovitis, acne, pustulosis, hyperostosis, osteitis)

Infective arthritides/spondylitis/spondylodiscitis
Pyogenic (bacterial arthritis, with *Staphylococcus aureus, Strept. pneumoniae*, streptococci, *Haemophilus
influenzae, Neisseria gonorrhoeae*), *Brucella spondylodiscitis*
Lyme disease (*Borrelia burgdorferi*)
Tuberculous (*Mycobacterium tuberculosis*, atypical mycobacteria)
Viral (AIDS, rubella, mumps, measles, hepatitis B, parvovirus)
Mycoses (*Actinomyces, Candida albicans, Sporotrichosis*)

Crystal-induced arthritides
Gouty arthritis (uric acid arthritis)
Pseudogout with chondrocalcinosis (calcium pyrophosphate hydrate crystals), idiopathic or secondary, especially
in Wilson's disease, haemochromatosis, hyperparathyroidism
Hydroxyapatite-induced arthritis
• Milwaukee shoulder (rapidly destructive shoulder arthropathy)
• With dialysis, milk-alkali syndrome, chondrocalcinosis
Corticosteroid injection

Arthropathies with endocrine and metabolic disturbances
Acromegaly, diabetes mellitus, hyper-/hypoparathyroidism, renal osteodystrophy, thyroid disorders, Cushing's
syndrome
Haemochromatosis, ochronosis

Neuropathic arthropathies (Charcot joint) in
Diabetes mellitus, tabes dorsalis, syringomyelia, hemiplegia

Arthropathies with haematological illnesses
Haemoblastoses, coagulopathies, haemolytic anaemias, haemochromatosis, reticuloses

Arthropathies with tumours
Paraneoplastic syndrome, villonodular synovitis, benign and malignant tumours, tumour metastases

Classification of degenerative illnesses

Osteoarthritis (arthrosis deformans)

Polyarthrosis of fingers (Heberden's nodes) (involvement of distal interphalangeal joints), Bouchard's arthrosis (involvement of proximal interphalangeal joints), rhizarthrosis (involvement of the basal thumb joint) Osteoarthritis of shoulder, hip, knee, etc.

Degenerative diseases of the vertebral column

(± associated with malformations and abnormal posture (static disturbances, scoliosis, juvenile kyphosis, Scheuermann's disease))

(Osteo-)chondrosis, spondylosis, spondylarthrosis

Disc prolapse ± root compression (including cauda equina syndrome, spinal stenosis (neurogenic intermittent claudication))

DISH (diffuse idiopathic skeletal hyperostosis; Forestier's disease)

Classification of extra-articular illnesses

(Soft-tissue rheumatism)

Fibromyalgia (generalized tendon myopathy)

Diseases of the subcutaneous connective tissue

• Panniculosis ('cellulitis')
• Panniculitis nodularis (Pfeifer–Weber–Christian disease)
• Panniculitis with pancreatic diseases
• Lipomatosis; erythema nodosum

Diseases of the tendons, tendon sheaths, ligaments, fasciae, bursae

• (Insertion) tendinitis, (insertion) tendinosis, tendomyositis, tendoperiostitis, tenosynovitis
• Progressive hardening and contracture of the palmar aponeurosis (Dupuytren's disease), or of the plantar fascia (Ledderhose's disease)
• Bursitis

Diseases of the musculature

• Functional myalgic syndrome (with overload, abnormal posture and static disturbances (spine))
• Myopathies of various causes
• Infectious myositis
• Polymyositis with collagenoses

Periarthropathies

• Hip periarthropathy (insertion tendinosis, possibly with bursitis of greater trochanter), periarthropathy of knee
• Humeroscapular periarthropathy (HSP) as collective term for periarticular pain and functional disturbances in the shoulder region:
  – HSP simplex
      Supraspinatus syndrome (with calcium deposits)
      Biceps tendinopathies
  – Acute HSP (acute inflammation in region of a calcium or hydroxyapatite deposit with shoulder mobility limited by pain
  – Pseudoparalytic/pseudoparetic HSP with rotator cuff injury (supraspinatus and long biceps tendon)
  – Ankylosing HSP (frozen shoulder) with capsule contracture following trauma, reflex (after cardiac infarct), with degenerative changes, diabetes mellitus

Peripheral nerve entrapment syndromes

Carpal tunnel syndrome (median nerve)
Ulnar compression syndrome (in ulnar groove at elbow)
Meralgia paraesthetica (lateral cutaneous nerve of thigh)
Tarsal tunnel syndrome (tibial nerve or its branches (medial or lateral plantar nerves) between medial malleolus and calcaneum)
Morton's metatarsalgia (digital branches of plantar nerves)

Neurodystrophic disturbances

Algoneurodystrophy (Sudeck's atrophy) at various sites

Classification of illnesses of bone (including osteogenic arthropathies)

Osteoporosis, osteomalacia
Paget's disease of bone (osteodystrophy deformans)
Fibrous osteodystrophy, osteosclerosis, osteonecrosis, (juvenile) osteochondritis dissecans, other osteopathies (such as osteomyelitis, benign and malignant tumours)

Laboratory investigations

Tests	Interpretation (selection)
Humoral inflammation parameters	
Sedimentation rate (ESR)	Important parameter for differentiation inflammatory/non-inflammatory rheumatic illness, indicator for activity
Others: C-reactive protein (CRP) Acute-phase proteins	Reacts more quickly than ESR in inflammatory conditions α_1-glycoprotein, α_1-antitrypsin, α_2-ceruloplasmin, α_2-haptoglobin, fibrinogen and others
Electrophoresis	p. 201
Blood count	Microcytic anaemia as parameter of inflammatory activity (DD: haemorrhagic complications of NSAIDs, steroids; autoimmune haemolytic anaemia in SLE, gold therapy) Leucocytosis/thrombocytosis in acute inflammatory illnesses Leucopenia/thrombocytopenia in SLE, Felty's syndrome
Clinical chemical laboratory findings	
Uric acid	Gout. Diuretics (hydrochlorothiazide, chlorthalidone, frusemide, ethacrynic acid) Myeloproliferative syndrome (p. 211)
Creatine kinase (CK) Aldolase Lactate dehydrogenase	Raised in (poly)myositis, dermatomyositis, inflammatory muscle involvement in SLE, rheumatoid arthritis, Sjögren's syndrome Drug-induced myopathy (triamcinolone, chloroquine, penicillamine)
Alkaline phosphatase Calcium, inorganic phosphate	Metabolic bone diseases (hyperparathyroidism, osteomalacia, Paget's disease), see p. 264
Serological–immunological investigations	
Rheumatoid factors (Latex test, Rose–Waaler test)	Occurrence: Rheumatoid arthritis (RA) 70–80%. Note: patients with juvenile RA are often seronegative. Collagenoses ca. 30%. Non-rheumatoid illnesses: often positive; also in subacute bacterial endocarditis, liver diseases, TB, syphilis, acute viral infections
Antinuclear factors/antibodies (ANF/ANA)	Collagenoses (especially SLE, systemic sclerosis, mixed connective tissue disease (MCTD)) Special antibody patterns
Complement tests	Serum complement as total haemolytic activity (CH50), individual complement components (C3, C4). Reduced in active SLE. Raised in acute-phase reaction
Circulating immune complexes (CIC), C1q binding	Measurements of progression and activity criteria in various inflammatory illnesses
Arthritis serology, bacterial antibodies in reactive arthritides	Demonstration of antibodies against: *Salmonellae*, shigellae, yersiniae, *Campylobacter*, gonococci, borreliae, chlamydiae, HIV, etc., antistreptolysin O titre (clearly positive in ca. 80% of patients with rheumatic fever); measurement of progression
Immunogenetic investigations	
Histocompatibility antigen (HLA typing)	HLA-B27 – ankylosing spondylitis, Reiter's syndrome, etc.

Joint aspirates

Basic aspirate characteristics	Normal values	Non-inflammatory (Group I)	Inflammatory (Group II)	Septic (Group III)	Haemorrhagic (Group IV)
Volume (knee joint)	< 3.5 ml	> 3.5 ml	> 3.5 ml	> 3.5 ml	
Turbidity	Transparent	Transparent	Cloudy	Cloudy	Cloudy/bloody
Colour	Colourless	Pale yellow	Yellow/white to xanthochromic	Yellow to greenish	Reddish
Viscosity	High	High	Reduced	Reduced/variable	Increased
Leucocytes (per µl)	< 20	200–2000	2000–100 000	> 100 000[b]	Erythrocytes
Polymorphonuclear leucocytes	< 25%	< 25%	50% and more	75% and more	Corresponding to blood count
Cultures	Negative	Negative	Negative	Often positive	Negative
Mucin coagulation	Firm	Firm	Deficient to absent	Fragile coagulum	
Glucose	Almost as blood glucose[a]	Almost as blood glucose[a]	More than 25% lower than blood glucose[a]	Mostly considerably lower than blood glucose[a]	Almost as blood glucose[a]
Possible aetiology		Degenerative (osteoarthritis)	Rheumatoid arthritis	Bacterial infections	Trauma
		Trauma (also haemorrhagic)	Reiter's syndrome		Haemorrhagic diathesis
		Osteochondritis dissecans	Acute crystal sinovitis (gout and pseudogout) Ankylosing spondylitis (Bechterew's disease)		Neuropathic joint illnesses (also Group I)
		Osteochondromatosis			Neoplasms
		Neuropathic joint illnesses (also Group IV)	Psoriatic arthritis		Haemangioma, synovioma
		Hypertrophic osteoarthropathy	Arthritis with ulcerative colitis and regional enteritis (Crohn's disease)		Pigmented villonodular synovitis (also Group I or II)
			Rheumatic fever (also Group I) SLE (also Group I) Progressive systemic sclerosis (scleroderma) (also Group I)		

[a] Simultaneously collected serum.   [b] Fewer on treatment or with organisms of low virulence.

Viscosity: normal (drop from syringe with tail longer than 6 cm); **reduced** (shorter or completely absent tail)
Turbidity: transparent (print can be read through synovial fluid in test tube); **cloudy** (print cannot be read through synovial fluid in test tube)

Further investigations: Demonstration of crystals (uric acid crystals, negative birefringence: gout)
Demonstration of phagocytes
Centrifuge ⊰ Sediment → Cytology
Supernatant → Immunological/biochemical examination

(After Rodman (1973))

Revised (1987) ARA criteria for the classification of rheumatoid arthritis (RA)

(American Rheumatism Association, 1988)

1. Morning stiffness > 1 h
2. Simultaneous swelling of > 3 joint regions
   (Joint regions: right and left PIP, MCP, wrist joints, elbow, knee, ankle joints or MTP joints)
3. Swelling of MCP, PIP or wrist joint
4. Symmetrical swelling
5. Rheumatoid nodules
6. Positive rheumatoid factor (any method is suitable which has a specificity >95%)
7. Typical radiological changes (definite osteoporosis near affected joints, periarticular erosions) in the P–A film of the hands and/or wrist joints

At least 4 of these 7 criteria must be fulfilled for the diagnosis of rheumatoid arthritis. Criteria 1 to 4 must be present for > 6 weeks.

Abbreviations: **PIP** proximal interphalangeal joint
 MCP metacarpophalangeal joint
 MTP metatarsophalangeal joint

ARA criteria (1982) for systemic lupus erythematosus (SLE)

(Tan *et al.*, 1982)

1. Butterfly erythema of face
2. Discoid lupus
3. Photosensitivity
4. Mucous ulceration in mouth and nasopharynx
5. Non-erosive arthritis
6. Pleurisy and/or pericarditis
7. Renal involvement: proteinuria > 0.5 g/day or urinary casts
8. CNS involvement: psychosis or fits
9. Haemolytic anaemia or leucopenia (< 4000/μl) (on at least 2 occasions) or lymphopenia (< 1500/μl (on at least 2 occasions)) or thrombocytopenia (< 100 000)
10. LE cells or anti-DNA antibodies or anti-Sm antibodies or false-positive serological tests for syphilis (twice within 6 months)
11. High antinuclear antibody (ANA) titre

Revised Jones criteria for diagnosis of rheumatic fever (RF)

(Stollermann *et al.*, 1965)

Main criteria
Carditis, polyarthritis, Sydenham's chorea, erythema (marginatum), subcutaneous nodules

Secondary criteria
Clinical
Previous rheumatic fever or rheumatic carditis, arthralgia, fever

Investigations:
Acute-phase reactions (raised sedimentation rate, raised C-reactive protein, leucocytosis, prolonged PQ interval (ECG))
plus
Indication of preceding streptococcal infection (raised antistreptolysin O titre or other streptococcal antibodies, throat swab positive for streptococci Lancefield Group A, preceding scarlet fever)

Rheumatic fever very probable:
2 main criteria or 1 main criterion and 2 secondary criteria, when preceding streptococcal infection confirmed

ARC criteria for fibromyalgia 1990

(Wolfe *et al.*, 1990)

1. History of widespread pains

Definition:
Pains are considered as widespread if they are present in both sides of the body above and below the waist. Axial skeletal pains (cervical, thoracic or lumbar spine or anterior chest wall) must also be present.

2. Pains in at least 11 of the 18 examined pressure pain points

Definition:
Pain on palpation must be present in at least 11 of the following examined pressure pain points:

Occiput: bilateral, at the insertion of the sub-occipital muscles.
Lower cervical spine: bilateral, on the anterior aspect between the transverse processes C5–C7.

Trapezius: bilateral, middle of upper border of trapezius.
Supraspinatus: bilateral, at origin, near the middle of the border, above the spine of the scapula.

2nd rib: bilateral, level of the 2nd chondrosternal junction.

Lateral epicondyle of humerus: bilateral, 2 cm distal to the epicondyles.

Gluteal: bilateral, in upper outer quadrant of buttock.

Greater trochanter: bilateral, dorsal to the trochanteric prominence.

Knee: bilateral, over the medial fat pad proximal to the joint cleft.

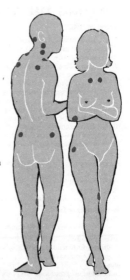

Finger pressure should be applied at about 4 kg. For a pressure point to be designated positive the patient must describe it as painful.
'Pressure sensitive' is not regarded as 'painful'.

> The diagnosis of fibromyalgia can be made if both criteria are fulfilled. The pains must be present for at least 3 months. The presence of another illness does not exclude the diagnosis of fibromyalgia.

Diagnostic criteria for the spondylarthropathies

(Dougados *et al.*, 1991)

| Pains from the spine with inflammatory characteristics | or | Synovitis asymmetric preferentially in the lower extremities |

and

one or more of the following criteria:

Positive family history:
Presence of the following conditions in first or second degree relatives:
(a) Ankylosing spondylitis, (b) psoriasis, (c) acute uveitis, (d) reactive arthritis, (e) inflammatory bowel disease

Psoriasis:
Previously diagnosed by a physician or present at the time of examination

Inflammatory bowel disease:
Crohn's disease or ulcerative colitis, previously diagnosed by a physician or present at the time of examination, and confirmed by endoscopy or radiology

Non-specific urethritis, cervicitis or acute diarrhoea:
Within 1 month of the appearance of the arthritis

Buttock pain, alternating between left and right gluteal region:
Previous, or present at the time of examination

Heel pain:
Spontaneously volunteered pain or tenderness at the insertion of the achilles tendon or the plantar fascia, previous or present at the time of examination

Sacroiliitis:
Bilateral grade 2–4 or unilateral grade 3–4 (grade 0 radiologically normal; grade 1 sacroiliitis possible; grade 2 minimal inflammatory changes; grade 3 moderately severe definite sacroiliitis; grade 4 ankylosis)

Principal symptoms of syndromes of vertebral origin

1. Soft-tissue rheumatic affections (including tendinoses, tendomyoses, e.g. chain tendinoses)

2. Pseudoradicular syndromes

3. Neurogenic syndromes (medullary, radicular, vegetative compression syndromes)

4. Vascular syndromes (intermittent circulatory disturbances)

5. Circumscribed postural changes (with kyphosis, lordosis, scoliosis, contracture)

6. Segmental disturbance of function (movement restriction with blockage, fixation; abnormal laxity)

Osteoporosis

I. Etiology: primary osteoporosis
(idiopathic, juvenile, postmenopausal, presenile and senile osteoporosis)

II. Etiology: secondary osteoporosis

1. Genetic (osteogenesis imperfecta; women > men, positive family history, slim configuration)

2. Endocrine (e.g. hyperthyroidism, Cushing's syndrome, gonadal insufficiency)

3. Gastrointestinal (e.g. after total or subtotal gastrectomy and small bowel resection, malabsorption*; liver, gall bladder, pancreatic diseases)

4. Dietary (malnutrition*, calcium deficiency)

5. Metabolic (e.g. diabetes mellitus; chronic alcoholism*)

6. Renal (e.g. with glomerular or tubular insufficiency)

7. Iatrogenic (e.g. steroids, heparin therapy)

8. Immobilization

*'Osteoporomalacia'

The radiologist's 'osteoporosis tree'
(After Haas (1983))

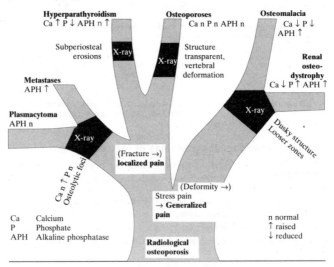

Non-steroidal anti-inflammatory drugs

Group	Substances	Plasma elimination half time
Fenamate	Mefenamic acid	ca. 1–2 h
Acetic acid derivatives	Acemetacin	ca. 2–6 h
	Diclofenac	1–2 h
	Etodolac	ca. 7–8 h
	Indomethacin	ca. 2 h
	Sulindac	7–16 h
	Tolmetin	ca. 2 h
Propionic acid derivatives	Ibuprofen	ca. 2 h
	Fenbufen	ca. 10 h
	Fenoprofen	ca. 3 h
	Naproxen	ca. 12 h
	Tiaprofenic acid	ca. 2 h
	Ketoprofen	ca. 2 h
	Flurbiprofen	ca. 3 h
Oxicams	Piroxicam	ca. 40 h
	Tenoxicam	ca. 70 h
Pyrazone derivative	Phenylbutazone	ca. 75 h
	Azapropazone	ca. 14 h
Salicylic acid derivative	Acetylsalicylic acid	ca. 15 min
	Benorylate	ca. 2 h
	Diflunisal	ca. 7.5 h
Naphthyl alkalone derivative	Nabumetone	ca. 24 h

Important pharmacokinetic interactions

I. **Anti-coagulants:** → In general, all NSAIDs can increase anticoagulation (haemorrhage!), including acetylsalicylic acid, azapropazone, oxyphenbutazone, phenylbutazone

II. **Anti-diabetics:** → Increased antidiabetic effect (hypoglycaemic shock!), especially acetylsalicylic acid, azapropazone, phenylbutazone, oxyphenbutazone

III. **Antihyper-tensives:** → In general, all NSAIDs can reduce the antihypertensive effect, especially indomethacin, naproxen, ibuprofen, piroxicam, salicylates in high dosage

IV. **Anti-convulsants:** → Increased phenytoin toxicity(!), especially phenyl-butazone

V. **Lithium:** → Lithium toxicity increased, especially diclofenac, indomethacin, naproxen, piroxicam, phenylbutazone

VI. **Metho-trexate:** → Increased MTX toxicity, especially azapropazone, diclofenac, indomethacin, naproxen, piroxicam, phenylbutazone, salicylate

VII. **Beta-blockers:** → Reduction of antihypertensive effect, especially indomethacin, naproxen

VIII. **Digitalis glycosides:** → Blood digoxin level increased, especially diclofenac, indomethacin

IX. **Diuretics:** → Reduced diuretic effect ± all NSAIDs in variable intensity

X. **Simultaneous administration of corticosteroids or other NSAIDs increases the risk of side effects!**

Differentiation of blood–CSF barrier disturbances and autochthonous IgG production in CNS

(Reiber and Felgenhauer, 1987)

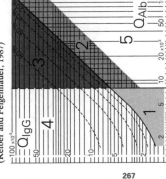

In order to characterize the blood–CSF barrier function, the quotient of CSF and serum concentrations of albumin (Q_{Alb}) is determined. The CSF/serum quotient for IgG is entered into the graph as a function of the albumin quotient and this permits the differentiation of five different situations:

1. Normal range;
2. Pure barrier disturbance without local IgG synthesis;
3. Barrier function disturbance with additional IgG synthesis in CNS;
4. Pure IgG synthesis in CNS without barrier function disturbance;
5. Empirically, no values have been found in this area, other than through errors in blood sample collection or in analysis.

As a rule, cases with local IgG synthesis in the CNS lie above the heavy line (hyperbolic function). Values below this usually represent CSF–serum IgG quotients which result from passive diffusion of serum IgG into the CSF. An isoelectric examination in this area can, through its greater sensitivity, differentiate fractions synthesized locally in the CNS (oligoclonal IgG). The logarithmic lines in areas 3 and 4 indicate the percentage of the total IgG which originates in the CNS.

Common CNS findings (cf. p. 178)

Cells	Glucose	Protein	Other findings	Diagnosis
Polymorphonuclear pleocytosis	↓ →	↑	Lactate ↑, possibly bacteria (cocci)	Bacterial meningitis, brain abscess
Mixed pleocytosis	↓		Spider's web clot	Tuberculous meningitis, chemical meningitis
Lymphomonocytic pleocytosis	Normal	(↑)	Perhaps specific antibody changes	Viral meningitis or encephalitis
Lymphomonocytic pleocytosis	→	–		Fungal, leptospiral, listerial, spirochetal meningitis; Mollaret's meningitis; carcinomatous or leukaemic meningitis
Discrete lymphomonocytic pleocytosis or normal	Normal	normal	Intrathecal IgG production	Multiple sclerosis
Normal	Normal	↑	–	Polyneuritis, Guillain-Barré syndrome

Visual pathway lesions and visual field defects

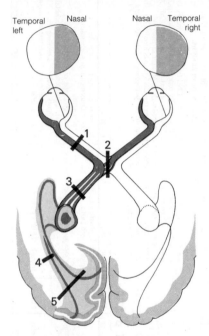

Left   Right

1 Left amaurosis

2 Bitemporal hemianopia

3 Right homonymous hemianopia

4 Upper quadrantic anopia

5 Right homonymous hemianopia with preserved central vision

Trigeminal nerve distribution

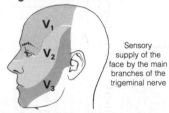

Sensory supply of the face by the main branches of the trigeminal nerve

V_1 ophthalmic division, V_2 maxillary division
V_3 mandibular division

Eliciting the corneal reflex

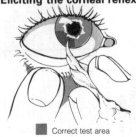

■ Correct test area

Neurological examination

	Upper limb	Lower limb	Trunk/Stature/Gait
General	Left/right handed, muscle tone, muscular atrophy, strength, mobility, position test	Lasègue's sign, muscle tone, muscular atrophy, strength, mobility, position test	Posture, configuration of spinal column, spinal pain, standing normally and on one leg, walking normally, on heels or toes, walking in a straight line
Pyramidal tract signs	Mayer reflex, Wartenberg's sign	Babinski's plantar sign, Gordon's sign, Oppenheim's reflex persistent clonus	Spastic gait

Pyramidal tract signs/reflexes

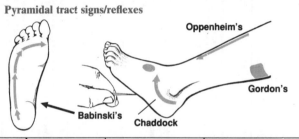

Superficial sensation	Touch, pain, temperature, two-point discrimination	Touch, pain, temperature two-point discrimination, figure writing appreciation	Walking with eyes shut (sensory ataxia?)
Deep sensation	Vibration sense, position sense of fingers (passive), astereognosis	Vibration sense, position sense of toes (passive)	
Coordination	Finger–nose test, diadochokinesia, rebound phenomenon, fine finger movements	Heel-knee test, rebound phenomenon	Walking in straight line, truncal ataxia, Romberg's sign, Unterberger's step test, walking with eyes shut
Proprioceptive reflexes	Brachioradialis jerk C_5, C_6 Biceps jerk C_5, C_6, Triceps jerk C_6, C_7, Trömner's sign C_8–T_1	Knee jerk $L_{3,4}$ Ankle jerk L_5, S_1	
Cutaneous reflexes		Plantar response L_5–S_2	Abdominal reflex T_{5-12} Cremaster reflex L_1, L_2 Anal reflex S_3–S_5

Cranial nerves

Cranial nerve	Function	Examination	Important causes of a lesion of the nerve	Remarks
I Olfactory n.	Sense of smell	Aromatic substances Trigeminal irritants	Trauma, olfactory meningioma, inflammation, drugs	Synaesthetic taste disturbance with anosmia
II Optic n.	Vision	Visual acuity, fundoscopy, visual fields (finger perimetry)	Papilloedema, retrobulbar neuritis, papillitis, ischaemic ophthalmopathy, optic n. glioma, trauma, Leber's optic atrophy, chiasmal compression (pituitary tumours)	Visual field defects with lesions of optic tract and visual cortex
III Oculomotor n.	Levator palpebrae, medial, superior, inferior rectus, inferior oblique muscles, pupillary sphincter	Eye following movements, pupil reactions, ptosis	Diabetic mononeuropathy, aneurysm of posterior communicating a., tumours, trauma, vascular causes	Pupil usually involved in pressure lesions; DD: internuclear ophthalmoplegia
IV Trochlear n.	Superior oblique m.	Eye movements	Trauma, vascular causes, tumours	Bielschowsky's phenomenon
V Trigeminal n.	Sensation of face and eyes, tongue, part of oral cavity and nasopharynx Muscles of mastication	Peripheral and central sensation Mouth opening (deviation towards affected side), chewing (palpation of the muscles) Corneal reflex, masseter reflex	Trigeminal neuralgia/-neuropathy, acoustic neuroma, Wallenberg's syndrome and other brain stem conditions, cerebral infarct Toxic, infective, tumours at base of skull, trigeminal neuroma, trauma	As accompanying symptoms with supratentorial conditions
VI Abducens n.	Lateral rectus m.	Eye following movements	Infections, increased intracranial pressure, skull/brain trauma, MS, parainfectious, vascular	Commonest isolated eye muscle paresis

Cranial nerve	Function	Examination	Important causes of a lesion of the nerve	Remarks
VII Facial n.	Facial innervation, tear and salivary glands, taste sensation to anterior 2/3 of tongue	Muscles of facial expression (frowning, eye closure, wrinkling of nose, showing teeth), Schirmer's test (tear secretion), stapedius reflex, taste examination	Cooling (idiopathic), otic zoster, fractures of petrous, borreliosis, Guillain-Barré syndrome, tumours, Melkersson–Rosenthal syndrome, perioperative lesion	Forehead not involved in central facial paresis and lid closure complete. Bell's phenomenon with peripheral facial paresis
VIII Auditory vestibular n.	Hearing, balance organ* (p. ••)	Hearing test (including Weber and Rinne tests), test for nystagmus, oculovestibular reflex	Sudden deafness, vestibulitis, petrous fracture, vestibular neuropathy, acoustic neuroma, benign positional vertigo (degeneration of otolith)	Central vertigo with vertebrobasilar ischaemia
IX Glosso-pharyngeal n.	Muscles of deglutition (swallowing), sensation (middle ear, pharynx, root of tongue), taste sensation to posterior 1/3 of tongue, secretion of saliva	Taste examination (bitter), salivary secretion, gag reflex, pharyngeal sensation	Wallenberg's syndrome, glossopharyngeal neuroma, glomus jugulare tumour, fracture of base of skull, tonsillectomy, glossopharyngeal neuralgia	Seldom affected in isolation
X Vagus n.	Vegetative parasympathetic innervation, laryngeal muscles, innervation of soft palate	Examination of soft palate, speech, larynx, vegetative function tests	Anomalies of craniocervical junction, Wallenberg's syndrome, diphtheria, poliomyelitis, bulbar paresis, thyroid surgery (recurrent laryngeal nerve)	Seldom involved in isolation
XI Accessory n.	Trapezius m. (in part), sternocleidomastoid m.	Turning of head Elevation of shoulder	Lymph node biopsy in lateral triangle of neck (only trapezius), lesions of skull base, poliomyelitis, pressure paralysis	Ipsilateral paresis of accessory n. with cerebral infarct and central haemorrhage
XII Hypoglossal n.	Tongue musculature	Protrude tongue (deviation towards affected side), inspection of tongue (atrophy), dysarthria	Tumours (Garcin's syndrome, chordoma of clivus, metastases, hypoglossal neuroma), tuberculous meningitis, after carotid surgery	Central pareses rapidly reversible

*Tests of labyrinthine function

Romberg's test:
Patient stands with eyes closed, feet together, arms extended forwards and supinated; tendency to fall is pathological.

Unterberger's step test:
Walking on the spot with eyes closed; normally not more than 45° deviation after 50 steps.
Barany's pointing test:
After pointing at target, patient raises arm, shuts eyes and slowly lowers arm vertically to the target.

Symptoms of autonomic involvement in polyneuropathies

(Occurrence in: diabetes mellitus, Guillain-Barré syndrome, porphyria, amyloidosis, toxic causes, e.g. alcohol, isoniazid, lead, quinoline, uraemia, hereditary illnesses)

	Symptom	Diagnostic tests
Cardio-vascular	Tachycardia at rest Silent myocardial infarct Orthostatic dysregulation	↓ Variability of heart frequency with hyperventilation, Valsalva test, drugs (atropine, betablocker) Schellong test
Gastro-intestinal	Nocturnal diarrhoea Bloating, heartburn, dysphagia Unrecognized hypoglycaemia Exocrine pancreatic insufficiency Gall bladder enlargement, gallstones, salivary gland inflammation	Small bowel biopsy (exclusion of coeliac disease) Barium meal and follow-through Absence of insulin tachycardia Secretin-pancreozymin test Ultrasound, palpation
Urogenital	Erectile impotence Retrograde ejaculation Residual urine with bladder dysfunction	Testicular analgesia Urinalysis Ultrasound
Trophic	Hypo-/anhydrosis of feet Vasomotor paresis Trophic oedema, alopecia Painless ulcer Disturbed nail growth Osteoarthropathy	Sweat test Histamine test (with noradrenaline) Sympathetic skin response with external stimulus (EMG lead) Plain X-ray

The principal neurological signs of polyneuritis (reduced vibration sense, stocking hypoaesthesia/-algesia and reduced ankle jerk) may be absent.

Red = Basic or screening test

Sensory dermatomes

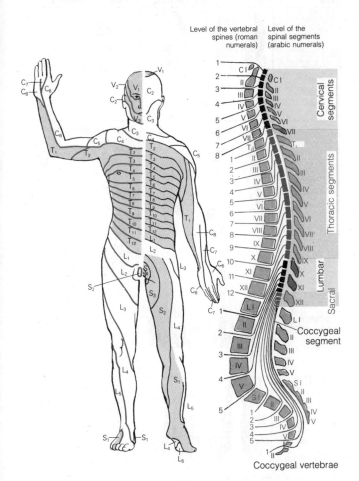

Level of the vertebral spines (roman numerals)

Level of the spinal segments (arabic numerals)

Cervical segments

Thoracic segments

Lumbar

Sacral

Coccygeal segment

Coccygeal vertebrae

Cervical root compression syndromes

Level	Pain	Hypoaesthesia	Pareses	Reflexes
C$_5$ (CV 4, CV 5)			Deltoid m.	Normal
C$_6$ (CV 5, CV 6)			Biceps, brachioradialis mm.	Biceps and brachioradialis reflexes ↓
C$_7$ (CV 6, CV 7)			Triceps m.	Triceps reflex ↓
C$_8$ (CV 7)			Hand muscles	Hoffmann's sign

CV = cervical vertebra
(Modified after Stöhr and Riffel (1988))

Lumbosacral root compression syndromes

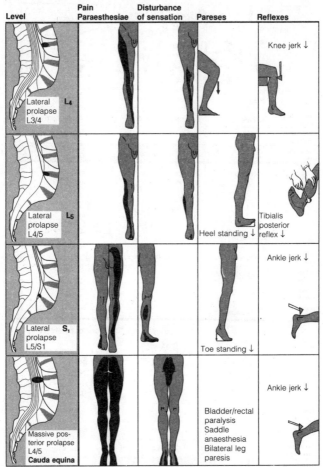

Level	Pain Paraesthesiae	Disturbance of sensation	Pareses	Reflexes
Lateral prolapse L3/4 L₄				Knee jerk ↓
Lateral prolapse L4/5 L₅			Heel standing ↓	Tibialis posterior reflex ↓
Lateral prolapse L5/S1 S₁			Toe standing ↓	Ankle jerk ↓
Massive posterior prolapse L4/5 Cauda equina			Bladder/rectal paralysis Saddle anaesthesia Bilateral leg paresis	Ankle jerk ↓

(Modified after Stöhr and Riffel (1988))

275

Muscle function testing

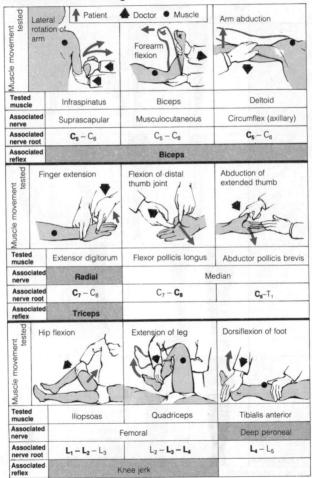

	Lateral rotation of arm	Forearm flexion	Arm abduction
Muscle movement tested	↑ Patient ▲ Doctor ● Muscle		
Tested muscle	Infraspinatus	Biceps	Deltoid
Associated nerve	Suprascapular	Musculocutaneous	Circumflex (axillary)
Associated nerve root	$C_5 - C_6$	$C_5 - C_6$	$C_5 - C_6$
Associated reflex	Biceps		

	Finger extension	Flexion of distal thumb joint	Abduction of extended thumb
Tested muscle	Extensor digitorum	Flexor pollicis longus	Abductor pollicis brevis
Associated nerve	Radial	Median	
Associated nerve root	$C_7 - C_8$	$C_7 - C_8$	$C_8 - T_1$
Associated reflex	Triceps		

	Hip flexion	Extension of leg	Dorsiflexion of foot
Tested muscle	Iliopsoas	Quadriceps	Tibialis anterior
Associated nerve	Femoral		Deep peroneal
Associated nerve root	$L_1 - L_2 - L_3$	$L_2 - L_3 - L_4$	$L_4 - L_5$
Associated reflex	Knee jerk		

			Muscle movement tested
Flexion of forearm between pronation and supination	Radial extension of hand	Forearm extension	
Brachioradialis	Extensor carpi radialis	Triceps	**Tested muscle**
Radial			**Associated nerve**
$C_5 - C_6$	$C_5 - C_6$	$C_6 - C_7 - C_8$	**Associated nerve root**
Brachialis		Triceps	**Associated reflex**
Opposition of metacarpal of thumb	Finger adduction and abduction	Abduction of little finger	Muscle movement tested
Opponens pollicis	Dorsal interosseus	Abductor digiti minimi	**Tested muscle**
Median	Ulnar		**Associated nerve**
$C_8 - T_1$	$C_8 - T_1$	$C_8 - T_1$	**Associated nerve root**
			Associated reflex
Extension of big toe	Plantar flexion of foot	Elevation of thigh while lying prone	Muscle movement tested
Extensor hallucis longus	Gastrocnemius	Gluteus maximus	**Tested muscle**
Deep peroneal	Tibial	Inferior gluteal	**Associated nerve**
$L_5 - S_1$	$S_1 - S_2$	$L_5 - S_1 - S_2$	**Associated nerve root**
	Ankle jerk		**Associated reflex**

277

Glasgow coma scale

(For prognosis in skull/brain trauma and secondary brain injury)
(Teasdale and Jennet, 1976)

	Points		Points
Eye opening		Motor response	
Spontaneous	4	On command	6
To speech	3	Localized pain response	5
To pain stimulus	2	Flexion to pain	4
None	1	Abnormal flexion response	3
		Extensor response	2
Verbal response		None	1
Orientated	5		
Confused conversation	4		
Single words	3		
Incomprehensible sounds	2	Maximal point count	15
None	1	Minimal point count	3

Definition of coma	Eyes	closed	1
	Verbal response	incomprehensible sounds	2 or fewer
	Motor response	localized pain response	5 or fewer
	Coma		8 or fewer

Scale for assessment of pupil size (mm)

2   3   4   5   6   7   8   9

Staging of subarachnoid haemorrhage

(preoperative clinical grading)

Grade	Symptoms and signs				
	State of consciousness	Neurological deficits	Headache	Meningism	Others
I A B	Alert	A^a: none B^b: present	Minimal	Slight	
II A B	Alert	A^a: none B^b: cranial nerve deficits (e.g. photophobia)	Moderate to severe	Definitely present	
III A B	Somnolent Disorientated	A^a: none B^b: mild focal deficits (mild paresis and/or dysphasia)			
IV	Soporific to comatose	Marked focal deficits (moderate to severe hemiparesis and/or dysphasia), early symptoms of decerebration			Pupil reactions present
V	Deep coma	Decerebration, possibly signs of coning			No pupil reactions, moribund

A^a without focal neurological deficits, B^b with focal neurological deficits.

Early operation within 72 h with grades I to III.

Somnolent	Patient wakes only on stimulation, but is completely orientated
Soporific	Patient can only be brought to consciousness briefly by strong stimuli

Disturbances of consciousness

		Slowly increasing disturbance of consciousness	Sudden loss of consciousness	Increasing confusion
Intracranial	Trauma:	Subdural haematoma	Extradural haematoma, contusion	Post-traumatic psychosis, subdural haematoma
	Tumour:	Oedema	Upper or lower impaction, haemorrhage, obstructive hydrocephalus	Oedema
	Vascular:	Space-occupying infarct(s), intracerebral haemorrhage	Brain stem infarct, hypertonic massive haemorrhage, subarachnoid haemorrhage	Oedema after infarct, haemorrhage, transitory global amnesia
	Infective:	Bacterial meningitis, encephalitis	Brain pressure with cerebral abscess, haemorrhage or oedema with (meningo)encephalitis	Encephalitis
	Toxic:	Central pontine myelinolysis, Wernicke's encephalopathy	Central pontine myelinolysis, Degeneration of corpus callosum	Wernicke's encephalopathy, delirium tremens, Korsakow syndrome, alcoholic hallucination
	Epilepsy:		Grand mal, temporal lobe 'faint'	Twilight states, psychomotor attacks
Extracranial	Metabolic:	Electrolyte disturbances (Na, K), acidosis/alkalosis uraemia, liver failure	Electrolyte disturbances (Na, K), porphyria	Electrolyte disturbances, dehydration
	Hormonal:	Hyperglycaemia, hypothyroidism, hypopituitarism	Hypoglycaemia	Hypo/hyperthermia, porphyria. Hyperglycaemia, thyrotoxicosis
	Heart/cardio-vascular, lungs:	Blood loss, anaemia, hypoventilation	Fall in blood pressure, cardiac arrhythmia, carotid sinus syndrome, pulmonary embolus	Anaemia
	Psychiatric:	Catatonia	Psychogenic faint	Dementias
	Toxic:	Sedatives, hypnotics, antidepressants, anticonvulsants, CO, heavy metals	Sedatives, hypnotics, CO, drugs	Heavy metals, drugs

(From Berlit (1992))

279

Anatomy of the cerebral arteries

Carotid system

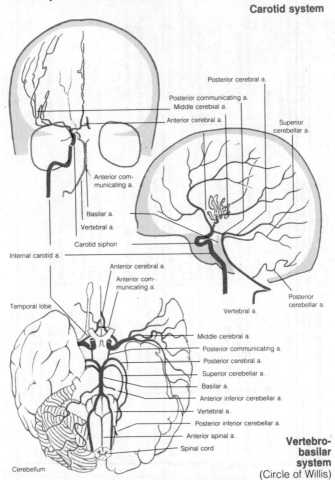

Posterior cerebral a.

Posterior communicating a.
Middle cerebral a.
Anterior cerebral a.

Superior cerebellar a.

Anterior communicating a.

Basilar a.

Vertebral a.

Carotid siphon

Internal carotid a.

Anterior cerebral a.
Anterior communicating a.

Temporal lobe

Posterior cerebellar a.

Vertebral a.

Middle cerebral a.
Posterior communicating a.
Posterior cerebral a.
Superior cerebellar a.
Basilar a.
Anterior inferior cerebellar a.
Vertebral a.
Posterior inferior cerebellar a.
Anterior spinal a.
Spinal cord

Cerebellum

Vertebro-basilar system
(Circle of Willis)

Classification of cerebral ischaemia

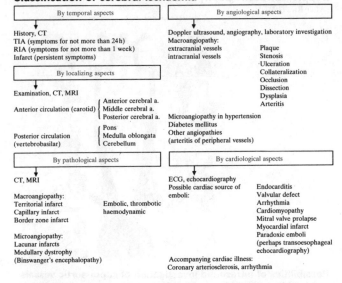

By temporal aspects

History, CT
TIA (symptoms for not more than 24 h)
RIA (symptoms for not more than 1 week)
Infarct (persistent symptoms)

By localizing aspects

Examination, CT, MRI

Anterior circulation (carotid) { Anterior cerebral a.
Middle cerebral a.
Posterior cerebral a.

Posterior circulation (vertebrobasilar) { Pons
Medulla oblongata
Cerebellum

By pathological aspects

CT, MRI

Macroangiopathy:
Territorial infarct
Capillary infarct   Embolic, thrombotic
Border zone infarct   haemodynamic

Microangiopathy:
Lacunar infarcts
Medullary dystrophy
(Binswanger's encephalopathy)

By angiological aspects

Doppler ultrasound, angiography, laboratory investigation
Macroangiopathy:
extracranial vessels   Plaque
intracranial vessels   Stenosis
                              Ulceration
                              Collateralization
                              Occlusion
                              Dissection
                              Dysplasia
                              Arteritis

Microangiopathy in hypertension
Diabetes mellitus
Other angiopathies
(arteritis of peripheral vessels)

By cardiological aspects

ECG, echocardiography
Possible cardiac source of   Endocarditis
emboli: Valvular defect
                                    Arrhythmia
                                    Cardiomyopathy
                                    Mitral valve prolapse
                                    Myocardial infarct
                                    Paradoxic emboli
                                    (perhaps transoesophageal
                                    echocardiography)
Accompanying cardiac illness:
Coronary arteriosclerosis, arrhythmia

Risk factors, accompanying illnesses and findings that increase the risk of cerebral infarction

Risk factors	Cerebral infarct risk
Hypertension	6-fold increase, rising with age
Diabetes mellitus	3-fold increase
Smoking	3-fold increase, with cigarette smoking
Hyperlipidaemia	2-fold increase
Oral contraceptives	2- to 3-fold increase
Alcohol abuse	2-fold increase (in young patients)
Accompanying illnesses	
Coronary artery disease	6-fold increase, with simultaneous arrhythmia up to 10-fold increase
Occlusive vascular disease of legs	2-fold increase
Migraine	Potentiated by existing risk factors (oral contraceptives, smoking)
Obesity	No definite effect
Findings	
History of TIA	4% per year
Extracranial asymptomatic carotid stenosis of 70% > 80%	2% per year 4–8% per year
Ulcerated plaque	4–8% per year
Polycythaemia	Up to 2-fold increase
Hyperuricaemia	No definite effect

Doppler ultrasonography of the extracranial cerebral arteries
(After Ries (1987))

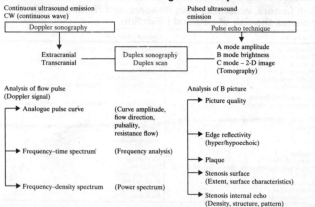

Anterior circulation   Posterior circulation

Supratrochlear a.

Internal carotid a.

External carotid a.

Carotid bifurcation

Common carotid a.

Vertebral a.

Atlas loop

Vertebral a.

Origin of vertebral a.

Distal subclavian a.

Proximal subclavian a.

Possibilities of ultrasound investigation of supra-aortic vessels

Continuous ultrasound emission
CW (continuous wave)

Pulsed ultrasound emission

| Doppler sonography |

| Pulse echo technique |

Extracranial
Transcranial

| Duplex sonography
Duplex scan |

A mode amplitude
B mode brightness
C mode – 2-D image
(Tomography)

Analysis of flow pulse
(Doppler signal)

→ Analogue pulse curve   (Curve amplitude,
flow direction,
pulsality,
resistance flow)

→ Frequency–time spectrum   (Frequency analysis)

→ Frequency–density spectrum   (Power spectrum)

Analysis of B picture

→ Picture quality

→ Edge reflectivity
(hyper/hypoechoic)

→ Plaque

→ Stenosis surface
(Extent, surface characteristics)

→ Stenosis internal echo
(Density, structure, pattern)

Doppler ultrasonographic criteria for quantification of carotid stenoses
(After Hennerici and Neuerburg-Heusler (1988))

	Non-stenosing plaque	Low-grade stenosis	Moderate-grade stenosis	High-grade stenosis	Subtotal stenosis	Occlusion
Narrowing of lumen	<40%	40–60%	60–70%	ca. 80%	>90%	100%
Indirect criteria	Normal	Normal	Normal	No or retrograde flow at edge of orbit Reduced flow in common carotid compared with other side		
Direct criteria in region of stenosis:						
Analogue pulse curve	Normal	Abrupt flow increase	Distinct flow increase, loss of pulsation, systolic slowing (turbulence)	Marked flow increase, systolic slowing	Variable stenosis signal with intensity reduction	Absent vessel
Frequency–time spectrum	Normal	Widened	Widened, increase in low-frequency components	Reduced, inverse frequency components	Reduced, inverse frequency components	Absent vessel
Post-stenotic findings	Normal	Normal	Normal	Reduced systolic flow rate	Reduced signal, difficult to detect	Absent signal
Peak systolic frequency of internal carotid (at 4 MHz)	<3 kHz	3–5 kHz	5–8 kHz	>8 kHz	Variable	Absent
Possibility of demonstration by B-mode	Very good	Very good	Good	Moderate	Moderate	Moderate

International classification of epileptic seizures

(International League against Epilepy, 1981, 1989)

I   **Focal (partial) seizures** (local onset, focal cerebral lesion)
- **A Simple focal seizures (without disturbance of consciousness):**
  1. with motor symptoms (e.g. Jacksonian fit: circumscribed muscle twitching with generalized evolution – march; adversive attack with turning of head/trunk, epilepsia partialis continua without march);
  2. with sensory symptoms (e.g. sensory Jacksonian fit: circumscribed wandering paraesthesiae) or other sensations (e.g. flashes of light, acoustic sensation, olfactory or gustatory hallucinations);
  3. with vegetative symptoms (pallor, nausea, sweating, isolated aura);
  4. with psychic symptoms (memory disturbance, cognitive or affective symptoms, e.g. déjà-vu experience, dreamy state, terror).
- **B Complex focal seizures (with disturbance of consciousness)**
  (psychomotor seizures)
  1. Simple focal seizure followed by loss of consciousness
  2. Disturbance of consciousness at onset (often with automatism such as fidgeting, lip smacking, chewing)
- **C Focal seizures with secondary generalization**
  (e.g. grand mal with focal onset)

II   **Generalized seizures** (convulsive or non-convulsive)
  (often idiopathic, certain forms also residual or symptomatic)
- **A 1. Absences** (brief disturbances of consciousness with spike-and-wave complexes in EEG)
     2. Atypical absences (with clonic, atonic or tonic components or automatism)
- **B Myoclonic seizures** (e.g. impulsive petit mal – brief twitching of proximal muscle groups with poly-spike-wave EEG)
- **C Clonic seizures**
- **D Tonic seizures**
- **E Tonic–clonic seizures** (grand mal)
- **F Atonic seizures** (including myoclonic–akinetic seizures)

III   **Unclassifiable seizures** (because of insufficient data, or unclassifiable seizures of infants)

Locality determined (focal) epilepsies
- **A Idiopathic:**
  Benign focal epilepsy in childhood
- **B Symptomatic:**
  Chronic progressive epilepsia partialis continua
  Temporal lobe epilepsy
  Extratemporal epilepsy

Generalized epilepsies
- **A Idiopathic:**
  Benign seizures of newborn
  Absence epilepsy of childhood
  Juvenile epilepsy with myoclonus (impulsive petit mal)
  Others
- **B Cryptogenic or symptomatic:**
  West syndrome (infantile spasms)
  Early myoclonic encephalopathy
  Lennox–Gastaut syndrome
  Progressive myoclonic epilepsy

Special syndromes (occasional seizures)
Febrile convulsions
Metabolic or toxic causes (e.g. alcohol)
Single seizure or status epilepticus

    Status epilepticus: Frequent epileptic seizures without intervening recovery: generalized (absence status, grand mal status) or focal (Jacksonian status, epilepsia partialis continua)

Anticonvulsants

Type of seizure	Aetiology	Treatment	Dose/day (mg)	Therapeutic blood level (μg/ml)	Steady state after:
Absences	Idiopathic epilepsy	1. Sodium valproate	1200–1800	80–100	5 days
Impulse petit mal		2. Phenobarbitone	200	10–40	3 weeks
Wakening grand mal		3. Primidone	750	5–15	4 days
		4. Ethosuximide	750–1500	40–100	7 days
Complex partial seizures	Residual epilepsy	1. Carbamazepine	800–1200	4–8	3 days
Sleeping grand mal		2. Phenytoin	300–400	10–20	10 days
Simple partial seizures	Symptomatic epilepsy	1. Phenytoin	300–400	10–20	10 days
Diffuse grand mal		2. Carbamazepine	800–1200	4–8	3 days
Status epilepticus	Mostly symptomatic	1. Clonazepam (i.v.) 2. Diazepam (i.v.) 3. Phenytoin (i.v.)	As required, with preparation for intubation; in case of failure, short anaesthetic		

(From Berlit (1992))

Syncope

Aetiology	Supportive investigations
Inadequate vasoconstriction	
Vasovagal	Retake history
Orthostatic	Posture test (Schellong test, cf. p. 93). Treatment with diuretics, vasodilators
Autonomic insufficiency	Diabetes, sympathectomy, look for primary forms
Reduced venous return	
Valsalva (cough, micturition)	Repeat Valsalva manoeuvre under controlled conditions
Late pregnancy	
Atrial myxoma	Echocardiogram
Disturbances of rhythm	
Carotid sinus syndrome	Monitored carotid sinus massage
SA, AV blocks (Stokes–Adams)	Long-term ECG monitoring
Sinus bradycardia	
Asystole, fibrillation	ECG
Ventricular/supraventricular tachycardia	
Reduced cardiac output	
Aortic stenosis, hypertrophic obstructive cardiomyopathy	Auscultation, echocardiogram (cf. pp. 62, 63)
Pulmonary stenosis	
Pulmonary embolus	Isotope lung scan
Cardiac infarct with heart failure	ECG
Pericardiac tamponade	Echocardiogram
Cerebrovascular	
TIA	
Carotid stenosis	Doppler ultrasonogram
Vertebrobasilar stenosis	Angiography (cf. p. 282)
Subclavian steal syndrome	
Others	
Epilepsy	EEG
Hypovolaemia	Neck veins, CVP, diuretics?
Hyperventilation, fear	Allow patient to hyperventilate under control
Hypoxaemia	Blood gas analysis
Anaemia	Blood count
Hypoglycaemia	Blood glucose, extended glucose tolerance test
Hysteria	History

Note: In up to 50% of patients no cause can be found.

Therapy for parkinsonism

Product group (Generic name)	Duration of action in hours	Daily dose	Effect on Tremor	Rigidity	Akinesia	Vegetative symptoms	Special indications	Side effects Acute	Chronic
Anticholinergics Benzhexol Biperiden Benztropine Orphenadrine Procyclidine	1–6	1–15 mg 2–12 mg 0.5–4 mg 150–400 mg 7.5–30 mg	++	+	0	+	Drug-induced parkinsonism – Depressive symptoms	Vomiting Mydriasis Dry mouth Urinary retention Constipation Confusion, psychosis Beware: prostatic hypertrophy and glaucoma	Dementia
Amantadine	1–8	100–200 mg	0	+	++	(+)	Parkinsonian crisis	Confusion, restlessness Psychosis, hypotension disturbances Nausea Beware: renal insufficiency	Sleep
L-Dopa (and decarb-oxylase inhibitors) Levodopa + benserazid (co-beneldopa) Levodopa + carbidopa (co-careldopa)	1–5	100–800 mg 300–1500 mg	(+)	+	++	(+)	Basic therapy	Vomiting Hypotension Tachycardia Arrhythmias Psychoses Beware: heart failure	Sleep disturbances Dyskinesias On-off phe-nomenon Hallucinations
Dopaminergics Bromocriptine Lysuride Pergolide	1–6 2–3	1–40 mg 0.2–5 mg 50–3000 µg	(+)	+	+	(+)	On-off phenomenon Late dyskinesias Early administration to spare L-dopa	Vomiting Hypotension Raynaud's symptoms Dyskinesias	Psychoses Sleep distur-bances
MAO-B-inhibitors Selegiline	24–48	5–10 mg	+	+	+	(+)	End-of-dose akinesia Wearing-off phenomenon Depressive symptoms	Hypotension Nausea Vertigo Sweating	Confusion Dyskinesias

Modified after *BNF*

Differential diagnosis of headache

Name	Age of onset and sex incidence	Temporal onset	Localization and character of pain	Accompanying symptoms	Triggers	Drug therapy
Migraine	Puberty: f > m In childhood more frequent in boys	Often starts in morning, duration 24–48h, recurs at weekly intervals	Unilateral or onset unilateral; mainly frontotemporal (side changes). Throbbing, boring pain. Patient withdraws (to bed)	Nausea, vomiting, sensitivity to light and noise. Possibly aura in form of flickering scotoma or focal neurological signs	Certain foods (cheese, chocolate) or drinks (red wine), premenstrual, relief of stress, alcohol, change of weather	Betablockers, calcium-channel blockers as interval therapy. Sumatriptan, ergotamine for treatment of attack
Cluster headache, Horton's syndrome, migrainous neuralgia	4th decade; 80% men	Mostly at night at fixed time; duration 30–120 min. Daily occurrence for some weeks – then gap of several months	Strictly unilateral periorbital. Piercing very severe pain which makes patient walk about	Reddening of eye and forehead; unilateral lacrimation and rhinorrhea. Horner's syndrome on affected side	None; possibly alcohol, histamine, nitrates	Corticosteroids, serotonin antagonists, lithium
Chronic paroxysmal hemicrania	4th to 5th decade; women > men	Day and night for 5–30min; no remissions	Unilateral piercing, boring	Lacrimation, swelling of lid, facial flushing	None; rarely head movements	Indomethacin
Trigeminal neuralgia	Mostly older age; commoner in women	Many attacks throughout day lasting seconds only; remissions for months or years	Unilateral, usually 2nd and 3rd trigeminal branches. Unbearably severe burning or piercing pain	Anorexia. Patient does not shave, does not speak for fear of attacks of pain	Touching of certain trigger points, chewing, swallowing, cold draughts	Carbamazepine, phenytoin, if necessary, surgery
Temporal arteritis	> 50 years	Day and night; persistent pain for weeks or months, no remissions	Mainly temporal, often bilateral; dull, heavy pain	Swollen, tender temporal artery; raised ESR; possibly loss of vision, joint symptoms	Chewing increases the pain (masticatory claudication)	Corticosteroids
Tension headache	Adults, women > men	Increasing during the day, persisting for weeks	Diffuse, sometimes accentuated occipitally; 'tight band around head'	Sleep disturbances, psychic symptoms, anxiety	Stress, psychic factors	Amitriptyline
Analgesic headache	Adults; 90% women	Morning to evening, over weeks and months	Diffuse, dull, heavy	Pallor, hair loss, anorexia, nausea	Analgesic withdrawal	Betablocker, amitriptyline

288

Differential diagnosis of vertigo

Type	Peripheral labyrinthine	Central vestibular
Positional vertigo		
Latent time to onset	Up to 20s	None
Duration of nystagmus	Up to 30s	Longer than 30s
Vertigo symptoms	Strong, directional	Less strong, non-directional
Direction of nystagmus	Towards lower-lying ear	Variable
Critical head position	Often single	Mostly several
Clinical syndromes	Benign positional vertigo	Acoustic neuroma (late)
	Alcoholic vertigo	Vertebrobasilar ischaemia
	Perilymph fistula	Multiple sclerosis
Persistent vertigo		
Nystagmus	Horizontal rotating	Variable, also downbeat, upbeat
Accompanying symptoms	Sometimes hearing loss, tinnitus	Often vestibular vertigo, pendular nystagmus, other focal signs
Clinical syndromes	Ménière's syndrome	Postmedullary brain stem
	Acute labyrinthine lesion	lesion – ischaemic,
	Vestibular neuronitis	tumour, inflammatory,
	(no hearing loss!)	malformation
	Acoustic neuroma (early – little vertigo!)	

Neurological syndromes of malignancy

(From Berlit (1989))

	Occurrence in
Brain	
Encephalomyelitis: limbic encephalitis, bulbar encephalitis, spinocerebellar degeneration, myoclonus–opsoclonus syndrome	Small cell carcinoma of bronchus Rarely: carcinoma of breast, ovary, colon
Progressive multifocal leucoencephalopathy (PML)	Lymphoma, leukaemias
Isolated angiitis of the CNS	Hodgkin's disease
Subacute cerebellar atrophy	Carcinoma of ovary, breast
Spinal cord	
Subacute necrotizing myelopathy	Small cell carcinoma of bronchus
Amyotrophic lateral sclerosis	Lymphomas, carcinoma of bronchus, breast, stomach, bowel
Peripheral nerve	
Subacute sensory neuropathy (often simultaneous encephalomyelitis)	Small cell carcinoma of bronchus
Paraproteinaemic polyneuropathy	Plasmacytoma, lymphomas
Sensorimotor polyneuropathy	Carcinoma of bronchus
Neuromuscular synapse	
Eaton–Lambert syndrome	Small cell carcinoma of bronchus
Myasthenia gravis	Thymoma
Muscle	
Polymyositis–dermatomyositis	Carcinoma of breast, bronchus, stomach, bowel, uterus, ovary

Pharmacokinetic formulae

1. Loading

(a) Loading dose$_{i.v.}$ = $(C_{target} - C_{actual}) \times V_d \times BW$
(mg/l)

C_{target}: desired plasma concentration
C_{actual}: actual plasma concentration   (mg/l)
V_d: distribution volume   (l/kg)
(see table pp. 298 to 326)

(b) Loading dose$_{oral}$ = $\dfrac{(C_{target} - C_{actual}) \times V_d \times BW}{F}$

F: bioavailability
(100% absorption = 1.0)
BW: body weight   (kg)

(c) Rapid estimation of loading dose from nomogram

1. Choose target concentration on left ordinate.
   (If loading does not proceed from zero, the target concentration is the difference between the desired and the actual concentration.)

2. Choose the corresponding distribution volume on right ordinate.

3. The intersection of the line joining the two points with the central ordinate gives the desired loading dose (mg/kg).

4. This is multiplied by the body weight.

(5. Divide by bioavailability for oral administration.)

2. Dose adjustment

$$C_0 = \frac{F \times dose_{bolus}}{V_d}$$

F: bioavailability (i.v. administration = 100% absorption = 1.0)
$Dose_{bolus}$: bolus dose   (mg/kg)
V_d: distribution volume   (l/kg)

3. Peak concentration after bolus administration

$$Dose_{new} = \frac{Dose_{previous} \times C_{target}}{C_{actual}}$$

C_{target}: desired plasma concentration   (mg/l)
C_{actual}: actual plasma concentration   (mg/l)

(This formula must not be used for drugs with non-linear kinetics. In these cases small dose increases can lead to disproportionate increases in the plasma concentration; beware toxicity.)

4. Time to achievement of steady-state concentration

Elapsed time since start of therapy	% Steady-state concentration achieved	Further increase in plasma concentration to be expected
Alternatively:		
Drug elimination		
Elapsed time since last dose	Amount of drug remaining in body	Amount of drug excreted
1 half life	50%	50%
2 half lives	75%	25%
3 half lives	88%	12%
4 half lives	94%	6%
4.3 half lives	95%	5%
5 half lives	97%	3%

Nomogram for calculation of loading dose

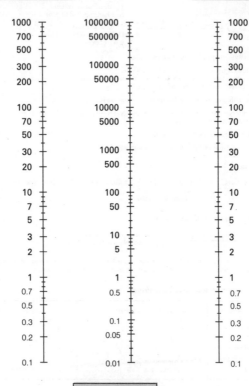

1. Target concentration

2. Distribution volume (l/kg)

1.		2.
1000	1000000	1000
700	500000	700
500		500
300	100000	300
200	50000	200
100	10000	100
70	5000	70
50		50
30	1000	30
20	500	20
10	100	10
7	50	7
5		5
3	10	3
2	5	2
1	1	1
0.7	0.5	0.7
0.5		0.5
0.3	0.1	0.3
0.2	0.05	0.2
0.1	0.01	0.1

3. Loading dose per kg

4. Multiplication by body weight

5. Estimation of individual half life (cf. illustration)

$$\text{Half life} = t_{\text{final-initial}} \times \frac{0.301}{\log C_{\text{initial}} - \log C_{\text{final}}}$$

$t_{\text{final-initial}}$: interval between C_{initial} and C_{final}
C_{initial}: initial concentration
C_{final}: final concentration

$$= t_{\text{final-initial}} \times \frac{0.693}{\ln C_{\text{initial}} - \ln C_{\text{final}}}$$

Nomogram for estimation of half life

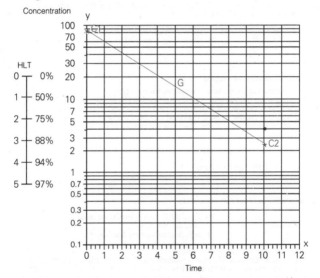

Time

Graphic determination of elimination half life time (HLT) using two plasma concentrations

1. Enter the initial (greater) concentration at time 0 (i.e. on the y-axis) of the graph (C1)
2. Enter the second concentration at the correct time interval (C2)
3. Connect the two points with a straight line (G)
4. The HLT can now be determined using the enclosed plastic measure:
   Lay the measure on the graph parallel to the x-axis so that the upper line ('C1') comes to lie on the initial concentration (C1).
5. Determine the intersection of the joining line (G) with the line '1 HLT'.
6. Slide the measure parallel to the x-axis until the arrow comes to lie on the intersection of G and '1 HLT'.
7. The arrow now points at the HLT of the drug under examination on the x-axis.
8. Similarly the duration of 2 (line '2 HLT') 3 or 4 HLT can be read off. Alternatively, the time required to attain a given concentration can also be estimated.

Drugs with variable HLT

- Drugs with non-linear kinetics (HLT dependent on concentration) (see below)
- Drugs with self-induction (induction of own metabolism)
- Hepatic, renal, cardiac failure, combination therapy (cf. table pp. 298–326)

6. Estimation of HLT in anuria

The following formula permits the approximate estimation of HLT in anuria. With prolonged renal insufficiency, however, the elimination can be modified by additional changes in distribution volume and plasma protein binding.

$$HLT_{anuria} = \frac{HLT_{normal}}{Q_0}$$

HLT_{normal}: HLT with normal renal function
Q_0: fraction of drug eliminated by extrarenal mechanisms

7. Dose adjustment in renal failure

(a) Determination of the individual elimination fraction (Q):
The elimination fraction with normal renal function (Q_0, cf. table pp. 298–326) is entered on the left vertical axis and joined to the right upper corner of the nomogram. The intersection of the line with the individual creatinine clearance (measured or estimated) is read off on the left vertical axis. This value corresponds to the individual elimination fraction Q.

(b) Determination of the individual renal function (creatinine clearance; $Cl_{creatinine}$):

$$Cl_{creatinine} = \frac{(150 - age) \times weight}{C_{creatinine}}$$

Men: +10%
Women: −10%
$C_{creatinine}$: creatinine serum concentration   (μmol/l)

(c) Determination of the individual HLT:

$$HLT_{individual} = \frac{HLT_{normal}}{Q}$$

HLT_{normal}: HLT with normal renal function
(cf. table pp. 298–326)
Q: individual elimination fraction

(d) Determination of the individual dose:
The initial loading dose of a drug is independent of its elimination and is not influenced by the renal function of the patient. Its calculation is therefore the same as in a patient with normal creatinine clearance. The maintenance dose, however, must be modified.

General rule

For **most** drugs:
Maintenance dose = Q × Maintenance dose$_{healthy}$.
The dose reduction can be achieved by increasing the dose interval or reducing the individual doses.

Exceptions

For many antibiotics (aminoglycosides, many cephalosporins and penicillins):
Maintenance dose = d × Maintenance dose$_{healthy}$, where d is decay fraction
The decay quotient can also be determined from the nomogram: the intersection of the relevant dose interval (dose interval/HLT$_{individual}$) with the dotted curve indicates the decay fraction d on the right vertical axis.

Removal of drugs by dialysis

Nomogram

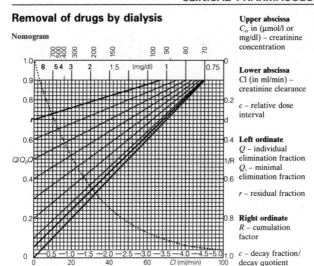

Upper abscissa
C_{cr} in (μmol/l or mg/dl) – creatinine concentration

Lower abscissa
Cl (in ml/min) – creatinine clearance

c – relative dose interval

Left ordinate
Q – individual elimination fraction
Q_i – minimal elimination fraction

r – residual fraction

Right ordinate
R – cumulation factor

c – decay fraction/decay quotient

8. Estimation of the dialysing ability of a drug

(a) Dialysing ability: Principles: The smaller the distribution volume, the smaller the binding to plasma protein and the lower the molecular weight (factor in the table > 2, i.e. molecular weight < 500), the more readily can the elimination of a drug be expected during a dialysis procedure.

(b) Clearance during a dialysis:

$$Cl_{dialysis} = \frac{\dot{V} \times (C_{arterial} - C_{venous})}{C_{arterial}}$$

$C_{arterial}$: drug concentration in arterial limb $\quad$ (mg/l)
C_{venous}: drug concentration in venous limb $\quad$ (mg/l)
V: blood flow through dialyser $\quad$ (ml/min)

$$Clearance_{total} = Cl_{patient} + Cl_{dialysis}$$

9. Distribution volume (cf. table)

$$HLT \quad = \quad \frac{Distribution\ volume}{Clearance_{total}}$$

Distribution volume:
51 $\quad$ (≈ 0.07 l/kg): $\quad$ Distribution in practice exclusively in blood
10–201 $\quad$ (≈ 0.15–0.3 l/kg): $\quad$ Distribution in total extracellular fluid
401 $\quad$ (≈ 0.6 l/kg): $\quad$ Distribution in total body water
> 401 $\quad$ (> 0.6 l/kg): $\quad$ Concentration outside the body water (e.g. in adipose tissue)

Drug interactions

(After Stockley, I.H. Reprinted with permission of Firma Boehringer Ingelheim KG)

How to use this schedule

An interaction between two products is indicated by a symbol where the vertical and horizontal columns intersect; e.g. for anticoagulants and phenylbutazone:

The **symbol** indicates the effect of the interaction. The **arrow** indicates the affected product.

The **colour** indicates its significance.

Thus the action of anticoagulants is enhanced by phenylbutazone, and the interaction is of great significance and potentially dangerous

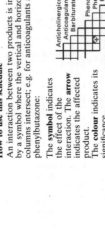

Arrow indicates the affected product

Explanation of symbols

☠ Contraindicated, dangerous
+ Enhanced activity
– Diminished activity
T Toxic reaction
O Occasional cases of interaction
? Danger! Possible interaction

Explanation of colours

■ Marked or potentially serious interaction
■ Moderate or minor interaction
■ Interaction the significance of which is difficult to estimate

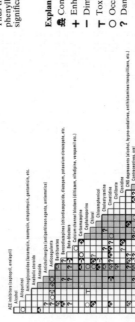

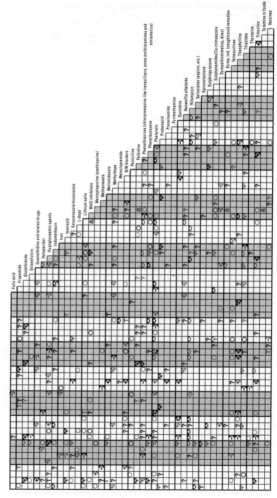

Pharmacokinetic and toxicological data

Drug	Factor	Plasma concentration (mg/l) Therap.	Toxic	Lethal	HLT	V_d l/kg
Acebutolol	2.97	0.5–2			2.9/11	2.9
Acemetacin	2.35				4.5/6	1
Acetazolamide	4.5	5–20			Nlin(6,3)	0.2
Acetylcysteine	6.13				1.5	
Acetylsalicylic acid	5.55	20–100	> 450	> 1200	Nlin(0.25)/Nlin(4)	0.25
Acyclovir	4.44	0.7–2			2.4 (N↑,I↑)	0.7
Acipimox	6.49				2	
Adenosine	3.74				0.008	
Alfentanil	2.4	0.1–0.3			π: 2 min, α: 10 min	
Allopurinol	7.35	10			0.8/40	0.6
Alprazolam	3.24	10–50	> 75		11(A↑,Ci↑)/1,5	0.9
Alteplase (t-PA)	0.017				0.05	0.1
Amantadine	5.33	0.2–0.9	>1	11.8	12(A↑)	3.5
Amikacin	1.71	Peak: 20–25 trough: 1–4	> 30 > 8		2.5(Ci=)	0.21
Amiloride	4.35				10(A↑)	5
Aminoglutethimide	4.31				12	
Amiodarone	1.55	0.8–2.5	(> 2.5)		14–1300/700	66
Amitriptyline	3.61	0.05–0.2	> 0.5	10–20	17(A↑)/27	15
Amlodipine	2.45				40–60(A↑,Ci↑)	21.4
Amoxapine	3.19	0.2–0.4	> 0.5	3	8/30	
Amoxicillin	2.74	2–8			1.2	0.47
Amphetamine	7.4	0.02–0.03	0.5	> 2	12.2	4
Amphotericin B	1.08	0.2–2	> 6–10		360	4
Ampicillin	2.86	2–8			0.9(N↑,S↑,A↑,Ci↑)	0.52
Amylobarbitone	4.42	1–8	10–30	> 30	8–42 (I↑)	1.1
Anistreplase (APSAC)	–				1.5	
Aprotinin	0.154				0.7	
Arsenic	13.35	<0.02	> 1	> 9		
Ascorbic acid	5.68	6–10			6(S↓)	0.5
Astemizole	2.18	0.00013			20/50	250
Atenolol	3.75	0.2–1.3			6.1(A↑,Ci=)	1
Atracurium	0.8	0.65	> 1.1		0.33/?	0.15

Q_0	Active metabolites Name	Potency	Extra dose after dialysis	Clinical application
0.6	Diacetolol	× 1	nH	β_1-antagonist, type II anti-arrhythmic
0.6	Indomethacin		?	Indole NSAID
0.1			? (unlikely)	Carbonic anhydrase inhibitor
0.99				Mucolytic
0.99	Salicylic acid	< × 1	H,P	Salicylate
0.23			H	Antiviral drug (herpes)
0.01	–		?	Lipid-lowering drug
0.99			?	Anti-arrhythmic
0.99			?	Opiate analgesic
0.85	Oxypurinol	Potent	H,Itx:H	Xanthine oxidase inhibitor
0.89	(OH-alprazolam)	× 0.5	? (unlikely)	Benzodiazepine
			? (unlikely)	Thrombolytic
0.1			nH,nP,Itx:H	Antiviral drug (influenza)
0.06	–		H,P	Aminoglycoside antibiotic
0.25			?	Potassium-sparing diuretic
0.9			?	Corticoid synthesis inhibitor
0.99	N-monodesethyl amiodarone		nH,nP	Type III anti-arrhythmic
0.95	Nortriptyline	> × 1	nH,nP,Itx:kP	Tricyclic antidepressant
0.9			? (unlikely)	Type II calcium-channel blocker
0.95	8-OH-A, 7-OH-amoxapine		?	Tricyclic antidepressant
0.06			H,nP	Aminopenicillin
pH↓ (0.79–0.45)			Itx:H,Itx:P	CNS stimulant
0.99			nH,nP	Antifungal
0.1			H,nP	Aminopenicillin
0.99			?	Barbiturate hypnotic
			?	Thrombolytic
0.99			?	Kallikrein inhibitor
			Itx:H	Heavy metal
0.3–0.98			H	Vitamin C
0.99	Demethyl-astemizole	× 1	? (unlikely)	Non-sedative antihistamine
0.06	–		H,nP	β_1-antagonist
0.99	Laudanosid		nH	Non-depolarizing muscle relaxant

Drug	Factor	Plasma concentration (mg/l)			HLT	V_d
		Therap.	Toxic	Lethal		l/kg
Atropine	3.46	0.035–0.2		> 0.2	2.5(I↑,A↑)	2
Auranofin	1.47				600	0.05
Azapropazone	3.33				13	0.16
Azathioprine	3.61	–			0.2/0.9	0.8
Azlocillin	2.17	50–500			Nlin(1)(I↑)	0.2
Aztreonam	2.3	0.01–20			1.6(Ci↑)	0.82
Bacampicillin	2.15				–/0.9	0.25
Baclofen	4.68	0.08–0.4			3.5	0.85
Beclomethasone	2.45				15	
Bendrofluazide	2.37				3.5	1.5
Betamethasone	2.55				5.6	1.4
Betaxolol	3.25				18(N↑,A↑)	7
Bezafibrate	2.76				1.7	0.3
Bisoprolol	3.07				12 (Ci↑)	3.2
Bleomycin	–				3.1	0.27
Boric acid	16.17	< 7	> 20	> 200	21	0.3
Bretylium	2.41	0.8–2.4			8.9	5.9
Bromazepam	3.16	0.08–0.17			16(A↑)/?	1
Bromide	12.52	<100	>500	>2000	24	> 40
Bromocriptine	1.53				3	3.4
Brompheniramine	3.13	0.008–0.015			25	11.7
Budesonide	2.32				2.7	4.4
Bumetanide	2.74				1.5(Ci=,HF↑)	0.3
Bupivacaine	2.92	1–4	> 1.6		2.4	0.9
Buprenorphine	2.14				2.5	2
Buspirone	2.59				2.4(Ci↑)/2	5.3
Busulphan	4.06				2.6	0.99
Butobarbitone	4.27	1–5	10–30	> 30	37.5	0.8
Cadmium	8.9	< 0.005	> 0.05			
Caffeine	5.15	5–10		>100	N1in(5)	0.61
Captopril	4.6	≤ 0.05			1.9	0.7
Carbamazepine	4.23	4–10	> 8	> 15	16–37(N↓)/7	1.2
Carbenicillin	2.64	10–125			0.8(N↑,I↑,Ci↑)	0.15
Carbenoxolone	1.75	–			16.3(A↑)	0.1
Carbimazole	5.37				0.5	
Carisoprodol	3.84	10–30	> 30	> 110	8	0.6
Carmustine	4.67				0.3	3.3
Carnitine	6.2	< 12			2–15	0.25

Q_0	Active metabolites Name	Potency	Extra dose after dialysis	Clinical application
0.6			nH,nP	Anticholinergic
0.9			nH	Antirheumatic
0.4			?	NSAID
0.99	6-Mercaptopurine		(H)	Immunosuppressant
0.35	–		H,nP	Antipseudomonal penicillin
0.33	–		H,(P)	Monobactam antibiotic
0.99	Ampicillin	Prodrug	H,nP	Aminopenicillin
0.2	–		?	Skeletal muscle relaxant
0.99			?	Glucocorticoid
0.7			?	Thiazide diuretic
0.95			?	Glucocorticoid
0.85	–		nH	β_1-antagonist
0.15			nP	Lipid-lowering drug
0.5	–		? (unlilkely)	β_1-antagonist
0.32			nH	DNA synthesis inhibitor
			?	Disinfectant
0.2	–		nH	III-Anti-arrhythmic
0.99	3-OH-bromazepam		? (unlikely) Itx:H	Benzodiazepine
0.99			?	Central dopamine agonist
0.95				Sedative antihistamine
			?	Glucocorticoid
0.5			?	Loop diuretic
0.98			?	Local anaesthetic
0.99			?	Opioid analgesic
0.99	1-(2-pyrimidiny)-piperazine	× 0.2	nH	Anxiolytic
0.99			?	Alkylating drug
0.92			?	Barbiturate hypnotic
	–		?	Heavy metal
0.99			Itx:kP	Analeptic
0.5	–		H	ACE inhibitor
0.99	Carb. 10,11 epoxide	(× 1)	(H),Itx:H	Anticonvulsant
0.2			H,P	Penicillin active against *Pseudomonas*
0.99			?	Ulcer-healing drug, mineralocorticoid
0.99			?	Antithyroid drug
0.99			?	Skeletal muscle relaxant
			?	Alkylating drug
0.2	–		H	Vitamin

Drug	Factor	Plasma concentration (mg/l)			HLT	V_d
		Therap.	Toxic	Lethal		l/kg
Cefaclor	2.72	–			0.8	0.24
Cefadroxil	2.75	< 35			1.3	0.15
Cefotaxime	2.2	0.2–8			1.2(A↑,Ci↑)/ 2.5(A↑)	0.38
Cefoxitin	2.34	1–10			0.7(I↑)	0.15
Cefsoludin	1.88				1.5	0.35
Ceftazidime	1.83	–			1.8(I↑,A↑)	0.25
Ceftizoxime	2.61	2–64			1.2	0.25
Ceftriaxone	1.8	0.2–8			·8(C↓,Ci=)	0.15
Cefuroxime	2.36	1–50			1.4(I↑,Ci↓)	0.28
Cephalexin	2.88	6–50			0.9	0.26
Cephamandole	2.16	0.5–5			0.8(I↑)	0.16
Cephazolin	2.2	< 200			1.6(I↑)	0.17
Cephradine	2.86	0.5–12			0.76	0.32
Celiprolol	2.64	0.2–0.8			5	
Chloral hydrate	6.05	2–10(−20)	> 100	> 250	–/8	0.6
Chlorambucil	3.29				1/2	0.86
Chloramphenicol	3.09	**5–20**	> 25	> 100	2.7(I↑,Ci↑)	0.57
Chlordiazepoxide	3.34	0.7–3	> 5	> 20	15(A↑,Ci↑)/ 80(A↑)	0.3
Chlormethiazole	6.19				4.1(A↑,Ci↑)	5.4
Chloroform	8.38	20–230	> 70	> 390		
Chloroquine	3.13	0.01–0.28		> 3	1000/360	115
Chlorothiazide	3.38	6			1.5	0.2
Chlorpheniramine	3.64	0.005–0.04			20/?	4.3

Q_0	Active metabolites Name	Potency	Extra dose after dialysis	Clinical application
0.4			H,P	Oral second generation cephalosporin
0.05	–		H,nP	Oral second generation cephalosporin
0.35	Desacetyl-cefotaxime		H,nP	i.v. third generation cephalosporin
0.15			H,nP	i.v. second generation cephalosporin
0.2			H	i.v. 3rd generation antipseudomonal cephalosporin
0.12			H,nP	i.v. 3rd generation antipseudomonal cephalosporin
0.05			H,nP	i.v. third generation cephalosporin
0.4			nH,nP	i.v. third generation cephalosporin
0.05			H,nP	Second generation cephalosporin
0.1			H,nP	Oral first generation cephalosporin
0.05			H,nP	i.v. second generation cephalosporin
0.15			H,nP	i.v. first generation cephalosporin
0.1	–		H,P	First generation cephalosporin
0.6			?	α_2,β_1-antagonist, β_2-agonist
0.99	Trichloroethanol	×1, Prodrug	H,nP:Itx:H,KP	Sedative
0.99			nH,nP	Alkylating agent
0.95	–		nH,nP	Antibiotic
0.99	Demethyl-chlordiazapine →demoxipam → nordazepam → oxazepam		nH	Benzodiazepine
			? (unlikely)	Hypnotic
			? (unlikely)	Inhalation anaesthetic
pH ↓ (0.4)	Desethyl-chloroquine		nH,nP	Antimalarial
0.05			?	Thiazide diuretic
0.77			H,nP	H_1-antagonist

| Drug | Factor | Plasma concentration (mg/l) | | | HLT | V_d |
		Therap.	Toxic	Lethal		l/kg
Chlorpromazine	3.14	0.05–0.5	> 0.75	> 3	30(C↓)/25	21
Chorpropamide	3.61	50–150	> 200		32/?	0.15
Chlorthalidone	2.95	0.02–7.7			53(A↑)	4.1
Chlortetracycline	2.09	0.5–6			5.6	1.74
Cholestyramine		Not absorbed				
Cilastatin	2.8				0.8	0.2
Cimetidine	3.96	0.5–4	> 1.25 (minimum value)		2(A↑,Ci=)	1.8
Cinnarizine	2.71				5	
Cinoxacin	3.81	<30			2.1	0.33
Ciprofloxacin	3.02				5/?	2.1
Cisapride	2.15	0.01–0.1			10(A↑)	1.9
Cisplatin	3.33				0.5	0.51
Clavulanic acid	5.02				0.9(I↑)	0.3
Clindamycin	2.35	<4			2.8(Ci↑)/?	1.1
Clobazam	3.33				11–77(A↑)/50	1.4
Clofazimine	2.11	0.5–1.5			240	
Clofibrate	4.12	80–150			−/15–54(Ci=)	
Clomipramine	3.18	0.05–0.4			24/50	17
Clonazepam	3.17	0.02–0.07			20–60	3.2
Clonidine	4.35	< 0.0005	> 0.001		Nlin(8)	3.5
Clorazepate	3.01	< 0.02			2/80(A↑)	0.33
Cloxacillin	2.29	7–14			0.6/?	0.35
Clozapine	3.06	0.1–0.7			10	
CO	35.7	< 6%	> 15%		> 50%	
Cocaine	3.3	0.05–0.15	0.9	> 1–20	0.71	2.1
Codeine	3.34	0.01–0.12	> 0.2	> 0.6	3.3/2.3	3.5
Colchicine	2.5	0.0003–0.03			19.4	10
Colestipol		Not absorbed				
Colistin	0.86	1–5			3	0.55
Copper	15–74	0.1–1.5		> 2.5		
Cortisone	2.77				0.5/1.75	
Cyclophosphamide	3.83	–			7.6/?(C↓)	0.8
Cycloserine	9.8				10	
Cyclosporin	0.83	0.2–0.5			6(C↓,Ci↑)	3.5

Q_0	Active metabolites		Extra dose after dialysis	Clinical application
	Name	Potency		
0.99	7-OH-chlorpromazine, N-desmethyl chlorpromazine	($\times 0.5$)	nH,nP	Phenothiazine sedative
PH$\uparrow$(0.05–0.85)	(3 Metab.)		nP,Itx:H	Sulphonylurea
0.35	–		?	Diuretic
0.82			? (unlikely)	Short-acting tetracycline
			nH,nP	Resin
0.3			H	Dihydropeptidase inhibitor
0.3	–		(H),(P)	H_2-antagonist
0.99			?	Vasodilator
0.2			?	Urinary antiseptic
0.5			nP,Itx:H	4-Quinolone antibiotic
0.99			?	Gastric motility stimulant
0.75			(H)	Cytotoxic drug
0.55			H	β-lactamase inhibitor
0.9	N-demethyl-clindamycin	$> \times 1$		Macrolide antibiotic
	Desmethyl-clobazam		? (unlikely)	Benzodiazepine
0.99			? (unlikely)	Antileprotic drug
0.85	Clofibrinic acid	Prodrug	nH	Lipid-lowering drug
0.99	Desmethyl clomipramine		nH,nP	Tricyclic antidepressant
0.99	7-amino-cl., 7-acetamino-cl.		?(unlikely)	Benzodiazepine
0.4			nH	Central α_2-agonist antihypertensive
0.99	Nordazepam → Oxazepam	Prodrug	nH	Benzodiazepine
0.25			nH	Penicillinase-resistant penicillin
0.99	(N-desmethyl-cl.)		nH	Antipsychotic
				Carbon monoxide
0.99			?	Local anaesthetic
0.99	Morphine	$\times 5$	?	Opiate analgesic
0.99			nH,Itx:H,P	Gout treatment
			nH,nP	Bile acid binder
0.2			nH,(P)	Polymyxin antibiotic
	–		?	Trace element
	Hydrocortisone	$\times 1.25$	nH	Glucocorticoid
0.9	Phosphoramide-nornitrogen mustard	Prodrug	H	Alkylating agent
0.4			H	Antitubercular agent
0.99	?		nH,nP	Immunosuppressant

| Drug | Factor | Plasma concentration (mg/l) | | | HLT | V_d |
		Therap.	Toxic	Lethal		l/kg
Cytarabine	4.11	0.01–0.1			2.3	2.2
Dacarbazine	5.49				0.7	0.63
Dactinomycin	0.8	–			36	
Danazol	2.96	0.1–0.15			29	
Dantrolene	3.18	0.3–3			9/?	
Dapsone	4.03	1–7			29	1.9
Demeclocycline	2.15	0.5–3			13.6	1.8
Desferrioxamine	1.68	< 100			6	
Desipramine	3.75	0.15–0.3	> 0.5	10–20	Nlin(17)(A↑)/?	41.9
Desmopressin	0.94				0.5–2	
Dexamethasone	2.55				3	0.82
Dexfenfluramine	4.32				18	
Dextromethorphan	3.68				2.7/6.5	1.1
Diamorphine	2.71				0.05	
Diazepam	3.51	0.1–1	> 5	> 20	33(I↑,A↑,Ci↑) /80(A↑)	2
Diazoxide	4.33	15–35	> 100		30	0.2
Diclofenac	3.54				1.5	0.2
Didanosine	4.23				0.63	1
Diethylcarbamazine	5.02				12	2.5
Diflunisal	4.0	9–90		> 600	11	0.1
Digitoxin	1.31	0.01–0.03	> 0.04	> 0.3	164(Ci=)/43(Ci=)	0.6
Digoxin	1.28	0.0008–0.002	> 0.002	> 0.015	43/(N↑,I↓,A↑, Ci=,HF=)	6.3
Diltiazem	2.41	0.03–0.4			4(A↑)/8	5.3
Diphenhydramine	3.92	0.01–1	> 5	> 10	5.2(Ci↑)	3.7
Diphenoxylate	2.21	0.01	–	–	2.5/13	4.6
Dipyridamole	1.98	< 1.5			0.8	
Disopyramide	2.95	2–5(–8)	> 9	> 26	7.8(HF=)/9	0.8
Disulfiram	3.37	2.5			7.3	8.2
Dobutamine	3.32	0.04–0.17			0.033(HF=)	0.2
Domperidone	2.35				8	
Dopamine	6.53	0.01–0.1			0.15(C↓)/0.03	0.93
Dothiepin	3.38	–			22	45
Doxapram	2.64	2.7–5.2			7	3.5
Doxazosin	2.21				13	1.3
Doxepin	3.58	0.01–0.25	> 0.5–2	10–20	18/35	20

| Q_0 | Active metabolites | | Extra dose after dialysis | Clinical application |
	Name	Potency		
0.9			?	Antimetabolite
0.3			?	DNA/RNA synthesis inhibitor
			? (unlikely)	mRNA synthesis inhibitor
			?	Gonadotrophin inhibitor
0.96	5-OH-dantrolene	($\times$ 0.5)	?	Skeletal muscle relaxant
0.85	Monoacetyl-dapsone		Itx:H	Antileprotic drug
0.6			H,nP	Medium-duration tetracycline
			Itx:H	Chelating agent
0.99	5-OH-desipramine		nH,nP	Tricyclic antidepressant
0.99			?	Vasopressin analogue
0.97			?	Glucocorticoid
0.9			? (unlikely)	Appetite suppressant
0.8	Dextrophan		?	Opiate analgesic
0.99			?	Opiate analgesic
0.99	Nordiazepam →	$\times$ 1	nH	Benzodiazepine
	oxazepam (temazepam)		? (unlikely)	Benzodiazepine
0.6			H,P	Antihypertensive
0.99	–		? (unlikely)	Acetoacetate NSAID
0.6			?	Antiviral (HIV)
0.15			?	Antihelminthic
PH↑ (0.94)	–		nH,nP	Salicylate
0.68	Digoxin		nH,nP	Digitalis alkaloid
0.24			nH,nP	Digitalis alkaloid
0.96	Desacetyl-diltiazem	$\times$ 0.4	nH,nP	Type I calcium-channel blocker,
				Type IV anti-arrhythmic
0.97			?	H_1-antagonist
0.99	Diphenolic acid	$\times$ 5	?	Antidiarrhoeal
0.99			nH	Antiplatelet drug
0.45	Nordisopyramide	($\times$ 0.25)	(H?)	Type Ia anti-arrhythmic
0.5			?	Alcohol-deterrent compound
0.99			?	β_1-agonist
0.99			?	Antiemetic
0.97	Noradrenaline		?	β_1-agonist
0.99	?		? (unlikely)	Tricyclic antidepressant
0.99			?	Analeptic
0.91	?		nH	α_1-antagonist
0.99	Desmethyldoxepin		nH,nP	Tricyclic antidepressant

| Drug | Factor | Plasma concentration (mg/l) | | | HLT | V_d |
		Therap.	Toxic	Lethal		l/kg
Doxorubicin	1.84				36/?	25
Doxycycline	2.26	1–2			20	1.5
Droperidol	2.64	–			2.2	1.75
Edrophonium	4.06	< 0.15			1.8	1.1
Enalapril	2.66/2.6	0.02–0.08 (Enalaprilat)			1.3/11(HF↑)	1.7
Enflurane	5.42	50–100				
Enoximone	4.03				1–20/2.2–25	2.5
Ephedrine	6.05	0.1			6	
Epirubicin	1.84				39/≤39	50
Epoetin	–				6	0.03
Ergotamine	1.72				1.9	1.8
Erythromycin	1.36	0.5–2.5			Nlin(2)(Ci↑)	0.6
Esmolol	3.39	0.2			0.15(Ci=)	3.4
Estramustine	2.27				1.3/15	
Ethacrynic acid	3.3				1	0.1
Ethambutol	4.89	2–5			3.5	2.3
Ethanol	21.7	–	> 1800	> 3500	Nlin(0.25)	0.54
Ether	13.49	500–1500		> 1400		
Ethinyloestradiol	3.37				13	2.9
Ethosuximide	7.08	40–100	> 150	> 250	50(C↓)	0.67
Etidronate disodium	4.85				6	1400
Etomidate	4.09				0.5–4.6	45
Etoposide	1.7				7	0.35
Etretinate	2.82	0.2–0.8			8(–2900)/50	2
Famotidine	2.96				2.2(A↑)	1.3
Felodipine	2.6				10.2(A↑)	9.7
Fenbufen	3.93				10/?	3
Fenfluramine	4.32	0.04–0.12	> 0.2	> 6	19/?	14
Fenofibrate	2.77	5–15 (Fenofibricacide)			–/22	0.9
Fenoprofen	4.13	20–65		> 700	2.2	0.09
Fentanyl	2.97	0.001–0.003		3.7	π: 2 min, α: 10 min 4(A↑,Ci=)	4
Flecainide	2.41	0.2–1	> 1		9–20(C↓,A↑,HF↑)	7.5
Flucloxacillin	2.2	0.4			0.8/?	0.12
Fluconazole	3.26				30	0.8
Flucytosine	7.75	35–70	> 100		4.8/0.25	0.6

Q_0	Active metabolites Name	Potency	Extra dose after dialysis	Clinical application
0.85	Doxorubicinol		? (unlikely)	DNA synthesis inhibitor
pH↑(0.45)			nH,nP	Long-acting tetracycline
0.99	?		? (unlikely)	Hypnotic
0.2			?	Cholinesterase inhibitor
0.1	Enalaprilat	Prodrug	H	ACE inhibitor
			? (unlikely)	Inhalation anaesthetic
0.99	Enoximone sulphoxide	(+)	?	Phosphodiesterase inhibitor
0.3			?	β_1-antagonist
0.99	13-OH-epirubicin		? (unlikely)	Cytotoxic antibiotic
0.9			nH	Erythropoietic hormone
0.5			Itx:H	Antimigraine drug
0.85			nH,nP	Macrolide antibiotic
0.99	–		?	β_1-antagonist, Type II anti-arrhythmic
0.99			?	Alkylating oestrogen
0.35			nH	Loop diuretic
0.15	–		H,P	Antituberculous drug
0.97			Itx:H	Hypnotic
			? (unlikely)	Inhalation anaestheic
			? (unlikely)	Sex hormone
0.7	–		H	Anticonvulsant
			? (unlikely)	Chelating agent
0.99	–		?	Intravenous anaesthetic agent
0.6			?	Antimetabolite
0.99	Etretin		? (unlikely)	Oral retinoid for psoriasis
0.3	?		nH	H_2-antagonist
0.99			? (unlikely)	Type II calcium-channel blocker
0.95	Biphenyl acetate, OH-biphenylacetate	Prodrug	? (unlikely)	Propionic acid NSAID
0.6	Norfenfluramine		?	Appetite suppressant
0.2	Fenofibrinic acid	Prodrug	nH	Lipid-lowering drug
0.95	–		nH	Propionic acid NSAID
0.92	–			Opioid analgesic
pH↓(0.75)	–		nH	Type Ic anti-arrhythmic
0.45	OH-flucloxacillin		nH	Penicillinase-resistant penicillin
0.2			H,P	Antifungal drug
0.02	5-Fluorouracil		H,P	Antifungal drug

Drug	Factor	Plasma concentration (mg/l)			HLT	V_d l/kg
		Therap.	Toxic	Lethal		
Flumazenil	3.3				0.9	0.95
Flunisolide	2.3				1.8/?	1.8
Flunitrazepam	3.19	0.003–0.006			30(A↑)/28	4.5
Fluoride	52.66				4.3	
Fluouracil	7.69				0.2/70	0.25
Fluoxetine	3.23				24–170/170	35
Flupenthixol	2.3				30	15
Fluphenazine	2.29	< 0.002	> 2		36/?	
Fluphenazine deconate	1.76	< 0.001			180–340	
Flurazepam	2.58	0.01–0.1	> 0.2	> 0.5	2(A↑)/40–100	22
Flurbiprofen	4.09				3.5	0.1
Flutamide	3.62	0.5–3 (2-OH-Flutamide)			7.8/Nlin(4–22)	
Fluvoxamine	3.14				17.5	
Folic acid	2.27				0.75	
Folinic acid	1.95				9.3	3.2
Foscarnet	5.21				β: 3,3,γ: 18	1.3
Fosfestrol	2.33				0.08/?	
Fosfomycin	7.24	< 400			2	0.3
Frusemide	3.02	0.1–0.3	> 25		1.5(I↑,A↑,Ci=, HF=)	0.2
Fusidic acid	1.94				6	
Gallamine	1.12				2.5	0.15
Ganciclovir	3.92	0.6–25			2.9	0.6
Gemfibrozil	3.99				1.5	
Gentamicin	ca. 2.1	peak: 6–10 trough: <2	> 12 > 2		2(N↑,I↑)	0.25
Glibenclamide	2.02	(< 0.007)			10	0.1
Gliclazide	3.09				12(A↑)	0.2
Glipizide	2.24	–			3	0.16
Gliquidone	1.9				17/?	
Glycerol	10.86				0.5	
Glyceryl trinitrate	4.4	0.001–0.01			0.04/0.8 0.04/0.8	3.3
Griseofulvin	2.83				0.3–1.3	
Guanethidine	5.04	> 0.008			43–150/?	
Haloperidol	2.66	0.002–0.02	> 0.025	–	20(C↓)/?	18
Halothane	5.07	80–260		> 200		
Heparin	–				Nlin(0.5)(Ci↑)	0.06

Q_o	Active metabolites Name	Potency	Extra dose after dialysis	Clinical application
0.99	–		?	Benzodiazepine antagonist
0.95	(6-β-OH-flunisolide)		?	Glucocorticoid
0.99	Desmethyl-flunitrazepam		nH	Benzodiazepine
0.96	Dihydro-fluouracil		H	Antimetabolite
0.98	Desmethyl-fluoxetin		nH	Antidepressant
	–		? (unlikely)	Antidepressant
0.99	7-OH-fluphenazine	(× 0.7)	nH	Antipsychotic
0.99			nH	Antipsychotic
0.99	Desalkyl-flurazepam OH-ethyl-flurazepam		nH	Benzodiazepine
0.9	–		? (unlikely)	Propionic acid NSAID
0.99	2-OH-flutamide		?	Anti-androgen
0.99	–		? (unlikely)	Antidepressant
			H	Vitamin
0.7			? (unlikely)	Antidote against folate antagonist
0.2			?	Antiviral (HIV)
0.95	Diethylstiboestrol	Prodrug	?	Mitosis inhibitor
0.01	–		H,P	Antibiotic
0.25			nH	Loop diuretic
0.99			nH	Antibiotic
0.05			H,P	Non-depolarizing muscle relaxant
0.1	Ganciclovir triphosphate		H	Antiviral (CMV)
0.99			?	Lipid-lowering drug
0.1	–		H,P	Aminoglycoside antibiotic
0.99			?	Sulphonylurea
0.99			?	Sulphonylurea
0.95	–		?	Sulphonylurea
0.99	p-OH-gliquidone		?	Sulphonylurea
0.8			?	Osmotic diuretic
	1,3-Glyceryl dinitrate 1,2-Glyceryl dinitrate		? (unlikely)	Vasodilator
0.99			?	Antifungal agent
0.5	Guanethidine-N-oxide	(< 0.1)	?	Antihypertensive
0.99	(reduced haloperidol)	× 0.1	nH, nP	Antipsychotic
			? (unlikely)	Inhalation anaesthetic
0.99			nH,nP	Parenteral anticoagulant

| Drug | Factor | Plasma concentration (mg/l) | | | HLT | V_d |
		Therap.	Toxic	Lethal		l/kg
Hexamine	7.13	20			20	0.6
Hydralazine	6.24	0.1–1.5			2.5(HF↑)	5
Fast acetylator					1	1.5
Slow acetylator					1	1.5
Hydrochorothiazide	3.36	0.07–0.45			10.2(A↑)	3
Hydrocortisone	2.76	0.05–0.25			Nlin(1.8)	0.3
Hydroflumethiazide	3.02	–			16.6	6.4
Hydroxychloroquine	2.98	0.01–0.02		> 60	72	50
Hydroxyurea	13.15				≤ 6	0.5
Hydroxyzine	2.67				14(A↑)/≤14	22.5
Hyoscine	3.3	0.00004			2.9	1.4
Ibuprofen	4.85	0.5–50	> 100	–	2.2(A↑)	0.1
Ifosfamide	3.83				Nlin(7)/?	
Imipenem	3.34	–80			1.0(I↑)	0.3
Imipramine	3.57	0.05–0.25	> 0.3–1.5	> 2	7–18(A↑)/17	15
Indapamide	2.73				18	1.6
Indomethacin	2.79	0.5–3	> 5		6(I↑)	0.9
Indoramin	2.88				4/?(A↑)	7.4
Insulin	7.18	10–20 mU/l			0.25–2	0.6
Interferon α_{2a}	0.0052				5.1	0.4
Interferon α_{2b}	0.0052				2	
Ipatropium bromide	2.42				1.6	
Iron	17.91	0.65–1.75	5–6	20–50		
Isocarboxazid	4.32	< 0.5			2	
Isoniazid	7.29	0.5–15	> 20		2.3(I↑,Ci↑)	0.6
Fast acetylator					1.1	0.6
Slow acetylator					3.6	0.6
Isoprenaline	4.73				5/?	
Isosorbide dintrate	4.23	0.003–0.2			1.3/2	1.5
					1.3/5(Ci=)	
Isotretinoin	3.33				14	7
Isradipine	2.69				3.2(A↑)	4
Kanamycin	2.06	peak: 20–25	> 30		2(N↑,I↑)	0.25
		trough: 1–4	> 8			
Ketamine	4.21	0.1–0.15			α: 0.2, β: 3.6/?	2.9
Ketoconazole	1.88				8	0.36
Ketoprofen	3.93				1.5(A↑)	0.11
Ketorolac	3.92				4.5(A↑)	0.1
Ketotifen	3.23	1–4			4–20/?	

Q_0	Active metabolites Name	Potency	Extra dose after dialysis	Clinical application
	Formaldehyde	Prodrug		Urinary antiseptic
0.9			nH,nP	Vasodilator
0.98				
0.9				
0.05			?	Thiazide diuretic
0.99			?	Glucocorticoid
0.5			?	Thiazide diuretic
pH↓(0.33)			? (unlikely)	Antimalarial
0.5			?	DNA synthesis inhibitor
	Cetirizine	Potent	? (unlikely)	H_1-antagonist
0.95			?	Anticholinergic
0.99	–		nH	Propionic acid NSAID
0.8	4-OH-ifosfamide		?	Alkylating agent
0.3			H	Carbapenem antibiotic
0.98	Desipramine → 2-OH-desipramine	> ×1	nH,nP	Tricyclic antidepressant
0.95			nH	Diuretic
0.85	–		nH	Indole NSAID
0.9	6-OH-indoramin		? (unlikely)	α_1-antagonist
0.95			nH	Hormone
0.99			nH	Immunostimulant
0.99			nH	Immunostimulant
0.4	–		?	Anticholinergic
			nH	Trace element
			?	Irreversible MAO inhibitor
pH↑(0.7)			H,P	Antituberculous drug
0.93				
0.7				
0.5	3-O-methyl-isoprenaline		?	β_{1+2}-agonist
0.99	2-mononitrate		nH	Nitrate vasodilator
	5-mononitrate			Nitrate vasodilator
0.99			?	Oral retinoid for acne
0.99	–		?	Type II calcium-channel blocker
0.19	–		H,P	Aminoglycoside antibiotic
0.97	Norketamine	× 0.3	? (unlikely)	Intravenous anaesthetic
0.97			nH,nP	Antifungal drug
0.99	–		Itx:H	NSAID
0.4	–		?	NSAID
0.99	Norketotifen	× 1	?	Mast cell stabilizer

Drug	Factor	Plasma concentration (mg/l)			HLT	V_d
		Therap.	Toxic	Lethal		l/kg
Labetalol	3.04	–			4(Ci=)	9
Lead	4.83	< 0.03	> 0.9	> 1.1		
Levodopa	5.07	0.2–4			1.4	12.7
Levonorgestrel	3.2				28	2.9
Lignocaine	4.27	2–5	> 8	> 25	1.8(I↑,A↑,Ci↑, HF↑)/2.1	1.5
Lisinopril	2.26				7(A↑)	
Lithium (mmol/l)	144.07	0.5–1.2	> 2	> 3	pH (22)(A↑)	0.79
Lofepramine	2.39	–			4.5/17(A↑)	
Loperamide	2.1	< 0.003			11	
Loprazolam	2.15				6(A↑)	
Loratadine	2.61				14.4	
Lorazepam	3.11	0.02–0.24	> 0.3		13(I↑,Ci↑)	1.5
Lormetazepam	2.98				12/8	
Loxapine	3.05	0.002–0.03	> 0.2	> 7.7	1.5–3.5	
Lysergide (LSD)	3.09	–	0.001– 0.004	–	3	
Lysuride	2.95				2	
Magnesium (mmol/l)	41.14	1.6–3.3	> 7	> 15		
Mannitol	5.49				0.25–1.5	0.18
Maprotiline	3.61	0.2–0.3	> 0.5	> 2	43/?	51.7
Mebendazole	3.39	–			1.1	2
Medroxyprogesterone	2.9				36	0.6
Mefenamic acid	4.14	2–20	> 25		4(Ci=)	
Mefloquine	2.41				530	19
Melphalan	3.28				1.4/?	0.45
Meprobamate	4.58	5–30	60–100	140–350	12(Ci↑)	0.7
Mercaptopurine	6.57				0.9/?	0.56
Mercury	4.99	< 0.08	> 0.2	> 6		
Metformin	7.74	0.5–4	> 45		1.5	3.1
Methadone	2.89	0.1–1.1	> 2	> 4	25(Ci↑)	3.9
Methanol	31.2	–	200–800	> 800	3	0.7
Methicillin	2.63	1–6			1(N↑,I↑)	0.3
Methocarbamol	4.15	–			1.2	0.5
Methohexitone	3.52	5			π: 5.5 min, α: 60 min	
					3.9(Ci=)	2.2
Methotrexate	2.2	–			8.4(C↓)	0.75
Methotrimeprazine	3.04	0.02–0.14			21	29.8

Q_0	Active metabolites Name	Potency	Extra dose after dialysis	Clinical application
0.95			nH,nP	α_1-β_{1+2}-antagonist
			?	Heavy metal
0.99			? (unlikely)	Antiparkinsonian drug
			?	Progestogen
0.95	MEGX, GX	$\times 1, \times 0.25$	nH	Ib anti-arrhythmic. Local anaesthetic
0.2			nH,nP	ACE inhibitor
0.05	–		H,P,Itx:H	Antipsychotic
0.99	Desipramine $\to$ 2-OH-d.		? (unlikely)	Tricyclic antidepressant
0.99			?	Anti-diarrhoeal
0.99			? (unlikely)	Benzodiazepine
0.99	Descarboethoxy-L.		?	H_1-antagonist
0.99	–		nH	Benzodiazepine
0.99			? (unlikely)	Benzodiazepine
0.99	8-OH-loxapine 8-OH-amoxapine		? (unlikely)	Antipsychotic
			?	CNS stimulant
0.99			?	Prolactin inhibitor
0.01	–		Itx:H,P	Anticonvulsant
0.05			Itx:H,P	Osmotic diuretic
0.98			? (unlikely)	Tetracyclic antidepressant
0.99			nH	Antihelminthic
0.55			?	Progestogen
0.95	–		nH	NSAID
0.9			? (unlikely)	Antimalarial
0.88			?	Alkylating agent
0.9			H,P,Ttx:H,KP	Anxiolytic
0.78	TIMP, MTIMP		nH,nP	Antimetabolite
	–		? (unlikely)	Heavy metal
0.01	–		Itx:H	Biguanide oral antidiabetic drug
pH↑(0.7)			nH,nP	Opiate analgesic
			Itx:H	Solvent
0.25			nH,nP	Penicillinase-resistant penicillin
0.99	–		?	Skeletal muscle relaxant
0.99			? (unlikely)	Intravenous barbiturate anaesthetic
pH↑(0.15–0.5)			(H),nP,Itx:KP	Dihydrofolate reducatase inhibitor
0.99			? (unlikely)	Analgesic, hypnotic

| Drug | Factor | Plasma concentration (mg/l) | | | HLT | V_d |
		Therap.	Toxic	Lethal		l/kg
Methyldopa	4.73	1–5	>7		1.4(I↑)/?	0.4
Methylprednisolone	2.67				2.5	0.84
Methysergide	2.83				0.75	
Metoclopramide	3.34	–			2.7	2.4
Metolazone	2.73				20	1.6
Metoprolol	3.74	0.025–0.3			3–6(Ci↑)/?	4.2
Metronidazole	5.84	1–2.5			8(Ci↑)/15	0.75
Metyrapone	4.42	0.5–4			0.4/?	
Mexilitine	5.58	0.8–2	>2		10(Ci↑,HF↑)	5.3
Mianserin	3.78	0.02–0.07	>0.1		Nlin(23)(A↑)/≤23	6
Miconazole	2.4	0.001–10			22.5	21
Midazolam	3.07	0.2–0.5			2.5(Ci↑)/1	0.7
Milrinone	4.73	0.05–0.3			1.5(HF↑)	0.3
Minocycline	2.19	0.5–3			12	0.43
Minoxidil	4.78				3.1/?	2.7
Misoprostol	2.61				–/157	
Mitomycin	2.99				Nlin(0.25)	
Moclobemide	3.72	0.2			2	1.1
Moracizine	2.34	–			2–8	12
Morphine	3.5	0.01–0.1	0.1–1	>(0.05)–4	π:1.5 min, α: 15 min	
					2.3(Ci=)/4	3.5
Nadolol	3.23	0.025–0.275			14.1	2.1
Nafarelin	0.76				2.7	
Nalbuphine	2.8				3.5(C↓)/?	3.8
Nalidixic acid	4.31	5–50			6(I↑,A↑)/?	1
Naloxone	3.05	0.01			1	2.8
Naltrexone	2.93				3.9/12.9	19
Naproxen	4.34	>50			14	0.09
Neomycin	1.63	5–10			2.5	0.2
Neostigmine	3.3				1.3	0.7
Netilmicin	2.1	peak: 6–10	>12		2.2	0.25
		trough:<2	>2			
Nicardipine	2.09				5(Ci↑)	1.1
Nickel	17.04	0.001–0.004			5	
Nicotine	6.16		>10	50–500	2(5↓)	2.6

Q_0	Active metabolites Name	Potency	Extra dose after dialysis	Clinical application
0.72	Dopamine		H,P	Central α_2-agonist
0.95			H	Glucocorticoid
0.9			?	Migraine prophylactic
0.83			nH,nP	Antiemetic
0.2			nH	Thiazide diuretic
0.9	α-OH-meoprolol	$< \times 0.1$	(H)	β_1-antagonist
0.92	OH-metronidazole		H,nP	Antibiotic
0.99	Metyrapol		?	Corticoid synthesis inhibitor
pH↓(0.9)	–		nH,nP	Type Ib anti-arrhythmic
0.95	Desmethyl-mianserin	($\approx \times 1$)	? (unlikely)	Tetracyclic antidepressant
0.99			nH,nP	Antifungal antibiotic
0.99	α-OH-midazolam	$\times 1$	?.	Benzodiazepine
0.2			?	Phosphodiesterase inhibitor
0.9			nH,nP	Long-acting tetracycline
0.88	Min.-N-O-sulphate	Prodrug	nH	Vasodilator
0.99	Misoprostolic acid	$\times 1$	?	Prostaglandin-E_1 analogue
0.9			?	DNA synthesis inhibitor
0.99	?		?	Reversible MAO inhibitor
0.99	?		? (unlikely)	Type I anti-arrhythmic
	Mo.-6-glucuronide			Opiate analgesic
0.3	–		H	β_{1+2}-antagonist
0.95			?	Gonadotrophin RH antagonist
0.95			? (unlikely)	Analgesic
0.95	OH-nalidixic acid	$\times 16$	?	Urinary antiseptic
0.99			?	Opiate antagonist
0.99	6-β-naltrexol	($< \times 0.08$)	? (unlikely)	Opiate antagonist
0.99	–		nH	Propionic acid NSAID
0.5	–		H	Aminoglycoside antibiotic
0.33			?	Cholinesterase inhibitor
0.05	–		H,P	Aminoglycoside antibiotic
0.99			nH	Type II calcium-channel blocker
	–		?	Trace element
pH↓(0.83)			? (unlikely)	CNS stimulant

Drug	Factor	Plasma concentration (mg/l)			HLT	V_d
		Therap.	Toxic	Lethal		l/kg
Nicotinic acid	8.12				0.75	
Nifedipine	2.89	0.015–0.1			1.7(Ci↑,HF=)	1.1
Nimodipine	2.39				1.5	1.5
Nitrazepam	3.56	0.03–0.18			22(A↑,Ci=)	2.1
Nitrofurantoin	4.2	1.8			0.33	0.8
Nitroprusside	3.82	6–29			0.1	
Nizatidine	3.02	0.07–0.7			1.3/4	1.2
N₂O (nitrous oxide)	22.72	17–22		> 350		
Noradrenaline	5.91				0.03	
Norethisterone	3.35				10	4
Norfloxacin	3.13	< 5			4(Ci=)/?	3.2
Nortriptyline	3.8	0.05–0.4	> 0.5	> 13	27(T↑)/> 27	20
Ofloxacin	2.77				4(Ci↑)	1
Omeprazole	2.9				1/1	0.35
Orciprenaline	4.73				2.1	7.6
Orphenadrine	3.71	0.4–1	> 1	4–8	18/25	6
Ouabain	1.71	0.0002			22/?	15.7
Oxatomide	2.34	0.1			14	
Oxazepam	3.49	0.2–2	> 2		12(Ci=)	1.2
Oxpentifylline	3.59				0.8/1	4.2
Oxprenolol	3.77	0.04–0.1			1.9	1.2
Oxytetracycline	2.17	0.05–3			9.2	1.9
Pancuronium	1.36	0.25–0.5		> 1.6	2.3(A↑, Ci↑)/1.1	0.26
Papaverine	2.95	0.1–4			1.6	0.2
Paracetamol	6.62	5–20	120–300	> 1500	2.5(I↑,A↑,S↓,Ci↑, HF=)	1.1
Paraldehyde	7.57	10–100	> 200	> 500	6	
Paraquat	5.37	–	> 1	> 2		2.8
PAS	6.53	0.6–4			1.5(Ci=)	0.11
Pemoline	5.68				11	
Penicillamine	6.7				2.5	
Penicillin G (Benzylpenicillin)	2.69	1.5–16			0.7(N↑,I↑)	0.5
Penicillin V (Phenoxymethylpenicillin)	2.85	3–5			0.6	0.4
Pentamidine	2.94				6.2	16
Pentazocine	3.5	0.1–0.6	2–5	> (1–)5	2.5(S↓,Ci↑)	4
Perindopril	2.71	0.003 (Perindoprilat)			2.9(Ci=)/11	
Perphenazine	2.48	0.005	> 1	–	10/?	25

Q_0	Active metabolites Name	Potency	Extra dose after dialysis	Clinical application
0.1			?	Lipid-lowering agent
0.98			nH,nP	Type II calcium-channel blocker
0.9	–		? (unlikely)	Type II calcium-channel blocker
0.99			? (unlikely)	Benzodiazepine
pH↑(0.6)			H	Urinary antiseptic
0.99			nH,CN-Itx:H	Vasodilator
0.4	(N2-monodesmethyl-N.)		nH, Itx:H	H_2-antagonist
0.99			? (unlikely)	Inhalation anaesthetic
0.99			?	$\alpha\beta_1$-agonist
			?	Progestogen
0.35	6 different metabolites		nH	4-Quinolone antibiotic
0.98	10-OH-nortriptyline		nH,nP,Itx:KP	Tricyclic antidepressant
0.25			?	4-Quinolone antibiotic
0.99	Omeprazole-sulphone		? (unlikely)	Proton pump inhibitor
0.9	–		? (unlikely)	β_2-agonist
0.92			nH	Skeletal muscle relaxant
0.63			nH,nP	Cardiac glycoside
0.99	?		?	H_1-antagonist
0.98	–		nH	Benzodiazepine
0.99	5-OH-pentoxifylline		? (unlikely)	Vasodilator
0.95	–		?	β_{1+2}-antagonist
0.5			nP	Short-acting tetracycline
0.33	3-OH-pancuronium	× 0.5	?	Non-depolarizing muscle relaxant
0.99			(H)	Vasodilator
0.95			(H),nP,Itx: H,KP	Analgesic
0.99			?	Anticonvulsant
	Paraoxone		Itx:KP	Herbicide
0.9			H	Antituberculous drug
0.6			?	CNS stimulant
0.85			?	Antirheumatic
0.2			H,nP	Natural penicillin
0.74			H,nP	Acid-resistant penicillin
0.95			? (unlikely)	Antiprotozoal
0.95			H	Opiate agonist/antagonist
0.9	Perindoprilat	Prodrug	?	ACE inhibitor
	(7−)H-perphenazine		nH	Antipsychotic

| Drug | Factor | Plasma concentration (mg/l) | | | HLT | V_d |
		Therap.	Toxic	Lethal		l/kg
Pethidine	4.04	0.3–1	> 5	10–30	α: 10 min	4.7
					6(N↑,A↑,Ci↑)/?	
Phenelzine	7.34	0.001–0.002		> 4	Nlin(1.5–4)	
Phenobarbitone	4.31	15–40	> 50	> 100	100(I↑,C↓,A↑,Ci↑)	0.7
Phenylbutazone	3.24	40–150	> 200	> 400	72(A↑,S↓)/48	0.1
Phenylephrine	4.91	0.03			2.5	
Phenytoin	3.96	10–20	> 20	> 40	Nlin(20)(I↑,C↓)	0.65
Physostigmine	3.63				1.5	
Phytomenadione	2.22				2	
Pimozide	2.17				53–111	24
Pindolol	4.03	0.05–0.15			2.2	2
Piperacillin	1.93	< 400			0.93	0.18
Pirenzepine	2.85				10	
Piretanide	2.76				1.4	0.3
Piroxicam	3.02	0.85–13.5			48	0.15
Pivampicillin	2.16				0.2/0.9	
Platinum	5.13	< 0.7			58–73	
Polymyxin B	–	0.5–4			4.4	
Polythiazide	2.27	2–7			26	
Pralidoxime	5.79				1.25	
Praziquantel	3.2				1.5	
Prazosin	2.61				2.9(HF↑)	0.6
Prednisolone	2.77				2.2(Ci=)	0.65
Prednisone	2.79				3.6(Ci=)	0.97
Prilocaine	4.54	1–5	> 8		2.1	
Primaquine	3.86				7	
Primidone	4.58	4–12	> 12	> 100	6.5/100(Ci↑)	0.8
Probenecid	3.87	100–200			Nlin(5)/?	0.15
Probucol	1.93	15–80			550	
Procainamide	4.25	4–10	> 16		3(C↓,HF=)/6	2
Procarbazine	4.52				0.17	
Prochlorperazine	2.67	–	> 1	> 5	23	
Promethazine	3.52	0.2–11			3–13	2
Propafenone	2.93	0.2–0.9	> 0.9		Nlin(7)/10	4.4
Propantheline	2.23				1.8	
Propofol	5.61	1–10			β: 0.8,γ: 10(A↑)	5

| Q_o | Active metabolites | | Extra dose after dialysis | Clinical application |
	Name	Potency		
	Normeperidine			Opiate analgesic
0.99	?		? (unlikely)	Irreversible MAO inhibitor
pH↑(0.75)	–		H,P,Itx:KP	Barbiturate hypnotic
0.99	Oxyphenbutazone	×1	nH,Itx:KP	NSAID
	τ-OH-phenylbutazone		?	NSAID
0.85			?	α-agonist
0.95	–		nH,nP,Itx:KP	Anticonvulsant, Ib-anti-arrhythmic
0.99			?	Cholinesterase inhibitor
0.95			?	Vitamin K_1
0.99	–		? (unlikely)	Antipsychotic
0.63			?	β_{1+2}-antagonist
0.29			H,nP	Broad-spectrum penicillin
0.8	–		?	Gastric secretion inhibitor
0.55			?	Loop diuretic
0.95	–		? (unlikely)	Oxicam NSAID
0.99	Ampicillin	Prodrug	H,nP	Aminopenicillin
			?	Heavy metal
0.4			nH,P	Polymyxin antibiotic
0.75			?	Thiazide diuretic
0.2			?	Cholinesterase reactivator
0.99	–		?	Antihelminthic
0.99			nH,nP	α_1-agonist
0.75	Prednisone		nH,nP	Glucocorticoid
0.97	Prednisolone	×1	H	Glucocorticoid
			?	Local anaesthetic
0.95	?		?	Antimalarial
0.9	Phenobarbitone	×1	H	Anticonvulsant
	Phenylethylmalonamide			Anticonvulsant?
0.98			?	Uricosuric
0.99	?		nH,nP	Lipid-lowering drug
0.5	NAPA		H,nP	Ia-anti-arrhythmic
0.95			?	Cytostatic
			nH	Antipsychotic
0.98			nH	H_1-antagonist
0.99	5-OH-propafenone	ca.×1	? (Unlikely)	Ic-anti-arrhythmic
0.85			?	Anticholinergic
0.99	?		?	Intravenous anaesthetic

Drug	Factor	Plasma concentration (mg/l)			HLT	V_d
		Therap.	Toxic	Lethal		l/kg
Propranolol	3.86	0.02–0.4	> 2	8–12	3.8(A↑,Ci↑)/?	4
Propylthiouracil	5.87				1.4	0.36
Protriptyline	3.8	0.1–0.2	> 0.5	> 1	78	22
Pseudoephedrine	4.96	0.5–0.8		> 19	6.9	2.8
Pyrazinamide	8.12	20–30			10	
Pyridostigmine	3.83	0.05–0.1			1.9	1.1
Pyrimethamine	4.02	0.07–0.2			96	2.2
Quinalbarbitone	3.84	1–5		> 3.5	28	1.5
Quinidine	3.08	2–5	> 10	30–50	6.3(A↑,Ci↑)/12	33
Quinine	3.08	7–17	> 10		16.4	1.2
Ramipril	2.4	0.001–0.01			−/3.5	
Ranitidine	3.18	0.1–0.2			2.3(A↑,Ci↑)	1.6
Rifampicin	1.22	0.5–10			3(Ci↑)/?	1
Salicylic acid	7.24	20–300	> 300	> 1200	Nlin(4)(I↑,A↑)	0.14
Sodium aurothiomalate		1–5			⩾ 600	0.26
Sodium cromoglycate	2.14				0.1	
Sotalol	3.67	0.5–4			7–14	1.85
Spectinomycin	3.01	7.5–20			1	0.12
Spironolactone	2.4				1.6(Ci=)/19	14
Streptokinase	−				1.4	0.016
Streptomycin	1.72	peak: 20–25	> 30		2.4	0.26
		trough: 1–4	> 8			
Sulfadoxine	3.22	100			184	
Sulindac	2.81				7/16	2
Sulphadiazine	4.0	100–150			7–17	0.9
Sulphamethoxazole	3.95	50–200			10(Ci=)	0.3
Sulphinpyrazone	2.47	−			4/18	0.74
Sulpiride	2.93	< 0.5			5.5	0.9
Tamoxifen	2.69	−			170/310	
Teicoplanin	0.53				30–100	0.6
Temazepam	3.33	0.4–0.9			13(Ci=)/12(Ci=)	1.1
Temocillin	2.41	50–250			5	0.27
Tenoxicam	2.96	10–15			70	
Terazosin	2.58				11	0.8
Terbutaline	4.43	0.003–0.007		> 0.04	16	1.4
Terfenadine	2.12				−/17	
Tetracycline	2.25	0.5–2			6.8	1.3
Thallium	4.89	< 0.005	> 0.1			

Q_0	Active metabolites		Extra dose after dialysis	Clinical application
	Name	Potency		
0.99	4-OH-propranolol	× 1	? (unlikely)	β_{1+2}-antagonist, II-anti-arrhythmic
0.9			? (unlikely)	Antithyroid drug
0.99			nH,nP	Tricyclic antidepressant
0.04			?	Sympathomimetic
0.99			?	Antituberculous drug
0.15			?	Cholinesterase inhibitor
0.99	?		? (unlikey)	Antimalarial
0.95			nH,nP	Barbiturate hypnotic
pH↓(0.8)	3-OH-quinidine	× 0.6	(H),(P),Itx:H	Ia-anti-arrhythmic
pH↓(0.85)			H.nP	Antimalarial
0.99	Ramiprilat	Prodrug	?	ACE inhibitor
0.3			H,p	H_2-antagonist
0.9	Desacetyl-rifampicin	× 1	nH,nP,Itx:H	Antituberculous drug
pH↑(0.98–0.7)			H,Itx:H	Salicylate
0.3			nH	Antirheumatic
0.6			?	Mast cell stabilizer
0.25	–		H,P	β_{1+2}-antagonist, II + III anti-arrhythmic
0.1			H	Antibiotic
0.99	Canrenone		?	Aldosterone antagonist
0.99			?	Thrombolytic
0.5	–		H,P	Aminoglycoside antibiotic
0.6			? (unlikely)	Antimalarial
0.99	Sulindac sulphide	Prodrug	? (unlikely)	Indole NSAID
0.4			?	Short-acting sulphonamide
0.65			H,nP	Medium-duration sulphonamide
0.6	N-OH-phenyl-S.	Active	nH	Uricosuric
0.12	–		?	Antipsychotic
0.99	N-desmethyl-tamox.	× 1.9	? (unlikely)	Anti-oestrogen
0.05	–		nH,nP	Antibiotic
0.98	(Oxazepam)		nH,nP	Benzodiazepine
0.3			H,nP	β-lactamase-resistant penicillin
0.99	–		?	Oxicam NSAID
0.9			? (unlikely)	α_1-antagonist
0.43	–		?	β_2-agonist
0.99		(× 0.3)	? (unlikley)	H_1-antagonist
0.4			nH,nP	Short-acting tetracycline
	–		Itx:H	Heavy metal

| Drug | Factor | Plasma concentration (mg/l) | | | HLT | V_d |
		Therap.	Toxic	Lethal		l/kg
Theophylline	5.55	10–20	> 20	> 30	Nlin(9)(N↑,I↓,C↓, S↓,Ci↑,HF↑)	0.5
Thiopentone	4.13	7–130		10–400	π: 3 min, α: 47 min Nlin(9)A↑)/22	2.3
Thioridazine	2.7	0.2–2.6	> 10	> (1–)13	20/?	
Thyroxine	1.29	0.04–0.13			110	0.15
Ticarcillin	2.6	50–350			1.2	0.21
Timolol	3.16	0.005–0.01			4–8	2.1
Tinidazole	4.04	< 25			15	0.75
Tobramycin	2.14	peak:6–10	> 12		2(N↑)	0.25
		trough:< 2	> 2			
Tocainide	5.2	4–10	> 10		12.5(Ci↑,HF=)	3
Tolazamide	3.21				7/?	
Tolbutamide	3.7	50–250	> 640		7(N↑,I↑)	0.12
Tolmetin	3.89	37	> 60		5	0.09
Tramadol	3.8				7/9	3.3
Tranexamic acid	6.36				2.3	
Tranylcypromine	7.51	0.01–0.04			2	
Trazodone	2.69	0.07–1.7	> 2		5(A↑)	1
Triamcinolone	2.54				1.4	1.8
Triamterene	3.95				4.2(Ci↑)/3	2.5
Tribavarin	4.09				β: 1, γ: 27	8.7
Trifluoperazine	2.45	< 0.8	> 1.2–3	> 3–8		
Triiodothyronine	1.54				≤ 48	0.5
Trimethoprim	3.44	0.5–12			8.8(C↓,Ci=)	2
Trimipramine	3.4				24	31
Tubocurarine	1.47	0.5–1.2			3.8	0.3
Urea	16.65					
Urokinase	–				0.3	
Ursodeoxycholic acid	2.55				100	
Valproate	6.93	50–100	> 200		12.2(Ci↑)	0.14
Vancomycin	0.67	peak: 30–40		> 80	6(Ci↑)	0.47
		trough: 5–10		> 20		
Vecuronium	1.57	0.2–0.4			1.5	0.21
Verapamil	2.2	0.02–0.8	> 2		Nlin(4.8)(Ci↑)/10	5.3

| Q_0 | Active metabolites | | Extra dose after dialysis | Clinical application |
	Name	Potency		
0.87			H,(P),Itx:KP	Bronchodilator
0.99	(Pentobarbitone)		? (unlikely)	Intravenous barbiturate anaesthetic
0.99	Mesoridazine	×2	? (unlikley)	Antipsychotic
0.99	Triiodothyronine	×4	?	Thyroid hormone
0.14			H,(P)	Penicillin active against *Pseudomonas*
0.8	–		nH	β_{1+2}-antagonist
0.8			H	Antiprotozoal, anti-anaerobic
0.02	–		H,P	Aminoglycoside antibiotic
pH↓(0.6)	–		H	Ib-anti-arrhythmic
0.85	3 weakly active		?	Sulphonylurea
0.99	OH-tolb., Carboxy-tol.		nH	Sulphonylurea
0.89	–		? (unlikely)	Indole NSAID
0.7			? (unlikely)	Opiate analgesic
0.03			?	Plasmin inhibitor
0.95			?	Irreversible MAO inhibitor
0.99			?	Antidepressant
0.99			?	Glucocorticoid
0.95	OH-triamterene		?	K⁺-sparing diuretic
0.65			? (unlikely)	Antiviral (RSV)
			nH	Antipsychotic
0.99			?	Thyroid hormone
0.4			H,nP,Itx:H	Antibacterial
0.99			? (unlikley)	Tricyclic antidepressant
0.37			H	Non-depolarizing muscle relaxant
			H,P	Osmotic diuretic
			nP	Thrombolytic
0.99			? (unlikely)	Cholesterol gallstone dissolvant
0.99	?		(H),nP	Anticonvulsant
0.05	–		nH,(P?)	Antibiotic
0.8	(3α-deacetyl-vecuronium)		?	Non-depolarizing muscle relaxant
0.97	Norverapamil	(×0.2)	nH,nP	Type I calcium-channel blocker

| Drug | Factor | Plasma concentration (mg/l) | | | HLT | V_d |
		Therap.	Toxic	Lethal		l/kg
Vigabatrin	7.74				7(A↑)	0.8
Vinblastine	1.23				25	27
Vincristine	1.21				85	8.4
Vindesine	1.33				24	8.8
Vitamin K	2.22	0.0004–0.0012			1.7/?	
Warfarin	3.24	1–10			46	0.11
Zidovudine (AZT)	3.74	0.27–1.5			1.1(Ci↑)	1.4
Zinc	15.3	0.5–1.5				
Zolpidem	3.25	< 0.2			1.7(A↑)	0.5
Zopiclone	2.57				5(A↑, Ci↑)/?	

Abbreviations:

A	Alteration of HLT in old age.
Ci	Alteration of HLT in cirrhosis.
HF	Alteration of HLT in heart failure.
H, P	During haemo- or peritoneal dialysis, the clearance of the substance increases by more than 30%; an additional dose after the dialysis is necessary; the administration of the substance after the dialysis is advisable.
HLT	Elimination half life; β-half life (if not stated otherwise).
Itx:H, Itx:P, Itx:KP	In intoxication with the relevant product the elimination can be substantially accelerated by haemo- or peritoneal dialysis or by charcoal perfusion.
C	Alteration of the HLT in children.
nH, nP	During a haemo- or peritoneal dialysis the clearance of the product increases by **less** than 30%; an additional dose after the dialysis is **not** necessary.
N	Alteration of the HLT in neonates.
Nlin	The kinetics of the substance are non-linear; doubling of the dose can therefore lead to a prolonged HLT and a disproportionate increase in the serum concentration. A typical 'HLT' is given in brackets.
NSAID	Non-steroidal anti-inflammatory drug.
pH	The pH reference in the Q_o column indicates a pH-dependent renal excretion of the product. Basic substances are generally eliminated better in an acid, and acid substances better in an alkaline urine. The arrow indicates the alteration of pH which leads to increased excretion.
Prodrug	Inactive substance that is metabolized in the body to the active substance.
Q_o	Fraction eliminated by non-renal mechanisms.
S	Alteration of the HLT in smokers.
I	Alteration of the HLT in infants.
↑, ↓, =	Increase, decrease, unchanged.
π	Initial (rapid) distribution HLT.
α	Distribution HLT.
/	Data after the oblique stroke refer to the active metabolites.

Q_0	Active metabolites Name	Potency	Extra dose after dialysis	Clinical application
0.35			?	Anticonvulsant
0.95			? (unlikely)	Antimetabolite
0.95			nH	Antimetabolite
			? (unlikley)	Antimetabolite
0.99	Vit.K-2,3,-epoxide		? (unlikely)	Coumarin antagonist
0.99	4 different ones	(+)	nH,nP	Oral anticoagulant
0.81	–		?	Antiviral (HIV)
	–		?	Trace element
0.99	–		nH	Hypnotic
0.95		$< \times 1$	nH	Hypnotic

Note:

1. The column marked 'Factor' gives the conversion factor from metric to SI units (conversion from mg/l to μmol/l). The calculation is derived from the following formula: 1000 (mg/l)/molecular weight (g/mol) = μmol/l. In combined preparations the factors vary for the individual components. Reversal of the formula permits the calculation of the molecular weight and thus gives an indication of the ability to remove the relevant substance by dialysis.

2. The data in general refer to healthy subjects.

3. Plasma concentrations are indicated as therapeutic, toxic and potentially life threatening ('lethal'). Values in the first column represent either clearly defined limits (for trough values = blood collection at lowest level) of an optimal effect (bold print) or concentrations found with conventional doses (normal print).

4. Known active metabolites are shown in the relevant column; their HLT, if known, is given after the HLT of the primary substance (cf. 5). The metabolite is given in brackets if under clinical conditions only small amounts of metabolite are present, or if the inactivation of the metabolite is so rapid that it does not have any clinical effect.

5. The column 'Potency' indicates the relative potency of the active metabolites compared with the primary substance; the value is given in brackets if the only data are from animal experiments. Irrelevant, weak activity is indicated by (+).

Drugs in pregnancy

The following list should not invalidate the general principle that drug administration during pregnancy should be kept to the absolute minimum.

Group A: Clinical studies have shown no evidence of an increased risk of fetal malformation in the first trimester. Similarly there is no evidence of any increased risk in the subsequent months of the pregnancy.

Digoxin, magnesium sulphate, nystatin (vaginal), pyridoxin (vitamin B_6), thiamin (vitamin B_1), thyroxine

Group B: No risk in animal studies, but adequate clinical studies not available; or no risk in clinical studies, but an increased risk has been demonstrated in animal studies.

Acebutolol, albumin, amiloride, azatadine, aztreonam, brompheniramine, buspirone, carnitine, cephalosporins, chlorhexidine, chlorpheniramine, cinoxacin, clemastine, clindamycin (topical), cromoglycate, cyclizine, desmopressin, dimenhydrinate, diphenhydramine, dipyridamole, doxapram, erythromycin, ethacrynic acid, etidronate, famotidine, fluoxetine, gemfibrozil, glibenclamide, gonadorelin, indapamide, insulin, ipratropium bromide, iron, ketoprofen, lindane (topical), lignocaine, maprotiline, metoclopramide, metolazone, metoprolol, mupirocin (topical), naloxone, naproxen, penicillins, permethrin (topical), pindolol, praziquantel, prilocaine, probucol, ranitidine, ritrodine, terbutaline, tranexamic acid, tretinoin (topical), triamterene, triprolidine, urokinase

Drugs and breast feeding
(not excreted in breast milk or not absorbed by the infant)

Ascorbic acid, antacids, antihistamines, barbiturates (in low dose), benzodiazepines (in low dose), bisacodyl, cephalosporins, clindamycin, clonidine, codeine, corticosteroids (in low dose), dextropropoxyphene, dichloralphenazone, digoxin, erythromycin, folic acid, heparin, ibuprofen, iron, ketoprofen, mefenamic acid, methyldopa, metronidazole, monoamine oxidase inhibitors, nitrofurantoin, paracetamol, penicillins, pentazocine, pethidine, phenothiazines (in low dose), rifampicin, salicylate (in low dose), tricyclics, B-vitamins

Drug metabolism

1. Genetic polymorphisms

Acetylator status

Enzyme:	Hepatic *N*-acetyltransferase
Inheritance:	Autosomal recessive
Test:	Sulphadimidine test
Drugs affected:	Aminoglutethimide, clonazepam, caffeine, dapsone, hydralazine, isoniazid, nitrazepam, phenelzine, procainamide, sulphadimidine, sulphasalazine, thymoxamine
% slow metabolizers:	Egyptians 83%, Americans (white) 58%, Americans (black) 50%, Canadian Eskimos 0–5%, Chinese 20%, Swiss 61%, Orientals 15%, South Africans (black) 41%

Hydroxylator status:

Enzyme:	Debrisoquine-4-hydroxylase (cytochrome P450 db_1; cytochrome P450 IID_6)
Inheritance:	Autosomal recessive
Test:	Dextromethorphan test
Drugs affected:	(Amitriptyline), (clomipramine), codeine, debrisoquine, desipramine, dextromethorphan, diltiazem, flecainide, (imipramine), indoramin, metoprolol, nortriptyline, phenformin, propafenone, propranolol, timolol
Pure inhibitors:	Cimetidine, diphenhydramine, methotrimeprazine, orphenadrine, quinidine, thioridazine
% slow metabolizers:	Egyptians 1%, Chinese 0.7%, Japanese 0%, Nigerians 0%, Saudi Arabians 1%, whites 3–10%

Mephenytoinpolymorphism

Enzyme:	*S*-mephenytoin-hydroxylase
Inheritance:	Autosomal recessive
Test:	Mephenytoin test
Drugs affected:	(Hexobarbitone), mephobarbitone, mephenytoin
Pure inhibitors:	Ketoconazole
% slow metabolizers:	White 5%, Japanese 20%, Cuna-Indians (Panama) 0%

Cholinesterase deficiency

Enzyme:	Serum cholinesterase (pseudocholinesterase)
Inheritance:	Autosomal recessive
Test:	Dibucaine inhibition test

Affected drugs:	Suxamethonium

% slow metabolizers:	Thais 0%, Japanese 0%, Koreans 0%, Indians 0%, blacks rarely, whites frequently

Glucose-6-phosphate dehydrogenase deficiency:

Enzyme:	G-6-P-D

Inheritance:	X-chromosomal, incomplete dominant

Haemolysis-inducing drugs:	Acetylsalicylic acid, chloramphenicol, dimercaprol, naphthalene, nitrofurantoin, primaquine, probenecid, quinidine, quinine, sulphonamides, vitamin K, analgesics, antimalarials

% slow metabolizers:	Africans 20%, Mediterraneans 35%, Chinese 20–30%, Thais 20%

2. Enzyme inducers

Enzyme inducers produce an increase in the amount and activity of a specific, generally hepatic, enzyme. They are usually lipophilic, often substrates of the induced enzyme, and commonly have a long half life. Enzyme induction usually appears after a few days and usually persists for 2–3 weeks, depending on the half life of the enzyme concerned. Increased enzyme activity frequently leads to a clinically significant reduction of the half life of the relevant substrate, necessitating dosage adjustments.

Substances that induce the metabolism of other substances:

a) **Foodstuffs, etc.:** Alcohol, grilled meat (barbecue), cabbage, cauliflower, tobacco

b) **Drugs**: Aminoglutethimide, amylobarbitone, ascorbic acid, carbamazepine, chloral hydrate, chlorpromazine, clofibrate, DDT, diazepam, diphenhydramine, fenofibrate, griseofulvin, meprobamate, nicotine, orphenadrine, phenobarbitone, phenylbutazone, phenytoin, progesterone, quinalbarbitone, rifampicin, spironolactone, testosterone, theophylline, tolbutamide, warfarin

Substances that induce their own metabolism (auto-inducers):

Carbamazepine, meprobamate, glyceryl trinitrate, phenobarbitone, phenylbutazone, phenytoin, probenecid, tolbutamide

Side effects of drugs: central nervous system

Drug-induced coma:
Antihistamines, barbiturates, benzodiazepines, betablockers, chloral hydrate, lignocaine, lithium, opiates, phenothiazines, salicylates, tricyclics, vitamin D

Hallucinations:
Amphetamine, anticholinergics, antihistamines, atropine, bromocriptine, cyclosporin, cocaine, LSD, mescaline, mexiletine, PCP, salicylates, tricyclics, yohimbine

Ophthalmic changes:
Mydriasis: Amphetamine, anticholinergics, (atropine, hyoscine), antihistamines, baclofen, barbiturates (in coma), cocaine, LSD, mescaline, methanol, neuroleptics, pethidine, phenylpropanolamine, sympathomimetics, tricyclics, yohimbine, withdrawal syndromes

Miosis: Baclofen, cholinergics (physostigmine), clonidine, (neuroleptics), opiates (except pethidine), organophosphates

Nystagmus: Alcohol, baclofen, barbiturates, carbamazepine, hydroxychloroquine, lithium, mexiletine, pemoline, phenytoin, vitamin A intoxication

Sweating (Poisoning):
Acetylcholinesterase inhibitors, amphetamine, barbiturates, cocaine, caffeine, LSD, mescaline, nicotine, organophosphates, phenylpropanolamine, mushroom poisoning, salicylates, sympathomimetics, withdrawal, hypoglycaemia

Drug-induced aseptic meningitis:
Azathioprine, carbamazepine, cytarabine, immunoglobulin, isoniazid, NSAID (ibuprofen, naproxen, sulindac, tolmetin), penicillin, sulphonamides (sulphamethizole, co-trimoxazole)

Promotion of convulsive phenomena:
Drug-induced epileptic attacks and epileptiform manifestations with therapeutic doses in non-epileptic patients:

Drug group	In therapeutic concentrations	In toxic doses
Anaesthetics	Enfluran, etomidate, ketamine	
Anti-asthmatics	Theophylline	
Antibiotics	Ciprofloxacin, cycloserine, imipenem/cilastatin, isoniazid, penicillins	Cephalosporins, nalidixic acid, (rifampicin)
Anticholinergics	Hyoscine	Anticholinergics
Antidepressants		
Tricyclics	Amitriptyline, amoxapine, clomipramine, desipramine, (doxepin), nortriptyline, imipramine	
Non-tricyclics	Amoxapine, (fluoxetine), (lithium), maprotiline, mianserin	Lithium (monoamine oxidase inhibitors)
Antiepileptics	Phenytoin (in high doses)	
Antihistamines		Dimenhydrinate, diphenhydramine
Antimalarial drugs	Chloroquine	Chloroquine, hydroxychloroquine, quinine
Antipyretics, NSAID		Mefenamic acid, ibuprofen, indomethacin, salicylates
Antiviral drugs	Acyclovir, amantadine	
β-blockers		Metoprolol
Cytostatic drugs	Busulphan, chlorambucil, methotrexate	Vinca alkaloids

Drug group	In therapeutic concentrations	In toxic doses
Illegal drugs		Amphetamine, cocaine, 'crack', pemoline
Local anaesthetics	Buvicaine, lignocaine, procaine	
Opiates	Alfentanil, fentanyl, pethidine	Morphine
Phenothiazines	Chlorpromazine, clozapine, promazine	
Others	Bismuth salts	Camphor, clonidine, CO, cyanide, dantrolene, lead, quinidine, strychnine, thiamin

Smaller risk of convulsive attacks: Doxepin, fluphenazine, haloperidol, pimozide, thioridazine, trazodone

Side effects of drugs: gastrointestinal tract

Drug-induced pancreatitis:

(Asymptomatic elevation of serum amylase and/or pancreatitis)
The prevalence of acute drug-induced pancreatitis is very low.
(Exceptions: azathioprine/mercaptopurine)
Incubation period: As a rule, days to weeks, occasionally years
Course: mostly benign, occasionally, however, fatal
Diagnosis: by exclusion. Note: Re-exposure can be dangerous

Drug	Symptom-free interval
Established relationship:	
Azathioprine	2–3 weeks
Chlorothiazide	1–4 months (rarely years)
Frusemide	3–5 weeks
Hydrochlorothiazide	1–4 months (rarely years)
Mercaptopurine	1–5 weeks
Methyldopa	1–7 days
Oestrogens	<3 months
Sulphonamides	1–2 weeks
Sulindac	1 month to 5 years
Tetracycline	<3 weeks
Valproate	Days to years

Probable relationship:

Asparaginase, cimetidine, cisplatin, cytarabine, glucocorticoids, pentamidine, rifampicin

Hiccups:
Drugs that can precipitate hiccup:
Chlordiazipoxide, dexamethasone, diazepam, fluconazole, methohexitone, methyldopa, methylprednisolone, mexiletine, midazolam, nicotine, nikethamide, phenobarbitone, propofol, thiopentone

Disturbances of temperature:
Drug fever
Definition: Development of raised body temperature related in time to administration of a specific drug and normalization of temperature after withdrawal of the drug.
Rechallenge with the same substance produces recurrence of fever.
Clinical picture: Often rigors, often indistinguishable from bacterial infection.
Pulse usually >100/min (no relative bradycardia); hypotension infrequent.

Accompanying symptoms: Myalgia > leucocytosis > (mild) eosinophilia > rash >
headache > others. Lag time: short with antineoplastic substances (on average 0.5
days); days to weeks for other substances
Resolution: as a rule within 48 h

Rule of thumb: Withdrawal syndromes lead to elevation of temperature, intoxications
more commonly to hypothermia.

Elevation of temperature
Frequently:
Amphotericin B, ampicillin, asparaginase, carboprost, dinoprost (prostaglandin E_2),
isoniazid, iodide, lisinopril, methyldopa, penicillin and derivatives, procainamide,
prostaglandin E_1 (alprostadil), quinidine, sulphonamides, co-trimoxazole

Occasionally:
Acetylsalicylic acid, adriamycin, allopurinol, antihistamines, azathioprine,
barbiturates, bleomycin, carbamazepine, cephalosporins, chlorambucil,
chlorpromazine, cimetidine, cisplatin, clofibrate, clozapine, colistin, cytarabine,
dacarbazine, dactinomycin, dantrolene, diazoxide, folic acid, haloperidol,
hydralazine, hydroxyurea, ibuprofen, interferon, levamisole, mebendazole,
mercaptopurine, methotrexate, metoclopramide, nifedipine, nitrofurantoin,
oxprenolol, PAS, penicillamine, pentazocine, plicamycin, prazosin, procarbazine,
propylthiouracil, ritodrine, streptokinase, streptomycin, sulindac, tetracycline,
terazosin, thioridazine, tolmetin, triamterine, vancomycin, vinblastine, vincristine

In intoxications with:
Amitriptyline, amphetamine, anticholinergics, atropine, cocaine, crack, doxepin,
LSD, MAO inhibitors, metal vapours, phenothiazines, salicylates,
sympathomimetics, thallium, thyroxine

Practically never:
Choramphenicol, digitalis glycosides, insulins

Temperature reduction
Intoxication:
Barbiturates, chloral hydrate, glutethimide, haloperidol, tricyclic antidepressants

Side effects of drugs: cardiac

Torsade de pointes
(polymorphic ventricular tachycardia with widening of QTc)

Anti-arrhythmics	Psychotropic drugs	Antibiotics
Quinidine	Thioridazine	Erythromycin
Mexiletine	Tricyclics	Pentamidine
Disopyramide		Co-trimoxazole
Procainamide		
Tocainide	**Others**	
Propafenone	Frusemide	**Intoxications**
Sotalol	Prednisolone	Chloral hydrate
Bretylium	Astemizole	

Side effects of drugs: genitourinary system

Discoloration of urine by drugs

Drug	Colour
Amitriptyline	Blue-green
Desferrioxamine	Reddish
Doxorubicin	Red
Doxycycline	Yellow
Methyldopa	Darkens on standing
Methylene blue	Dark green-blue
Metronidazole	Darkens on standing
Mitozantrone	Blue-green
Nitrofurantoin	Darkens on standing
Phenothiazine	Darkens on standing
Riboflavin (vitamin B_2)	Yellow-green
Rifampicin	Red
Sulphasalazine	Red
Triamterene	Blue-green

Precipitation of drugs in urine

Procedure with appearance of unusual crystalluria:

Obtain history of drug intake over preceding 48 h, consider change of drug therapy, infrared spectrophotometry of the urinary crystals.

Drug	Crystal appearance
Acetazolamide	
Acyclovir	
Allopurinol	Xanthine crystals
Amiloride	
Amoxicillin	Long colourless needle-formed rods of different lengths
Ampicillin	Fine rods with square cross-section
Co-trimoxazole	Rhomboid, hexagonal, greyish
Methotrexate	
Nitrofurantoin	Purple, irregular
Norfloxacin	
Sulphadiazine	Sea-urchin-shaped aggregation of fine rods (wheat sheaves)
Sulphasalazine	
Triamterene	Large aggregates: centrifuged deposit: yellow

Intoxications

Ethylene glycol	Needles and envelopes
Primidone	

References

ACTG (1992) *N. Engl. J. Med.*, **326**, 213.

American Diabetes Association (1985) *Diabetes*, **34** (Suppl. 2), 123.

American Psychiatric Association (1987) *DSM-III-R*. Quick Reference, Washington.

American Rheumatism Association (1988) The American Rheumatism Association 1987 revised criteria for the classification of rheumatoid arthritis. *Arthritis Rheum.*, **31**, 313.

Anacker, H. and Löffler, A. (1989) In *ERCP Atlas* (eds G. Potz and B. Schrameyer), Schattauer, Stuttgart.

Berlit, P. (1989) Paraneoplastische syndrom in der neurologie. *Zentralbl. Neurol.*, **252**, 3.

Berlit, P. (1992) *Klinische Neurologie*, Edition Medizin, Weinheim.

Berne, R.M. and Levy, M.N. (1977) *Cardiovascular Physiology*, Mosby, St Louis.

Biouv *et al.* (1987) *Gastroenterol. Clin. Biol.*, **11**.

Bubenheimer, P. (1982) *Herz und Gefäße*, **2**, 251.

Bubenheimer, P. (1990) *Herz und Gefäße*, **10**, 2.

Bubenheimer, P. and Kneissl, G.D. (1990) *Dopplerechokardiographie*, Edition Medizin, Weinheim.

Bundesamt für Gesundheitswesen (1985) *Infektionskrankheiten, Diagnose und Bekämpfung*, Bundesamt für Gesundheitswesen, Berne.

Burgener, A. and Kormano, M. (1985) *Differential Diagnosis in Conventional Radiology*, Thieme, Stuttgart.

Burroughs and McIntyre (1990) How to insert a Sengstaken-Blakemore tube. *Br. J. Hosp. Med.*, **43**, 274.

Chamberlain, D.A. (1989) *Br. Med. J.*, **299**, 446.

Child, C.G. and Turcotte J.G. (1964) Surgery and portal hypertension, in *The Liver and Portal Hypertension* (ed. C.G. Child), Saunders, Philadelphia, p. 50.

Chun, C.H. *et al.* (1986) Brain abscess. A study of 45 consecutive cases. *Medicine (Baltimore)*, **65**, 415.

Colonna, J.O. II *et al.* (1988) *Arch. Surg.*, **123**, 360.

Copeland, J.G. *et al.* (1987) Selection of patients for cardiac transplantation. *Circulation*, **75**, 1.

Csapo, G. and Kalusche, D. (1989) *Konventionelle und intrakardiale Elektrokardiographie*, Documenta Geigy, Basle.

Dannemann, B. *et al.* (1992) *Ann. Intern. Med.*, **116**, 33.

Deom, A. (1992) *Schwiez Ges. Klin. Chem.*

Deutsche Gesellschaft für Thorax und Gefässchirurgie, Deutsche Gesellschaft für Pneumologie und Tuberkulose (1988) Empfehlungen zur Diagnostik,

Stadieneinteilung und operativen Therapie des Bronchialkarzinoms. *Thorac. Cardiovasc. Surg.*, **36**, 295.

Deutsche Liga zur Bekämpfung der Atemwegserkrankungen (1988) *Dtsch Med. Wochenschr.*, **41**, 1609.

Deutsche Liga zur Bekämpfung des hohen Blutdrucks (1990) e. V., Heidelberg, 9th edn.

Dougados M. *et al.* (1991) The European Spondylarthropathy Study Group preliminary criteria for the classification of spondylarthropathy. *Arthritis Rheum.*, **34**, 1218.

Du Bois and Du Bois (1916) *Arch. Intern Med.*, **117**, 863.

Ekelund, L.D. and Holmgren, A. (1967) Central hemodynamics during exercise. *Circ. Res.*, **20/21**, 1.

Ellestad, M.H. *et al.* (1979) American Heart Association Committee Report: Standard for adult exercise testing laboratories. *Circulation*, **59**, 421A.

Empfehlungen der Arbeitsgruppe Lipide. Schweizerische Stiftung für Kardiologie (1989) *Schweiz Ärztezeitg.*, **70**, 1.

Empfehlungen zur Basisdiagnostik des Hochdrucks, Deutsche Liga zur Bekämpfung des hohen Blutdrucks (1990) e. V., Heidelberg.

Esposito, X. *et al.* (1979) *Arch. Intern. Med.*, **139**, 575.

Forrest, J.A.H. (1974) Endoscopy in gastrointestinal bleeding. *Lancet*, **2**, 394.

Franklin Bunn, H. (1983) In *Harrison's Principles of Internal Medicine*, 10th edn (eds R.G. Petersdorf *et al.*), McGraw-Hill, New York.

French-American-British Cooperative Group (1976) *Br. J. Haematol.*, **33**, 451.

Freye, K. and Lammers, W. (1982) *Radiologisches Worterbuch*, De Gruyter, Berlin.

Goldmann, N. *et al.* (1977) *N. Engl. J. Med.*, **297**, 845.

Görnandt, L. (1989) Rechtsherzeinschwemmkatheteruntersuchung, in *Herzkrankheiten* (eds H. Roskamm and H. Reindell), Springer, Berlin, p. 322.

Grossman, W. (ed.)(1980) *Cardiac Catherization and Angiography*, Lea & Febiger, Philadelphia.

Haas, H.G. (1983) *Klin. Prax.*, **37**, 6.

Haden, R.L. (1935) *Am. J. Clin. Pathol.*, **5**, 354.

Handschuh, M. and Diehl, V. (1986) In *Kompendium Internistische Onkologie* (eds H.-J. Schmoll *et al.*), Springer, Berlin.

Harrison, E.C. *et al.* (1988) *Ann. Emerg. Med.*, **17**, 194.

Haslbeck, M. (1989) Diagnostik und therapie des coma diabeticum. *Dtsch Med. Wochenschr.*, **114**, 385.

Haynes, R.C., and Murad, F. (1985) Adrenocortical steroids, in *The Pharmacological Basis of Therapeutics* (eds A. Goodman-Gilman, L.S. Goodman, T.W. Rall and F. Murad), 7th edn, Macmillan, New York.

Health Departments of Great Britain and Northern Ireland (1983) *Cadaveric organs for transplantation: A code of practice, including the diagnosis of brain death*, HMSO, London.

Hennerici, M. and Neuerburg-Heusler, D. (1988) *Gefäßdiagnostik mit Ultraschall*, Thieme, Stuttgart.

Horsburgh, C.R. Jr (1991) *N. Engl. J. Med.*, **324**, 1332.

Hughes, W.T. *et al.* (1990) Guidelines for the use of antimicrobial agents in neutropenic patients with unexplained fever. *J. Infect. Dis.*, **161**, 381.

International League against Epilepsy (1981) *Epilepsia*, **22**, 489.

International League against Epilepsy (1989) *Epilepsia*, **30**, 389.

International Nomenclature commission (1970) Leningrad.

Jarvis, M.J. *et al.* (1986) *Thorax*, **41**, 886.

Japanese Society for Gastroenterological Endoscopy (1962).

Johannesson, T. *et al.* (1990) *Jcl. Med. J.*, **76**, 203.

Joint National Committee (1988) The 1988 Report of the Joint National Committee on detection, evaluation and treatment of high blood pressure. *Arch. Intern. Med.*, **148**, 1023.

Kaiser, H. (1977) *Cortisonderivate in Klinik und Praxis*, Thieme, Stuttgart.

Kaltenbach, M. and Roskamm, H. (eds) (1980) *Vom Belastungs–EKG zur Koronarangiographie*, Springer, Berlin.

Keith, N.M., Wagener, H.P. and Barker, N.W. (1939) *Am. J. Med. Sci.*, **197**, 332.

Kennedy, H.L. (1988) *Eur. Heart J.*, **9**, 70.

Kielholz, P. (1966) *Psychiatrische Pharmakotherapie*, Huber, Bern.

Kielholz, P. (1971) *Diagnose und Therapie der Depressionen für den Praktiker*, 3rd edn, Lehmanns, Munich.

Kienast, J. and van de Loo, J. (1991) *Dtsch Ärztebl.*, **88**, B905.

Killip, T. and Kimball, J.T. (1967) Treatment of myocardial infarction in a coronary care unit. *Am. J. Cardiol.*, **20**, 457.

Krebs, J. and Otto, H. (1986) Komata bei diabetes mellitus, in *Differentialdiagnose der Komata*, Thieme, Stuttgart.

Lamerz, R. (1986) Tumormarker, Prinzipien und Klinik. *Dtsch Ärztebl.*, **15**, B771.

Larson *et al.* (1982) *Medicine (Baltimore)*, **61**, 269.

Lawton, A.R. and Cooper, M.D. (1983) Laboratory evaluation of host defense defects, in *Harrison's Principles of Internal Medicine* (eds R.G. Petersdorf *et al.*), 10th edn, McGraw-Hill, New York.

Lentner, C. (ed.) (1977) *Scientific Tables Geigy*, vol. 1, 8th edn, Ciba-Geigy, Basle.

Lissner, J. and Seiderer, M. (1990) *Klinische Kernspintomographie*, Enke, Stuttgart.

Löllgen, H. and Ulmer, H.V. (eds) (1985) Empfehlungen zur Durchführung und Bewertung ergometrischer Untersuchungen. *Klin. Wochenschr.*, **63**, 651.

Marsden, A.K. (1989) *Br. Med. J.*, **299**, 442.

McMorran, M. and Paraskevas, F. (1981) Methods of examining the immune system, in *Clinical Hematology* (eds M.M. Wintrobe *et al.*), 8th edn, Lea & Febiger, Philadelphia.

Mehnert, H. (1990) *Stoffwechselkrankheiten*, 4th edn, Thieme, Stuttgart.

Miller, A.B., Hoogstraten, B., Staquet, M. and Winkler, A. (1981) Reporting results of cancer treatment. *Cancer*, **47**, 207.

Mosteller, R.D. (1987) *N. Engl. J. Med.*, **317**, 1098.

Müller, W. and Schillung, F. (1982) *Differentialdiagnose rheumatischer Erkrankungen*, 2nd edn, Aesopus, Basle.

National Diabetes Data Group (1979) *Diabetes*, **28**, 1039.

Oh, C.-S. *et al.* (1988) Transplantation, **45**, 68.

Parsonnet, V. *et al.* (1981) A revised code for pacemaker identification. *Circulation*, **64**, 60A.

Pfreundschuh, M. and Diehl, V. (1986) In *Kompendium Internistische Onkologie* (eds H.-J. Schmoll *et al.*), Springer, Berlin.

Pichlmayer, R. (1987) *Hepatologie – Innere Medizin der Gegenwart*, Urban & Schwarzenberg, Munich.

Quanjer, P.H. (ed.) (1983) Standardised lung function testing. *Bull. Eur. Physiopathol. Respir.*, Suppl., 5.

Redfield, R.R. *et al.* (1986) The Walter Reed staging classification for HTLV–III/LAV infection. *N. Engl. J. Med.*, **314**, 131.

Reiber, H. and Felgenhauer, K. (1987) Protein transfer at the blood cerebrospinal fluid barrier and the quantitation of the humoral immune response within the central nervous system. *Clin. Chim. Acta*, **163**, 319.

Ries, F. (1987) Dopplersonographie der extrakraniellen Hirnarterien, in *Hirninfarkt*, (eds A. Hartmann and H. Wassmann), Urban & Schwarzenberg, Munich.

Rigo, P. *et al.* (1980) *Circulation*, **61**, 973.

Ring, J. and Messmer, K. (1977) Incidence and severity of anaphylactoid reactions to colloid volume substitutes. *Lancet*, **I**, 466.

Rodman, G.P. (ed.) (1973) Primer on the rheumatic diseases. *JAMA*, **224**, 662.

Sandoz, P. (1988) Abklärung der Hämaturie Heute. *Schweiz. Rundsch. Med. Prax.*, **77**, 38.

Sanford, J.P. (1991) *Guide to Antimicrobial Therapy*. Antimicrobial Therapy, West Bethesda.

Schaad, U.B. (1986) Treatment of bacterial meningitis. *Eur. J. Clin. Microbiol.*, **5**, 492.

Scheld, W.M. and Sande, M.E. (1990) Endocarditis and intravascular infections, in *Principles and Practice of Infectious Diseases* (eds G.L. Mandell *et al.*), Livingstone, New York, p. 670.

Schinz, H.R. *et al.* (1979) *Lehrbuch der Röntgendiagnostik*, vol. 3, Thieme, Stuttgart.

Schulze-Werninghaus, G. and Debelic, M. (eds) (1988) *Asthma. Grundlagen, Diagnostik, Therapie*, Springer, Berlin.

Schüpbach, J. (1991) Retroviren und AIDS, Part II. *DIA-GM*, **3**, 228.

Shah, P.M., Slodki, S.J. and Luisada, A.A. (1964) A review of the 'classic' areas of auscultation of the heart. *Am. J. Med.*, **36**, 293.

Siggaard-Andersen (1963) *Scand. J. Clin. Lab. Invest.*, **15**, 211.

Spech *et al.* (1982) *Leber. Magen. Darm.*, **12**, 109.

Stamm, W.E. *et al.* (1989) Urinary tract infections: from pathogenesis to treatment. *J. Infect. Dis.*, **159**, 400.

Stöhr, M. and Riffel, B. (1988) *Nerven- und Nervernwurzelläsionen*, Edition Medizin, Weinheim.

Stollermann, G.H. *et al.* (1965) Jones criteria (revised) for guidance in the diagnosis of rheumatic fever. *Circulation*, **32**, 664.

Study Group European Atherosclerosis Society (1987) Strategies for the prevention of coronary heart disease. *Eur. Heart. J.*, **8**, 77.

Talan, D.A. *et al.* (1988) Role of parenteral antibiotics prior to lumbar puncture in suspected meningitis: state of the art. *Rev. Infect. Dis.*, **10**, 365.

Tan, E.M. *et al.* (1982) The 1982 revised criteria for the classification of SLE. *Arthritis Rheum.*, **25**, 1271.

Teasdale, G. and Jennet, B. (1976) *Acta Neurochir. (Wien)*, **34**, 45.

Thiel, G. *et al.* (1986) Glomeruläre Erythrocyten im Urin, Erkennung und Bedeutung. *Schweiz. Med. Wochenschr.*, **116**, 790.

Thulesius (1976) *Cardiology*, **61**, Suppl. 1, 180.

UICC (1982) *TNM Classification of Malignant Tumors*, 3rd edn, UICC, Geneva.

Vanhoutte, P.M. (1987) *Am. J. Cardiol.*, **59**, 3A.

Vanuxem, D. *et al.* (1980) *Respiration*, **40**, 136.

Vaughan-Williams, E.M. (1975) *Pharmacol. Ther. B*, **1**, 115.

Voegeli, E. (1981) *Grundelemente der Skelettradiologie*, Huber, Berne.

Whitley, R.J. (1990) Viral encephalitis. *N. Engl. J. Med.*, **323**, 242.

WHO (1978) Arterial Hypertension. *WHO Tech. Rep. Ser. 628.*

WHO Expert Committee on Diabetes Mellitus (1980) *WHO Tech. Rep. Ser. 646*, p. 9.

WHO/ISFC (1980) Task Force on definition and classification of cardiomyopathies. *Br. Heart J.*, **44**, 672.

WHO/ISFC (1981) Task Force on definition and classification of cardiac myopathies. *Circulation*, **64**, 437A.

WHO/ISH (1989) Guidelines for the management of mild hypertension. *Clin. Exp. Hypertens., [A]*, **11**(5/6), 1203.

Wintrobe, M.M. *et al.* (1981) *Clinical Hematology*, 8th edn, Lea & Febiger, Philadelphia.

Wolfe, F. *et al.* (1990) The American College of Rheumatology 1990 criteria for the classification of fibromyalgia. *Arthritis Rheum.*, **33**, 160.

Zimmerli, W. (1990) Harnwegsinfekt: Was untersuchen? Wie behandeln? *Ther. Umsch.*, **47**, 675.

Zimmerli, W. *et al.* (1991) *Blood*, **77**, 393.

Index

O_2 delivery eqⁿ.

$$CO \times Hb \times Arterial\ saturation \times 1.34 \times 10$$

$$= ml/mm\ O_2.$$